T4-AHH-529

MALNUTRITION: DETERMINANTS AND CONSEQUENCES

CURRENT TOPICS IN NUTRITION AND DISEASE

Series Editors

Anthony A. Albanese
The Burke Rehabilitation Center
White Plains, New York

David Kritchevsky
The Wistar Institute
Philadelphia, Pennsylvania

MALNUTRITION: DETERMINANTS AND CONSEQUENCES

Proceedings of the Western Hemisphere Nutrition Congress VII
held in Miami Beach, Florida, August 7–11, 1983

Editors

PHILIP L. WHITE
and
NANCY SELVEY
American Medical Association
Chicago, Illinois

Alan R. Liss, Inc., New York

Library of Congress Cataloging in Publication Data

Western Hemisphere Nutrition Congress (7th : 1983 :
    Miami Beach, Fla.)
    Malnutrition, determinants and consequences.

    (Proceedings / Western Hemisphere Nutrition Congress ;
7) (Current topics in nutrition and disease ; v. 10)
    Includes bibliographies and index.
    1. Malnutrition—America—Congresses. 2. Nutrition
disorders—Congresses. 3. Food habits—America—Congresses. 4. Nutrition—America—Congresses. I. White,
Philip Louis, 1922-   . II. Selvey, Nancy.
III. Title. IV. Series: Western Hemisphere Nutrition
Congress. Proceedings ; 7. V. Series; Current topics
in nutrition and disease ; v. 10. [DNLM: 1. Nutrition
disorders—Congresses. 2. Nutrition disorders—Occurrence
—America—Congresses. 3. Nutrition—In pregnancy—Congresses. 4. Infant nutrition—Congresses. 5. Food
preferences—Congresses. 6. Urbanization—America—Congresses. W1 CU82R v.10 / WD 100 W527 1983m]
TX345.W4   no. 7   [RA645.N87] 338.1'9'1812S   83-24391
ISBN 0-8451-1609-6   [616.3'9]

Western Hemisphere Nutrition Congress VII
August 7–11, 1983
Miami Beach, Florida

ORGANIZERS

The American Medical Association's
Food and Nutrition Program,
The American Institute of Nutrition,
La Sociedad Latinoamericana de Nutrición,
The Canadian Society for Nutritional Sciences,
and The American Society for Clinical Nutrition

WHNC-VII COMMITTEE MEMBERS

G. Harvey Anderson
Howard Appledorf
   (deceased)
Stephanie Atkinson
John G. Bieri
Carlos H. Daza
Janet L. Greger
Charles H. Halsted
Alfred E. Harper

H. David Hurt
Frank L. Iber
Mary F. Picciano
Merrill S. Read
Mary Ann Sestili
J. Cecil Smith, Jr.
Noel W. Solomons
Herta Spencer
Willard J. Visek

WHNC-VII SECRETARIAT

American Medical Association
Philip L. White
Therese Mondeika
Nancy Selvey

American Institute of Nutrition
Max Milner
Sharon Rettenberg
Jennifer Hedlund

Contents

THE SEARCH FOR SOLUTIONS

Contributors

Lindsay H. Allen, PhD, RD, Department of Nutritional Sciences, University of Connecticut, Storrs, CT 06268 **[101]**

María A. Allen, MD, Hospital San Juan de Dios, Caja Costarricense de Seguro Social, San José, Costa Rica **[123]**

José R. Aráya, MD, Hospital San Juan de Dios, Caja Costarricense de Seguro Social, San José, Costa Rica **[123]**

M. Araya, MD, PhD, Division of Gastroenterology, Institute of Nutrition and Food Technology, University of Chile, Santiago 11, Chile **[259]**

Richard L. Atkinson, MD, Department of Internal Medicine, School of Medicine and Clinical Nutrition Center, University of California at Davis, Davis, CA 95616 **[405]**

M. Barac-Nieto, MD, PhD, Department of Physiology, University of Rochester, Rochester, NY 14642, and Universidad del Valle, Cali, Colombia **[165]**

R.P. Bates, PhD, Food Science and Human Nutrition Department, University of Florida, Gainesville, FL 32611 **[355]**

George H. Beaton, PhD, Department of Nutritional Sciences, Faculty of Medicine, University of Toronto, Toronto, Ontario, Canada M5S 1A8 **[61]**

José María Bengoa, MD, Nutrition Unit, World Health Organization, Geneva, Switzerland **[477]**

Dorothy Blake, MD, MPH, Project for Development of Health Services, Bureau Sanitaire Panamericain, Port-au-Prince, Haiti **[369]**

Malcolm C. Bourne, PhD, New York State Agricultural Experiment Station, and Institute of Food Science, Cornell University, Geneva, NY 14456 **[327]**

O. Brunser, MD, Division of Gastroenterology, Institute of Nutrition and Food Technology, University of Chile, Santiago 11, Chile **[259]**

Nancy Butte, PhD, Department of Pediatrics, Baylor College of Medicine, Houston, TX 77030 **[253]**

Juan J. Carvajal, MD, Instituto de Investigaciones en Salud (INISA), Universidad de Costa Rica, San Pedro, Costa Rica **[123]**

Maria Teresa Cerqueira, RD, MS, Direccion General de Educacion Para la Salud, Secretaria de Salubridad y Asistencia, Mexico City, Mexico **[189]**

Ranjit Kumar Chandra, MD, FRCP(C), Department of Pediatrics, Medicine, and Biochemistry, Memorial University of Newfoundland, St. John's Newfoundland, Canada A1B 3V6 **[245]**

The boldface number in brackets following each contributor's affiliation is the opening page number of that author's article.

J.E. Chappell, BASc, Department of Nutritional Sciences, Faculty of Medicine, University of Toronto, Toronto, Ontario, Canada M5S 1A8 **[85]**

Rolando Chateauneuf, Instituto de Nutrición y Tecnología de los Alimentos (INTA), University of Chile, Santiago 11, Chile **[29]**

Rajender K. Chawla, PhD, Department of Medicine, Emory University School of Medicine, Clinical Research Center, Atlanta, GA 30322 **[389]**

M.T. Clandinin, PhD, Department of Nutritional Sciences, Faculty of Medicine, University of Toronto, Toronto, Ontario, Canada M5S 1A8 **[85]**

Patricia Coleman, MS, Department of Nutritional Sciences, Faculty of Medicine, University of Toronto, Toronto, Ontario, Canada M5S 1A8 **[221]**

Susanna Cunningham-Rundles, PhD, Laboratories of Clinical Immunology and Human Immunogenetics, Memorial Sloan-Kettering Cancer Center, New York, NY 10021 **[233]**

Carlos Hernán Daza, MD, MPH, Pan American Sanitary Bureau, Pan American Health Organization, WHO, Washington, DC 20037 **[447]**

Hernán Delgado, MD, MPH, Institute of Nutrition of Central America and Panama (INCAP), Guatemala City, Guatemala **[3]**

A.J. D'Souza, MBBS, DPH, DIH, Ministry of Health and Local Government, Castries, St. Lucia, West Indies **[383]**

J. Espinoza, MD, Division of Gastroenterology, Institute of Nutrition and Food Technology, University of Chile, Santiago 11, Chile **[259]**

G. Figueroa, RT, Division of Microbiology, Institute of Nutrition and Food Technology, University of Chile, Santiago 11, Chile **[259]**

Marina Flores, MS, Pan American Sanitary Bureau, Guatemala City, Guatemala **[207]**

Rafael Flores, MAP STAT, Institute of Nutrition of Central America and Panama (INCAP), Guatemala City, Guatemala **[3, 207]**

William Fougère, MD, Ministry of Health, Port-au-Prince, Haiti **[379]**

Mark I. Friedman, PhD, Monell Chemical Senses Center, Philadelphia, PA 19104 **[295]**

María E. García, RN, Instituto de Investigaciones en Salud (INISA), Universidad de Costa Rica, San Pedro, Costa Rica **[123]**

Paul E. Garfinkel, MD, FRCP(C), Department of Psychiatry, University of Toronto and Toronto General Hospital, Toronto, Ontario, Canada M5G 1L7 **[305]**

David M. Garner, PhD, Department of Psychiatry, University of Toronto and Toronto General Hospital, Toronto, Ontario, Canada M5G 1L7 **[305]**

Cutberto Garza, MD, PhD, Department of Pediatrics, Baylor College of Medicine, Houston, TX 77030 **[253]**

Randall M. Goldblum, MD, Department of Pediatrics, The University of Texas Medical Branch, Galveston, TX 77550 **[253]**

Armond S. Goldman, MD, Department of Pediatrics, The University of Texas Medical Branch, Galveston, TX 77550 **[253]**

George G. Graham, MD, Instituto de Investigacion Nutricional, Miraflores (Lima), Peru and Johns Hopkins University, Baltimore, MD 21205 **[197]**

Carlyle Guerra de Macedo, MD, MPH, Pan American Sanitary Bureau, Pan American Health Organization, WHO, Washington, DC 20037 **[447]**

Mauricio Herman, PhD, Social Development Division, Inter-American Development Bank, Washington, DC 20577 **[471]**

Eva Hertrampf, MD, Institute of Nutrition and Food Technology (INTA), University of Chile, Santiago 11, Chile **[139]**

Nina Hrboticky, MSc, Department of Nutritional Sciences, Faculty of Medicine, University of Toronto, Toronto, Ontario, Canada M5S 1A8 **[221]**

Joseph H. Hulse, International Development Research Centre, Ottawa, Canada K1G 3H9 **[457]**

Juan José Hurtado V., MD, MA, Puesto de Socorro de San Juan Sacatepequez, Guatemala, and, Bethel College, North Newton, KS 67117 **[273]**

William T. Jarvis, PhD, Department of Public Health Science, School of Allied Health Professions, Loma Linda University, Loma Linda, CA 92354 **[415]**

Norge W. Jerome, PhD, Department of Community Health, Community Nutrition Division, University of Kansas College of Health Sciences, Kansas City, KS 66103 **[367, 385]**

Hilary Creed Kanashiro, BSc, SRD, MPhil, Instituto de Investigacion Nutricional, Miraflores (Lima), Peru **[197]**

Magdalena Krondl, PhD, Department of Nutritional Sciences, Faculty of Medicine, University of Toronto, Toronto, Ontario, Canada M5S 1A8 **[221]**

David H. Lawson, MD, VA Medical Center, Atlanta, GA 30322 **[389]**

Alexander R. Lucas, MD, Section of Child and Adolescent Psychiatry, Mayo Clinic and Mayo Foundation, Rochester, MN 55905 **[315]**

Francisco Mardones-Santander, MD, Institute of Nutrition and Food Technology (INTA), University of Chile, Santiago 11, Chile **[139]**

Leonardo Mata, ScD, Instituto de Investigaciones en Salud (INISA), Universidad de Costa Rica, San Pedro, Costa Rica **[123]**

Buford Nichols, MD, Department of Pediatrics, Baylor College of Medicine, Houston, TX 77030 **[253]**

Arnulfo Noguera, MD, MPH, Institute of Nutrition of Central America and Panama (INCAP), Guatemala City, Guatemala **[3]**

Luis A. Ordóñez, PhD, Section of Neurochemistry and Behavior, Instituto de Medicina Experimental, Universidad Central de Venezuela, Caracas, Venezuela **[179]**

Gretel H. Pelto, PhD, Department of Nutritional Sciences, University of Connecticut, Storrs, CT 06268 **[285]**

Mary Frances Picciano, PhD, Department of Foods and Nutrition, Division of Nutritional Sciences, College of Agriculture, University of Illinois, Urbana, IL 61801 **[111]**

David Picou, MB, PhD, Mount Hope Medical Complex Task Force, Port of Spain, Trinidad **[19]**

John R.K. Robson, MD, Department of Family Medicine, Medical University of South Carolina, Charleston, SC 29425 **[433]**

María E. Rodríguez, BS, Hospital San Juan de Dios, Caja Costarricense de Seguro Social, San José, Costa Rica **[123]**

Haydée Rondón, MD, University Autonoma of Santo Domingo, and Nutrition Department, Public Health Ministry, Santo Domingo, Dominican Republic **[373]**

Daniel Rudman, MD, Department of Medicine, Emory University School of Medicine, Clinical Research Center, Atlanta, GA 30322 **[389]**

Patricia Sáenz, MD, Instituto de Investigaciones en Salud (INISA), Universidad de Costa Rica, San Pedro, Costa Rica **[123]**

Nancy Selvey, RD, Food and Nutrition Program, American Medical Association, Chicago, IL 60610 **[xv]**

Ethan A.H. Sims, MD, Metabolic Unit, Department of Medicine, College of Medicine, University of Vermont, Burlington, VT 05405 **[151]**

Abraham Stekel, MD, Institute of Nutrition and Food Technology (INTA), University of Chile, Santiago 11, Chile **[139]**

Frederick L. Trowbridge, MD, Division of Nutrition, Center for Health Promotion and Education, Centers for Disease Control, Atlanta, GA 30333 **[45]**

Ricardo Uauy, MD, PhD, Instituto de Nutrición y Tecnologia de los Alimentos (INTA), University of Chile, Santiago 11, Chile **[29]**

Sergio Valiente, MD, Instituto de Nutrición y Tecnología de los Alimentos (INTA), University of Chile, Santiago 11, Chile **[29]**

Victor Valverde, PhD, Institute of Nutrition of Central America and Panama (INCAP), Guatemala City, Guatemala **[3]**

Luis Alberto Vargas, MD, PhD, Instituto de Investigaciones Antropológicas, National University of Mexico, 04510 México DF, Mexico **[423]**

Philip L. White, ScD, Division of Personal and Public Health Policy, American Medical Association, Chicago, IL 60610 **[xv]**

Douglas W. Wilmore, MD, Department of Surgery, Harvard Medical School and Brigham and Women's Hospital, Boston, MA 02115 **[403]**

Sylvan H. Wittwer, PhD, Agricultural Experiment Station and Department of Horticulture, College of Agriculture and Natural Resources, Michigan State University, East Lansing, MI 48824 **[337]**

Peter D. Wood, DSc, Stanford Heart Disease Program, Palo Alto, CA 94304 **[149]**

Anthony Wylie, PhD, Department of Food Technology, Fundación Chile, Santiago, Chile **[347]**

Preface

Study of the determinants and consequences of malnutrition should not be confined to the countries in great economic need. Examples of malnutrition can be found anywhere, although the effects of malnutrition may be more subtle in economically developed countries. Emerging nations may experience the nutritional problems found in the more affluent nations even as they undergo transition toward economic stability.

The consequences of malnutrition among impoverished people are poor performance in pregnancy and lactation, an alarmingly high infant mortality rate, anemias, stunted growth, and probably decreased work capacity. More affluent populations may experience obesity and nutritional anemias that debilitate without serious threat to life. Diet and other aspects of the life-style of the affluent may contribute to the development of certain diseases and disorders, e.g., coronary heart disease, obesity, adult-onset diabetes, hypertension, osteoporosis, and perhaps even some kinds of cancer. Whether there are direct cause and effect relationships between diet and chronic diseases is always going to be difficult to determine.

There is value in the simultaneous review of the varying nutritional problems among and within countries, regardless of their state of economic development.

The Honorable Billie Miller, Minister of Education of Barbados, in her WHNC banquet address, described the fate of those who, after years of subsistence by hard physical labor, made the successful transition to gainful urban employment. Dietary patterns changed as the rural migrants succumbed to the commercial promotion of food and labor-saving devices. An almost immediate effect was obesity, first among children and later among adults. Many of these people now experience the hypertension and diabetes associated with obesity. The initial thought was that richer foods, now readily available, were responsible for the rapid weight gain. It is equally possible that decreased energy expenditure contributes more to the obesity than does the increased intake of high calorie foods.

This example of inappropriate acceptance of an urban way of life described by Ms. Miller differs from the usual. Generally when families migrate from impoverished rural life to a city in search of something better, they regress instead of progress. Poverty and unemployment prevent them from enjoying a more varied urban food supply. Too often the result is a combination of a little of their rural diet with the worst aspects of the urban diet. Malnutrition is the result. Cycles of poverty, cycles of malnutrition.

The committee planning the WHNC discussed the many causes of malnutrition that range from inadequate and improper food to iatrogenic malnutrition that may result from a specific course of therapy. Special attention was given to the particular problems that arise in the Caribbean Islands where the quality of life varies from mere borderline existence for many citizens to pure escape for tourists.

These proceedings open with a survey of the major problems of food scarcity and malnutrition by regions of the Western Hemisphere and close with discussion of the search for solutions. In between are nine sections that cover in considerable detail the determinants and consequences of malnutrition of pertinence to the entire Hemisphere.

The U.S. Department of Agriculture honored the WHNC by presentation of the 1983 W.O. Atwater Memorial Lecture. Professor George H. Beaton's Atwater Lecture, *Energy in Human Nutrition: Perspectives and Problems*, is published with this volume. Having participated in four previous WHNCs, Professor Beaton is no stranger to those who enjoy the Congresses and their proceedings.

Many members of the cosponsoring organizations willingly gave of their time and talent to assure the quality of the Congress. We thank them and acknowledge their contributions in the front of this book. In addition we express our gratitude to the many companies and to the governments of the United States and Canada for generous financial support. The American Medical Association is grateful for the opportunity to participate in these efforts to help assure a better quality of life for many and hope for the millions who struggle in search of a meaningful future.

Philip L. White
Nancy Selvey

Acknowledgments

The generous financial support of the following organizations is deeply appreciated.

American Institute of Nutrition
American Medical Association
Best Foods–CPC North America
Canadian Government, Department of
    National Health and Welfare
Canadian Society for Nutritional Sciences
The Coca-Cola Company
Gerber Products Company
Hershey Foods Corporation
Hoffmann-La Roche Inc.
Kraft Inc.
McCormick & Company, Inc.
Mead Johnson Nutritional Division
National Dairy Council
National Live Stock & Meat Board
Nestle Coordination Center for Nutrition, Inc.
The Procter & Gamble Company
The Quaker Oats Company
Ross and Abbott Laboratories
Swift & Company/Esmark, Inc. Foundation
Thomas J. Lipton, Inc.
United States Government
    Bureau of Foods, Food and
        Drug Administration
    National Institutes of Health:
        Fogarty International Center
        National Cancer Institute
        National Institute of Child Health
            and Human Development

OPENING PLENARY SESSION: MALNUTRITION IN THE WESTERN HEMISPHERE

Moderator

Irwin H. Rosenberg, MD
Professor of Medicine
Director, Clinical Nutrition Research Center
Co-Director, Section of Gastroenterology
Department of Medicine
University of Chicago
Chicago, Illinois

Malnutrition: Determinants and Consequences, pages 3–17
© *1984 Alan R. Liss, Inc., 150 Fifth Avenue, New York, NY 10011*

Malnutrition in Tropical America

**Víctor Valverde, PhD, Hernán Delgado, MD, MPH,
Arnulfo Noguera, MD, MPH, and Rafael Flores, MAP STAT**
Institute of Nutrition of Central America and Panama (INCAP), Guatemala,
Guatemala

INTRODUCTION

The concepts about the causes of and the solutions to the food and nutrition problems in Third World nations have been substantially modified during the last two decades [Joy and Payne, 1975]. It is now generally accepted that chronic malnutrition in children results from inadequate access to and utilization of health and educational services and/or from the low purchasing power of families. Therefore, if malnutrition is to be effectively dealt with, governments should strengthen those programs oriented to reducing significantly the existing levels of poverty.

This chapter discusses the present nutritional and health conditions in Tropical America (TA) and the changes that have occurred in the principal health indicators over time. TA includes 17 countries that include approximately 16 million km² of national territory and 297 million inhabitants. It is subdivided into Continental Middle America (CMA), including Belize, Costa Rica, El Salvador, Guatemala, Honduras, Mexico, Nicaragua, and Panama, with 93 million people; and Tropical South America (TSA), which comprises Brazil, Bolivia, Colombia, Ecuador, Guyana, Paraguay, Peru, Suriname, and Venezuela, with 204 million inhabitants [PAHO, 1982a]. TA in general has a hot and humid climate, although temperature and rainfall vary dramatically by altitude. A mixture of indigenous and Spanish-speaking cultures forms the majority of the populations. The remaining, predominantly indigenous populations are found in the highlands or in bordering isolated communities. African-American populations are mostly concentrated on the Atlantic coasts. Approximately 43% of the population of the region is under 15 years of age. The adult literacy rates range from 47% in Guatemala to 90% in Costa Rica and Mexico [PAHO, 1982a]. Poverty affects 71% of the population in Guatemala and 65% in Honduras [MIDEPLAN, 1983]. Less than 40% of households in eight countries (Bolivia, Ecuador, El Salvador, Guatemala, Honduras, Mexico, Paraguay, and Peru) have access to adequate water supply systems [PAHO, 1982b].

MALNUTRITION IN TROPICAL AMERICA

The data available in TA since the 1940s had identified protein-energy malnutrition, anemias associated with iron and folate deficiencies, hypovitaminosis A, and iodine deficiency as the most pressing nutritional problems of the area.

In the following section, the most recent data related to nutritional and health conditions are reviewed. Most data sources consulted are derived from national nutrition surveys that did not provide details about sampling procedures, the validity and reliability of the data, the methods of data collection, the growth standards used, or the procedures for data editing and processing. Thus, in most countries it was not possible to estimate or adjust for the confounding effects imposed by different methodologies. However, for some countries, the changes observed in rates cannot be attributed solely to methodologic differences in the data sets. Despite those difficulties of interpretation it is important to get a general notion of trends in light of the health goals proposed for the year 2000.

National Prevalence and Changes Over Time

Mortality. Mortality and indicators of growth retardation to a large extent reflect prevailing deficiencies of energy and protein. The mortality figures reported in this chapter are derived from national health statistics. While infant and child deaths are underestimated by official statistics, the present trend in most countries is towards improving the reporting system. Thus, if reductions in mortality are observed, these are generally underestimations of the true changes occurring over time. The information on infant mortality (IM) in TA in the 1970s is presented in Table I. The most important annual declines in IM are seen in Paraguay (5.7 deaths of children under 1 year of age per 1,000 live births), Costa Rica (4.2/1,000), Peru (3.8/1,000), and Mexico (3.6/1,000). Belize (2.5/1,000), Ecuador (2.2/1,000), Guatemala (1.9/1,000) and Panama (1.9/1,000) have also shown important reductions in IM during the 1970s. Some countries in Central America report IM that underestimate the true figures. In spite of that, five countries in TA still have IM above 50/1,000, the maximum acceptable figure established in health for all in the year 2000.

The 1- to 4-year mortality figures (1–4 YM) for the year 1970 and the period 1977–1981 in TA are shown in Table II [PAHO, 1982a; OPS, 1981; MS, 1983; Baum and Arriaga, 1981]. Marked annual reductions in this indicator are reflected in all countries, particularly in Guatemala (1.46/1,000) and El Salva-

TABLE I. Infant Mortality in Tropical America in 1970 and 1977–1981

Country	Years		Average annual reductions[a]
	1970	1977–1981	
Paraguay	93.8	48.1	5.7
Costa Rica	61.5	19.0	4.2
Peru	65.1	35.1	3.8
Mexico	68.5	39.7	3.6
Belize	50.7	27.5	2.5
Ecuador	76.6	61.0	2.2
Panama	40.5	21.5	1.9
Guatemala	87.1	70.2	1.9
Venezuela	49.2	32.1	1.7
Colombia	50.5	39.5	1.6
El Salvador	66.7	53.0	1.5
Brazil[b]	92.0	85.2	1.0
Honduras	33.2	24.9	0.9
Guyana	34.7	28.5	0.6
Suriname	36.7	35.1	0.2
Bolivia[b]	151.6	151.0	0.1
Nicaragua	42.8	42.9	0.0

[a]Reference period varies from 6 to 11 years.
[b]From Baum and Arriaga [1982], and based on census and household surveys.

TABLE II. Mortality for Children 1–4 Years of Age in Tropical America in 1970 and 1977–1981

Country	Years		Average annual reductions
	1970	1977–1981	
Guatemala	27.0	12.4	1.46
El Salvador	13.0	4.1	1.11
Mexico	10.6	3.3	0.91
Peru	12.5	5.2	0.91
Ecuador	14.9	8.1	0.85
Nicaragua	9.5	3.6	0.84
Honduras	11.4	4.3	0.79
Panama	7.6	2.1	0.55
Belize	4.3	1.6	0.45
Venezuela	5.2	2.6	0.35
Colombia	6.8	4.5	0.33
Costa Rica	4.4	0.9	0.32
Suriname	4.3	1.4	0.31
Paraguay	6.7	4.1	0.26
Guyana	3.2	1.9	0.08

dor (1.11/1,000), where previous rates were among the highest in the region. The less dramatic annual reductions are seen in countries with previously low levels of 1-4 YM in 1970. With the exception of Colombia, Ecuador, Guyana, and Paraguay, all countries had a drop of at least 50% in the 1-4 YM during the period of analyses.

Incidence of growth retardation. A child with a weight for age below 75% of the median of an internationally accepted reference pattern is defined here as suffering from weight retardation (Gómez II and III) [Gómez et al, 1956]. The latest reports of incidence of growth retardation in children are shown in Table III. The highest rates of second- and third-degree malnutrition in children are found in Guatemala (30.5%) [Valverde et al, 1981], and Honduras (29.5%) [INCAP/CDC, 1972]; while in Colombia and Costa Rica the respective figures are 8.3% and 4.8% [Mora, 1982; Jaramillo, 1983]. The rates of growth retardation, 15% or less, reported from Nicaragua, Panama, El Salvador, and Venezuela [Parillón, 1982; INCAP, 1983; PAHO, 1982c] are also low compared to rates observed in other developing nations.

Comparable data on weight for age are not available for other countries. Nevertheless, the nutrition survey of Bolivia, conducted in 1981 [INAN, 1983], disclosed that 49% of children 6-59 months old had heights below two standard deviations of the reference pattern, as compared to only 22.4% of Colombian children [Mora, 1982]. Other countries, such as Peru and Ecuador, have reported rates of growth retardation based on growth patterns or reference values (25th percentile) that underestimate the true incidence of growth retardation [Amat and Cunurisy, 1981; PAHO, 1982c].

The information on changes in the incidence of weight retardation in TA countries is shown in Table IV. Important improvements occurred in El Salva-

TABLE III. Percentage of Children Under 5 Years of Age Weighing Below 75% of Standard Weight for Age (W/A) in Tropical America

Country	Year	Incidence (%)
Costa Rica	1982	4.8
Colombia	1977–1980	8.3
El Salvador	1978	10.4
Panama	1980	11.6
Venezuela	1974	13.6
Nicaragua	1966	15.0
Belize	1973	19.2
Brazil	1968	19.9
Honduras	1967	29.5
Guatemala	1977	30.5

TABLE IV. Percentage of Children Under 5 Years of Age Weighing Below 75% of Standard Weight for Age in Tropical America, 1965–1968 and 1974–1982

Country	Years		Average annual reductions
	1965–1968	1974–1982	
El Salvador	27.5	10.4	1.32
Venezuela	19.0	13.6	0.68
Colombia	15.7	8.3	0.62
Costa Rica	13.5	4.8	0.54
Guatemala	33.6	30.5	0.28
Panama	11.9	11.6	0.02

dor, Costa Rica, Colombia, and Venezuela. Panama maintained in 1980 [Parillón, 1982] the same low prevalence as that observed in 1967 [INCAP/CDC, 1972]. Guatemala showed a slight decline in the proportion of children with growth retardation, 33.6% in 1965 [INCAP/CDC, 1972] and 30.5% in 1977 [Valverde et al, 1981]. Data from Brazil that compare results from surveys conducted in the 1960s and 1970s also demonstrate a decline from 68.3% to 46% in the percentage of children under 5 years of age who are below 90% of appropriate weight for age [Dutra et al, 1981].

Incidence of vitamin A deficiency. Vitamin A deficiency is defined here as any case with a serum retinol level below 20 μg/dl (low and deficient levels). The latest reports of rates for children and for the total population in TA countries are presented in Table V. In El Salvador 33.3% of children below 60 months of age had low or deficient levels of serum retinol [MSPAS/INCAP, 1977]. Panama reported a vitamin A deficiency incidence in children of 18.4% [INCAP/CDC, 1972]. The more recent figures for children from Costa Rica (1.6%) [Novygrodt, 1983], Guatemala (9.2%) [Arroyave et al, 1979] and Honduras (less than 2.8%) [CID, 1980] indicate that vitamin A deficiency is no longer a public health problem in these three countries.

The proportions of the total population exhibiting vitamin A deficiency in Bolivia and Brazil are extremely high, being 45.1% and 43.0%, respectively [OPS, 1981]. The national nutrition survey conducted in Bolivia in 1981 reported a national incidence of night-blindness of 2.1% in children aged 6 to 59 months, confirming the existence of a severe deficiency of vitamin A in that country [INAN, 1983].

Table VI presents data on changes in vitamin A deficiency in children in the 1960s and from 1976 to 1980 [INCAP/CDC, 1972; MSPAS/INCAP, 1977; Novygrodt, 1983; Arroyave et al, 1979; CID, 1980]. The results show a marked decline in the incidence of vitamin A deficiency in all countries. Fur-

TABLE V. Incidence of Vitamin A Deficiency (20 μg/dl) in Children Under 5 Years of Age and in the Total Population in Tropical America

Country	Year	Incidence (%)
Children		
Costa Rica	1981	1.6
Honduras[a]	1980	2.8
Guatemala	1977	9.2
Panama	1967	18.4
Nicaragua	1966	19.8
El Salvador	1976	33.3
Total population		
Venezuela	—	4.9
Paraguay	—	6.6
Guyana	—	9.5
Colombia	1977–1980	12.4
Brazil	—	43.0
Bolivia	—	45.1

[a]The latest information from Honduras [CID, 1980] reported a percentage of cases below 30 μg/dl of 2.8%. Therefore, no more than 2.8% of cases are below 20 μg/dl.

(−) No information about the year was available [OPS, 1981].

TABLE VI. Incidence of Vitamin A Deficiency (20 μg/dl) in Children Under 5 Years of Age in Tropical American Countries During the 1960s and 1976–1980

Country	Period	Incidence (%) Previous survey (1960s)	Incidence (%) Latest survey (1976–1980)	Average annual reductions
Honduras	1967–1980[a]	39.5	2.8	2.82
Costa Rica	1966–1981	32.5	1.6	2.06
El Salvador	1966–1976	50.0	33.3	1.67
Guatemala	1965–1977	26.2	9.2	1.42

[a]For 1967, information from INCAP/CDC [1972]. Regarding figure for 1980, see footnote a, Table V.

thermore, two surveys conducted in children under 5 years of age in six communities of rural Honduras—one in 1978 prior to the initiation of a program designed to fortify sugar with vitamin A and one in 1980 after 2 years of sugar fortification—showed that the proportion of children with serum retinol levels below 30 μg/dl was reduced from 35% to 2.8% [CID, 1980]. In Honduras, Guatemala, and Costa Rica, national programs fortifying sugar with retinol palmitate were implemented in the 1970s.

TABLE VII. Incidence of Endemic Goiter in the Total Population
of Tropical America

Country	Year	Incidence (%)
Colombia	1965	2
Costa Rica[a]	1979	4
Panama	1975	6
Mexico	1972	8
Guatemala[a]	1979	10
Venezuela[a]	1966	13
Brazil[a]	1976	14
Peru	1975–1976	15
Honduras	1966	17
Paraguay	1976	18
Nicaragua	1981	20
El Salvador[a]	1973	24
Bolivia	1981	61

[a]School-age children.

Incidence of iodine deficiency. The incidence of iodine deficiency has
been evaluated by either the percentage of the total population or of the
school-age population with any clinical evidence of goiter.

The latest reports documenting the incidence of endemic goiter in the total
population in TA are presented in Table VII. Bolivia, Ecuador, Peru, Paraguay, Brazil, Guyana, Venezuela, El Salvador, Honduras, Guatemala, and
Nicaragua have rates above 10% [INCAP/CDC, 1972; OPS, 1981; INCAP,
1982; DeMaeyer et al, 1979; Quezada, 1979]. Colombia and Costa Rica have
successfully eliminated clinical cases of iodine deficiency, as less than 5% of
the populations have goiters. In Suriname, Mexico, and Panama the latest reported figures on incidence of goiter are less than 10% [DeMaeyer et al, 1979;
Flores et al, 1981; Parillón, 1979].

The changes in the incidence of endemic goiter have been well documented
in TA countries as reflected in Table VIII. With the exception of Paraguay and
Brazil, dramatic improvements have been seen in endemic goiter rates in most
countries.

Incidence of anemia. No current national statistics on the magnitude of
iron- and folate-related anemias are available for TA countries. The data
available by the end of the 1960s describing the proportion of pregnant women
with hemoglobin levels below the World Health Organization (WHO) norm
(less than 11.0 gm/liter) in different regions or cities of TA countries are
shown in Table IX [Royston, 1982]. The Pan American Health Organization
collaborative study, conducted in the early 1970s in cities of Brazil, Colombia,
Guatemala, Mexico, Peru, and Venezuela, showed anemia rates of 28.5% in
pregnant women, 17.3% in nonpregnant women, and 3.9% in adult males

TABLE VIII. Incidence of Endemic Goiter in Different Periods in Tropical American Countries

Country	Period	Incidence (%)		Average annual reductions
		First survey	Latest survey	
Nicaragua	1978–1981	33	20	4.3
El Salvador	1967–1973	48	24	4.0
Colombia	1945–1965	45	2	2.2
Panama	1967–1975	16	6	1.2
Costa Rica	1966–1979	18	4	1.1
Guatemala	1954–1979	38	10	1.1
Peru	1967–1976	22	15	0.8
Mexico	1950–1972	20	8	0.5
Brazil	1956–1976	18	14	0.2
Paraguay	1965–1976	18	18	0.0

TABLE IX. Estimates of Percentage of Pregnant Women With Levels of Hemoglobin Below the Norm* in Tropical American Countries

Country	Year	(%)
El Salvador	1969	15
Brazil	1968	20
Colombia	1968	22
Guatemala	1965	34
Peru	1968	35
Mexico	1968	38
Venezuela	1968	54
Guyana	1971	55

*Less than 11 gm/liter.

[Cook et al, 1971; Royston, 1982]. Iron-deficiency anemia was widespread in both high and low socioeconomic groups. Serum folate deficiency was found in 10% of women. Serum B_{12} deficiency was identified but only in pregnant women [Royston, 1982].

Variation in Mortality and Malnutrition Within Countries

The following analyses of variation in mortality and in the nutritional status of children within TA countries are based on data available from Costa Rica, Guatemala, and Panama.

A survey of schoolchildren's height conducted by Costa Rican teachers in 1979 showed dramatic differences among the 80 "cantones" in the numbers of children with attained height below 90% of the expected height for age. Five cantones had a rate of height retardation above 22%, and in another five, the proportion of children with heights below 90% ranged from 4.4 to 6.3% [Valverde et al, 1980b].

A survey of schoolchildren's height was conducted in Panama in 1982 [MS/ME, 1983]. The information was disaggregated for the 514 municipalities into which the country is divided. The percentage of children with a height more than two standard deviations below the median height of the (US) National Center for Health Statistics (NCHS) reference pattern [Hamill et al, 1979] was 21.8%. However, a total of 14 municipalities had rates of height retardation (> 2 SD below the NCHS median) above 70%, whereas in 34 municipalities, no children were found whose height was > 2 SD below the reference median. Similar data are available from other countries [Mora, 1982; SGCNPE/INCAP, 1980].

Data documenting differentials in the nutritional status of children according to the occupation of the head of household also have been reported. Information available from a national nutrition survey conducted in Guatemala in 1980 showed that in families whose heads of household were farmers with less than 0.7 hectare of land, 57.1% of children were reported with height retardation, as compared to 34.7% in those families where the head of household was a skilled employee [SGCNPE/INCAP, 1980]. Similar findings have been communicated from other TA countries [SIN/MS, 1980; Franklin et al, 1982].

Variation in IM in 1978, at the canton level, in Costa Rica is illustrated in Figure 1. The hatched areas represent cantones with IM above 35/1,000; areas

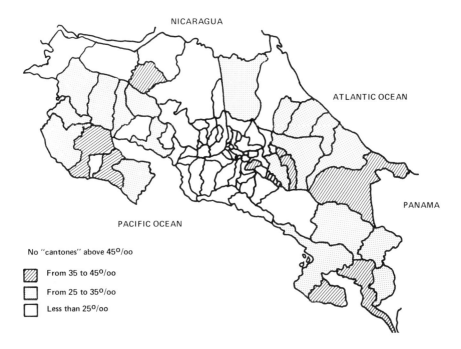

NICARAGUA

ATLANTIC OCEAN

PANAMA

PACIFIC OCEAN

No "cantones" above 45⁰/oo

From 35 to 45⁰/oo

From 25 to 35⁰/oo

Less than 25⁰/oo

Fig. 1.   Infant mortality by canton, Costa Rica, 1978.

in white are cantones exhibiting IM below 25/1,000 [Bermúdez, 1980]. Similar data describing differentials in IM in the 66 districts of Panama for 1982 have been reported [MS, 1983].

The probability of dying during the first 24 months of life has been reported by region in Guatemala [Haines et al, 1981]. The probability ranged from 92/1,000 children in the Central Region to 176/1,000 children in the Southern Region. During the period 1964–1973 the annual decline was observed mostly in nonindigenous populations (4.0/1,000) and to a lesser extent in indigenous groups (1.2/1,000).

Ecology dictates the differentials described. Poverty and malnutrition are concentrated mostly in rural communities. For example, the prevalences of height retardation in different ecological regions of El Salvador have been reported elsewhere [Valverde et al, 1980a]. Half of the children in coffee-growing areas are height-retarded, whereas in the urban slums only 33% are found in the same category. On the other hand, data gathered on schoolchildren in Costa Rica and Panama have shown that the areas inhabited by a higher proportion of Indians exhibit the highest levels of malnutrition [Valverde, 1980a; MS/ME, 1983]. Coincidentally these are also the most deprived regions within countries.

The coastal regions and lowlands are dedicated to banana, cotton, sugar, and other cash crops, which are grown on large plantations employing full-time or part-time laborers. The low-quality land is left for small farmers cultivating staple foods.

The high-quality land on the mountain slopes or the highlands is dedicated to coffee or other cash export crops, which are also grown on large plantations employing permanent and seasonal laborers. The poor land in the highlands also is left to subsistence farmers cultivating staple foods. These populations also form the seasonal labor force employed in the cotton and coffee harvests. Seasonal migration also entails family disruption and greater exposure to diseases.

DISCUSSION

The data show that nutritional deficiencies still exist in several TA countries. Within countries, important variation was identified in mortality and in the nutritional status by geographical location and occupation of the head of household.

Significant improvements in the incidence of protein-energy malnutrition and vitamin A and iodine deficiencies have occurred in several TA countries. These changes may be the result of the extension of health service coverage, improvements in agricultural production and local marketing systems and/or the efficient operation of food fortification programs.

Another contribution to improving the nutritional status of the region has been the decision to conduct periodic diagnoses of food and nutrition conditions and set up permanent nutrition information systems. These efforts have promoted political concern, both internationally and nationally, and facilitated the more rational allocation of existing resources to those families and/or communities in greatest need of social, health, and nutrition services.

The improvements in vitamin A status observed in Costa Rica, Guatemala, and Honduras can be attributed directly to the implementation of national programs adding vitamin A to sugar. However, in Colombia and El Salvador, where fortification of this type has not been implemented, the major contribution to improvements in vitamin A status and other nutritional deficiencies may be the extension of social services to dispersed communities. For example, in El Salvador a nationwide program, operating in 1973 and 1974, distributed vitamin A capsules through the health infrastructure [Sommer, 1976]. In many countries iron supplements are routinely distributed to pregnant women.

The analyses of changes in the nutritional conditions of the population of TA were based on incidence rates. However, population growth occurring during the study period may overshadow the nutritional improvements measured by these rates. In some countries in which national figures report less severe health and nutritional problems than in the past, more individuals are currently suffering from malnutrition in spite of the reductions in overall rates. For planning purposes and action programs the total number of persons at risk is often more useful than incidence.

Some CMA countries are now more exposed to man-made disasters owing to the rapid depletion of natural resources and to regional political conflicts. The latter has caused the displacement of entire communities and greater difficulties of access to basic services. Significant declines in the production of basic foods are also occurring in the same areas. Refugee problems are reported in Mexico, Guatemala, Honduras, and Costa Rica, and to a lesser extent in Panama.

The international crisis has also limited the capacity of governments to extend the coverage of social and nutritional services. Priority has been given again to direct government investments in productive activities, as opposed to the allocation of additional resources to social services. The deterioration of the purchasing power of national currencies has also imposed constraints on the normal operation of programs such as the fortification of salt and sugar, since the potassium iodate and the retinol palmitate are imported.

On the other hand, in almost all countries, governments have made efforts to identify and locate geographically the most deprived families and communities so that action programs can be better targeted. This has led to a more efficient provision of basic health and nutrition services to regions and communities that were traditionally excluded from these benefits. Still the lack of current valid and reliable health and nutritional data evidence the need for providing more support to the development of permanent food and nutrition information systems. At the same time, the likely impact of economic crises on health and nutrition indicators should not be overestimated. In spite of a severe economic crisis that occurred in Costa Rica from 1980 to 1982, the important improvements in health and nutrition conditions observed during the 1970s were maintained in the 1980–1982 period [Jaramillo, 1983]. The results of the 1977–1980 national survey in Colombia [Mora, 1982] provide similar evidence. Likewise, poor Guatemalan communities have not suffered a deterioration in health and nutritional conditions, in spite of the economic crisis and/or more limited access to social services [Delgado et al, 1983].

What changes in nutritional conditions can be expected from government interventions? This question is discussed in Gwatkin et al [1980], Delgado et al [1983] and Valverde et al [1983]. Undoubtedly, efficient food fortification programs have eradicated iodine and vitamin A deficiencies in many countries [Arroyave et al, 1979; DeMaeyer et al, 1979]. To estimate the expected nutritional effects of social and economic interventions by government, let us examine data from coffee plantations located in Western Guatemala. Families in these plantations were afforded a medical care program, an increase in minimum wages, and the distribution of an improved protein corn, Opaque-2, for 17 months [Valverde et al, 1983]. The overall incidence of weight retardation declined from 32.4% to 22.2% one year after a new wage scale was enacted. In those populations receiving the Opaque-2 corn, a medical care program, and an increase in wages, children's growth was better than in comparison populations with only medical care and improvements in wages.

The provision of medical care alone has been reported to produce declines in IM and 1–4 YM [MOH/INCAP, 1982; Delgado et al, 1983], but the effects are not immediately reflected in children's growth. In spite of dramatic declines in IM and 1–4 YM in Western Guatemala [Delgado et al, 1983] no reductions were seen in the percentage of children weighing less than 75% of standard weight for age after the communities were exposed for 3 years to an effective simplified medical care program [Valverde et al, 1983].

The variety of lifestyles should be a major consideration in designing interventions for deprived groups. For example, an increase in minimum wages will improve the purchasing power of laborers in coffee plantations but will not affect subsistence farmers or other laborers whose salaries are "above" minimum wages. On the other hand, small farmers will be positively affected by programs distributing land and credit, which to a much lesser extent may also affect other poor groups. Subsidies, through low-price shops, will not benefit populations residing in isolated communities, as these services are usually located in cities or in concentrated semiurban areas.

To conclude, mortality, anthropometric, and other data reflecting vitamin A, iodine, iron, and folate deficiencies indicate that nutritional problems still persist in TA countries. These deficiencies are often more dramatic when the data are analyzed by region and family type. Finally, nutritional problems in TA are not going to be eradicated by "a program" but rather by the operation of a set of programs of an economic and social nature under the responsibility of personnel who understand the behavior and the likely responses of communities to the proposed program activities. Furthermore, there is not — and let's not keep looking for — a single technological solution to overcome food and nutritional problems. It has to be accepted that if resources available are not directed efficiently to poor families, and if decisions of policy makers to implement effectively the proposed actions are not taken, malnutrition will continue to affect an important proportion of the population residing in Tropical American countries.

REFERENCES

Amat C, Cunurisy D (1981): "La Alimentación en el Perú." Lima, Perú.

Arroyave G, Aguilar JR, Flores M, Guzmán MA (1979): "Evaluation of Sugar Fortification with Vitamin A at the National Level." Scientific Publication No. 384. Washington, DC: PAHO.

Baum S, Arriaga E (1981): Levels, trends, differentials and causes of infant and early childhood mortality in Latin America. World Health Stat Q 34(3):147–167.

Bermúdez A (1980): La mortalidad infantil por cantón 1972–1977. In "Informe del Sistema de Información en Nutrición." San José, Costa Rica: Oficina de Información de la Casa Presidencial.

CID (Centro de Investigación y Desarrollo) (1980): Evaluación del programa de enriquecimiento de azúcar blanca de mesa con vitamina A en Honduras (unpublished).

Cook JD, Alvarado J, Gutnisky A, Jamra M, Labardini J, Layrisse M, Linares J, Loria A, Maspes V, Restrepo V, Reynafarje C, Sánchez-Medal L, Velez H, Viteri F (1971): Nutritional deficiency and anemia in Latin America: A collaborative study. Blood 38:591–603.

Delgado H, Valverde V, Hurtado E (1983): "Case studies on infant mortality, primary health care and nutrition in rural Guatemala." Guatemala City: INCAP (mimeograph).

DeMaeyer EM, Lowenstein FW, Thilly CH (1979): "The Control of Endemic Goitre." Geneva: WHO, pp 55–59.

Dutra de Oliveira J, de Souza W, Arteaga Pachecho H, Giarola LC (1981): Nutritional status in South America. Prog Clin Biol Res 7:283–291.

Flores M, López ME, Santisteban I, de Céspedes C (1981): Epidemiología del bocio endémico en Costa Rica. Bol Sanit Panamer 531:539.

Franklin D, Harrell ML, Parillón C, Valverde V (1982): Nutritional functional classification study in Panama. Raleigh, NC: Sigma One Corporation (mimeograph).

Gómez F, Ramos-Galván R, Frenk S, Muñoz JC, Chávez R, Vásquez J (1956): Mortality in second and third degree malnutrition. J Trop Pediatr 2:77–83.

Gwatkin D, Wilcox JR, Wray JD (1980): "Can Health and Nutrition Interventions Make a Difference?" Overseas Development Council Monograph No. 13. Washington, DC: ODC.

Haines MR, Avery RC, Strong MA (1981): "Differentials in infant and child mortality and their change over time. Guatemala 1959–1983." Paper presented at the annual meeting of the Population Association of America, Washington DC, March 25–28.

Hamill PV, Drizd T, Johnson R, Reed R, Roche A, More WM (1979): Physical growth: National Center for Health Statistics Percentiles. Am J Clin Nutr 32:607–629.

INAN (Instituto Nacional de Alimentación y Nutrición) (1983): Encuesta Nacional de Nutrición de Bolivia, 1981 (unpublished data).

INCAP (1982): "Informe anual 1 de enero–31 de diciembre de 1981." Guatemala City: INCAP.

INCAP (Instituto de Nutrición de Centro América y Panamá) (1983): "Diagnóstico Alimentario-Nutricional de El Salvador." Guatemala City: INCAP, Vol 1, Cuadro 2I-1.

INCAP/CDC (1972): "Nutritional Evaluation of the Population of Central America and Panama. Regional Summary." Washington, DC: DHEW Publication (HSM).

Jaramillo J (1983): "Los Problemas de la Salud en Costa Rica: Políticas y Estrategias." San José, Costa Rica: Litografía Ambar.

Joy L, Payne PR (1975): Nutritional and national development planning. Food Nutr 1(4):2–17.

MIDEPLAN (Ministerio de Planificación Nacional y Política Económica) (1983): "El deterioro de la condición social de los costarricenses." San José, Costa Rica: MIDEPLAN.

MOH/INCAP (Ministry of Public Health and Social Welfare and Institute of Nutrition of Central America and Panama) (1982): "Integrated Systems of Nutrition and Primary Health Care (SINAPS)." Guatemala City: INCAP.

MS (Ministerio de Salud) (1983): "Defunciones de menores de 1 año y de 1–4 años y tasas de mortalidad en la República de Panamá, según provincia y distrito. Año de 1982." Panamá City: Ministerio de Salud (mimeograph).

MS/ME (Ministerio de Salud y Ministerio de Educación) (1983): "Resultados del primer censo de talla en niños de primer grado escolar en Panamá: 1982." Guatemala City: INCAP.

MSPAS/INCAP (Ministerio de Salud Pública y Asistencia Social/Instituto de Nutrición de Centro América y Panamá) (1977): "Evaluación de la adecuación de vitamina A en la población salvadoreña." Guatemala City: INCAP.

Mora JO (1982): "Situación Nutricional de la Población Colombiana en 1977–1980." Vol 1. "Resultados Antropométricos y de Laboratorio. Comparación con 1965–1966." Bogotá: Instituto Nacional de Salud.

Novygrodt R (1983): Encuestas séricas de vitamina A en población infantil costarricense: 1966, 1979 y 1981. (submitted for publication).

OPS (Organización Panamericana de la Salud) (1981): "Salud para todos en el año 2000: Estrategias." Washington, DC: OPS, pp 63–71.

PAHO (Pan American Health Organization) (1982a): Demographic and socioeconomic background. In PAHO (1982): "Health Conditions in the Americas, 1977–1980." Scientific Publication No. 427. Washington, DC: PAHO, pp 1–16.

PAHO (Pan American Health Organization) (1982b): Environmental health. In PAHO (1982): "Health Conditions in the Americas, 1977–1980." Scientific Publication No. 427. Washington, DC: PAHO, pp 159–166.

PAHO (Pan American Health Organization) (1982c): Health studies measures. Total population. In PAHO (1982): "Health Conditions in the Americas, 1977–1980." Scientific Publication No. 427. Washington, DC: PAHO, pp 17–68.

Parillón C (1982): "Alimentación y nutrición en Panamá: La situación actual." Panamá City: Ministerio de Salud.

Parillón C (1979): "El bocio ya no es un problema de Salud en Panamá." Panamá City: Ministerio de Salud (mimeograph).

Quezada M (1979): "Evaluación del impacto del programa de yodización de la sal en Guatemala a través de una encuesta de prevalencia de bocio endémico y yoduria en una muestra de escolares de la República de Guatemala." Monografía (Magister Scientificae). Guatemala City: INCAP.

Royston E (1982): The prevalence of nutritional anaemia in women in developing countries: A critical review of available information. World Health Stat Q 35(2):52–91.

SGCNPE/INCAP (Secretaría General del Consejo Nacional de Planificación Económica/Instituto de Nutrición de Centro América y Panamá) (1980): Regionalización de problemas nutricionales en Guatemala. Guatemala City: INCAP, pp 51–64.

SIN/MS (Sistema de Información en Nutrición/Ministerio de Salud((1980): "Aspectos socioeconómicos de la nutrición." San José, Costa Rica: SIN, pp 45–48.

Sommer A (1976): Assessment of xerophthalmia and the mass vitamin A prophylaxis program in El Salvador (September 1973–December 1974). J Trop Pediatr 22:136–148.

Valverde V, Nieves I, Sloan N, Pillet B, Trowbridge F, Farrell T, Beghin I, Klein RE (1980a): Styles of life and nutritional status of children from different ecological regions of El Salvador. Ecol Food Nutr 9:167–177.

Valverde V, Vinocur P, Salazar S, Rojas Z (1980b): Relación entre la prevalencia de retardo en talla en escolares e indicadores socio-económicos a nivel de cantón en Costa Rica. Bol Inf SIN 2(10):4–10.

Valverde V, Arroyave G, Guzmán M, Flores M (1981): Nutritional status in Central America and Panama. Prog Clin Biol Res 67:271–282.

Valverde V, Delgado H, Belizán JM, Martorell R, Mejía-Pivaral V, Bressani R, Gonzaga-Elías L, Molina MR, Klein RE (1983): "The Patulul Project: Production, storage, acceptance and nutritional impact of Opaque-2 corn in Guatemala." Guatemala City: INCAP (mimeograph).

Malnutrition: Determinants and Consequences, pages 19–27
© *1984 Alan R. Liss, Inc., 150 Fifth Avenue, New York, NY 10011*

Malnutrition in the Western Hemisphere: Caribbean Islands

David Picou, MB, PhD
Mount Hope Medical Complex Task Force, Port of Spain, Trinidad

The Caribbean Islands comprise a chain of beautiful and mostly independent countries that encircle the Caribbean Sea and link the North and South American continents. I will deal with most of the English-speaking Caribbean; many important countries, including Spanish-speaking Cuba and the Dominican Republic, French-speaking Haiti, Martinique, and Guadeloupe, the U.S. Virgin Islands and Puerto Rico, and the Netherland Antilles, regrettably have been omitted from this presentation. However, both Guyana and Belize, which are on mainland South and Central America, respectively, and which border the Caribbean Sea, have been included. Table I contains the list of countries that form the basis of my presentation.

The objective of this chapter is to define the major problems of malnutrition and food scarcity in the Caribbean.

THE ENGLISH-SPEAKING CARIBBEAN: VITAL STATISTICS AND HEALTH STATISTICS

For more than 30 years many studies have been conducted in the Caribbean, particularly in Jamaica, on the prevalence, clinical features, and biochemistry of malnutrition in infants and young children. Notable institutions at which much of this work was and is done are the Tropical Metabolism Research Institute, the Caribbean Food and Nutrition Institute, the Medical Research Council's Epidemiology Research Unit, the University of the West Indies (Jamaica), and the Nutrition Unit in Barbados.

The data used to define malnutrition problems have been compiled from two main sources: vital statistics and health statistics. Most of the data are for

TABLE I. Vital and Health Statistics for 13 English-Speaking Caribbean Countries

| Country | Population | | Birth rate, 1975–1979 (average)[3] | Mortality | | % Low birth weight (≤2.5 kg) | % Pediatric admissions for malnutrition/ gastroenteritis | Gomez classification | | |
	Total	Under 5 years		Infant, 1975–1979 (average)[3]	1–4 years			I	II	III
Antigua (year)	75,000[1] (1978)	11.7	19.5	30.8	1.0[1] (1978)	12.4[1] (1979)	24.2[1] (1979)	25.5[1c] (1979)	2.9	0.75
Barbados (year)	247,300[1] (1975)	8.9	18.4	27.8	1.2[1] (1975)	19.0[1] (1975)	–	36.1[1n] (1975)	3.1	0.3
Belize (year)	128,327 (1973)	19.1	39.8[1] (1973)	33.7[1] (1972)	4.5[1] (1973)	–	–	33. 1c (1976)	11	2
Cayman Is (year)	15,013[4] (1974)	10.8	21.6[4] (1974)	17.8[4] (1974)	0.9[4] (1974)	7.9[4] (1973–1975)	27.7[4] (1973–1974)	14.1[4c] (1975)	2.0	–
Dominica (year)	81,000[1] (1978)	13.0	21.9	23.8	1.4[1] (1978)	10.5[1] (1978)	23.4[1] (1976)	38.6[1] (1976)	10.3	1.8
Grenada (year)	110,390[1] (1978)	13.4	24.8	22.4	1.9[1] (1972)	12.2[4] (1974–1975)	19.6[4] (1974–1975)	19.2[1c] (1979)	4.4	1.3
Guyana (year)	825,414[4] (1979)	14.7	35.5[4] (1970)	50.8[1] (1975)	3.8[1] (1975)	12.2[1] (1974–1975)	17.0[1] (1979)	30.4[1c] (1979)	8.3	0.7

Jamaica (year)	2,200,000[5] (1980)	15.8	28.7	17.5	5.5[5] (1971)	11–14[1]	25[9] (1968–1973) 0–2 years	31.1 (1976)	6.9	0.9
Montserrat (year)	13,292[4] (1975)	13.5	18.3	43.6	1.5[6] (1976)	17.9[1] (1975–1976)	13.5[1] (1972–1975)	19.8[1]c (1975)	2.3	0.2
St Kitts (year)	47,400[4] (1974)	14.7	23.8	41.7	2.0[4] (1975)	13.4[1] (1975)	20.8[1] (1975) <5 years	32.5[1]c (1976)	6.6	0.3
St Lucia (year)	110,800[1] (1974)	17.6	35.7	27.1	2.3[1] (1974)	9.3[1] (1975–1976)	14.4[1] (1975)	32.8[1] (1974)	8.9	1.9
St Vincent (year)	100,427[1] (1975)	16.7	30.1	49.1	4.3[1] (1975)	10.4[1] (1976)	40.9[1] (1976) <5 years	22.7[1]c (1976)	6.2	1.6
Trinidad & Tobago (year)	1,059,200[2] (1980)	11.2	21.0	24.0	1.5[1] (1974)	10.8[7] (1981–1982)	10.8[8] (1976)	36.8[1] (1976)	11.1	1.4

*Superscript symbols: c = clinic survey; n = national survey. Arabic numerals designate references: 1. CFNI (Caribbean Food and Nutrition Institute) [1980]. 2. Annual Statistical Digest, Trinidad and Tobago, 1980 [1983]. 3. Mc Glashan [1982]. 4. CFNI (Caribbean Food and Nutrition Institute) [1977]. 5. FAO Production Yearbook [1982]. 6. Guerney [1982]. 7. Ali [1983]. 8. Annual Report, Ministry of Health, Trinidad and Tobago [1977]. 9. Ashworth and Picou [1974].

the mid-1970s and caution should be exercised in attempting comparison between countries, since the sources of the data are not necessarily comparable.

The vital statistics reviewed are total population, population under 5 years old, birth rate per 1,000 population, infant mortality rate (IM) or number of deaths in the first year of life per 1,000 live births, and mortality for the age group 1–4 years or the number of deaths in the age group 1–4 years per 1,000 at risk.

Vital Statistics

Total population. The majority of these countries are small and so are their populations. Nine of the 13 countries have populations of less than 200,000 and two have populations between 1 million and 2 million. The estimated total population for the 13 countries in 1980 is 5.3 million [FAO, 1982].

Population under 5 years old. The average percentage of the total population aged < 5 years was 13.9%, with a range of 8.9%–19.1%, which is the same as that found in selected areas in eight Latin American and Caribbean countries by Burke [1979].

Birth rate. Only three of the 13 countries had a birth rate less than 20 births per 1,000 population, whereas five countries had birth rates in excess of 25.

Infant mortality. In the Caribbean infant mortality is a fair indicator of malnutrition, which occurs mainly in the first and second year of life. In 6 of 13 countries IM exceeded 30. One of the minimum health goals adopted by the regional governments for the year 2000 is that no country in the region will have an IM of more than 30 deaths per 1,000 live births [PAHO, 1982].

Mortality in the 1- to 4-year age group. This is a less sensitive indicator of malnutrition in the Caribbean because malnutrition is seldom seen after 2 years of age. Nine of the 13 countries have a rate less than 2.4 and have therefore already achieved one of the minimum health goals for the region [PAHO, 1982].

Health Statistics

Low birth weight. Low birth weight (2.5 kg or less) or malnutrition was an underlying or associated cause of death in about 57% of children under 5 years of age in one Caribbean and eight Latin American countries [Puffer and Serrano, 1975; Klein et al, 1976]. In 10 of 13 countries, the percentage of infants born weighing 2.5 kg or less was more than 10%.

Undernutrition in children 0–59 months of age. During the past two decades there have been several nutritional surveys in young children in the Caribbean. More representative data on nutritional status have been obtained from national surveys (Barbados, Dominica, Guyana, Jamaica, St. Lucia, and Trinidad and Tobago) than from clinic surveys, which underestimate the percentage of undernourished children. Gueri [1982] estimates that between 25% and

50% of children under age 5 years are malnourished on a weight-for-age basis. From the six national surveys cited above, it was found that averages of 35%, 8%, and 1.3% of children under 5 years of age were classified as Gomez I, II, and III grades of malnutrition, respectively. Gueri [1982] estimates that there are about 75,000 malnourished children in the English-speaking Caribbean.

Hospital admissions for malnutrition and gastroenteritis. Malnutrition often coexists with gastroenteritis and infections, and a malnourished infant is commonly admitted to hospital with a diagnosis of gastroenteritis or acute respiratory infection. In many hospitals in the Caribbean, pediatric admissions are reported for the age group 0–11 years, with no breakdown into smaller age groups. In eight Caribbean countries the percentage of pediatric admissions for malnutrition, gastroenteritis, or both ranged from 10.8 to 27, which amounts to 7% of all pediatric admissions (0–11 years). When data were gathered for percentage of admissions of children under 2 years or under 5 years of age, the figures were of course much higher. With the increasing use of oral rehydration therapy on an outpatient basis, eg, in Trinidad and Tobago, the number of hospital admissions for gastroenteritis has decreased. Taking into consideration these various factors, a likely estimate is that malnutrition accounts for 20–25% of all admissions of children under age 5 years in the English-speaking Caribbean.

Overnutrition. It is paradoxical that adult overnutrition coexists with childhood undernutrition. *Obesity* (more than 20% excess over ideal body weight) is more common in female than male adults. Surveys in five Caribbean countries show that between 24% and 39% of females are obese as compared to 2.4–13% of adult males [Fraser, 1980].

Two other nutrition-related problems of some magnitude in the Caribbean should be mentioned. *Anemia* is common in the preschooler and in pregnant and lactating females and is usually due to iron deficiency [Guerney, 1982]. *Diabetes mellitus* is an important cause of morbidity and mortality especially in the older female. The percentage of all deaths due to diabetes averaged 4.2% and 7.1% for males and females, respectively, in 10 of the 13 countries [McGlashan, 1982].

DETERMINANTS OF CHILDHOOD MALNUTRITION IN THE CARIBBEAN

The occurrence and development of malnutrition in the Caribbean have been attributed to several factors that operate in and interact with varying economic, social, and political events and systems. There is general agreement that the immediate, physiologic cause of malnutrition is a food intake that is inadequate in quantity or quality to meet the requirements for normal growth and development. There is less agreement on the underlying or associated factors and events that result in a deficient food intake. Poverty was identified as a significant underlying factor in studies in St. Vincent [Grenier and Latham, 1981; Antrobus, 1971] and Jamaica [Desai et al, 1968, 1970; Marchione and Prior, 1980; Guerney, 1982], but it was either not mentioned [Jenkins, 1982] or not considered a major factor [Marchione, 1980; Gueri, 1982] in other studies.

Other significant factors that have been reported to correlate with poor nutritional status were family type (size, number of children alive or deceased, dependency ratio, maternal and paternal age, paternal absence, short birth intervals, and age, birth weight, and birth rank), food availability and feeding practices (dependence on self-produced foods, duration of breast feeding, introduction of solids, intrafamilial sharing of food), occurrence of illness (diarrhea or previous malnutrition) or death in a sibling, and lack of education. It is clear that many of these factors are interrelated and are in turn influenced by local sociocultural practices (eg, use of herbal infusions during infant illness), national policies (eg, agricultural policy, food subsidies, the food-marketing system), and international events (price for primary products and imported food items). It is the complexity of local and external factors that has led to more in-depth studies (eg, see Marchione [1980]) and the proposal of a holistic approach to studies of this problem [Jonsson, 1981]. While a better understanding of the determinants of childhood malnutrition may emerge from such studies, there must be continuing government, community, and individual action, based on available relevant action plans [CFNI, 1974].

FOOD AVAILABILITY

At the national level, the amount and variety of available foods are determined by many factors including the amount, types, and cost of food imports, the amounts and types of locally produced foods, land use, the internal food distribution systems, and food-pricing policies and subsidies, as well as fluctuations in world food prices and levels of production. It is not the intention here to discuss these important issues in any detail. Le Franc [1981] has discussed the possible impact of social structure, land use, and food availability in the Caribbean, and there are two recent reports on food price and subsidy policies in Trinidad and Tobago [Mc Intosh, 1980] and Jamaica [Allen, 1980].

National food availability studies show three features that are common to the Caribbean. 1) There is heavy dependence on food imports, which account for about 46% of food energy supplies and 62% of protein supplies [Guerney, 1982]. 2) Cereals, in particular wheat products, account for about one-third of both energy and protein available and they are all imported, save rice in certain countries [Guerney, 1982]. 3) Many basic foods are heavily subsidized by governments.

A heavy price is paid for this dependence on food imports; the price increased from US$185 million in 1970 to an estimated US$740 million at present. Food subsidies are also an increasing drain on national treasuries and amounted to US$107 million in Trinidad and Tobago for 1981.

FOOD AVAILABILITY AND NUTRITIONAL STATUS

Estimates of percapita availability of protein and energy for the Caribbean were obtained from the FAO Production Yearbook [1982] for the years 1978–1980, and reference standards of 2,130 kcal for energy and 47 gm protein [Sukhatme and Basu, 1972] were arbitrarily chosen to assess the adequacy of percapita food availability. There are inherent risks in this analysis; one must bear in mind the continuing controversy that surrounds the correctness of protein and energy requirements in man and how these estimates are used or misused in relating them to population data [FAO, 1981].

There were three countries in which the percapita energy available was a little above or below the reference standard. In the other eight countries, the energy available ranged from 4% to 43% (mean 19%) above the reference standard. This is clearly a precarious situation, if the reference standard is valid for these countries. With regard to protein availability one country was at about the reference value, whereas there was a range 118–181% (mean 138%) for the other nine countries. As is well recognized, these aggregate data reflect the theoretical amount of energy or protein that is available to each person if the food were equally distributed. In this imperfect world this is clearly not such an accurate representation. Household food consumption data for five countries indicate that only about 44% of households get enough dietary energy and 56% get adequate dietary protein [Guerney, 1982]. Clearly there is a maldistribution of food among families. The picture is even more complicated when one looks at the data on overnutrition. Obesity (body weight 20% or more above ideal weight) is common in Caribbean females, ranging from 24% to 39% in five countries and is less common in Caribbean males (2.4%–13%).

This maldistribution of food among families is also seen within families [Marchione, 1981; Gueri, 1982] and has been identified as an important contributing cause of childhood malnutrition.

OUTLOOK AND REGIONAL STRATEGIES

One Caribbean territory has already banned certain food imports and another has begun to reduce food subsidies. Both measures appear to have been taken for economic reasons and the impact on food availability and nutritional status is not known. Caribbean governments are emphasizing the need to increase local production of food both for consumption and export individually and collectively through a Regional Food Plan, and to coordinate and rationalize regional food production with a view to meeting 70% of the region's food requirements by 1990. Failure to effectively implement these measures will result in a worsening of the nutritional status of Caribbean populations, especially those in which childhood malnutrition is already a major public health problem.

REFERENCES

Ali Z (1983): Personal communication.

Allen V (1980): Problems in implementing programmes to control or stabilize staple food prices in Jamaica. In Solimano G, Taylor L (eds): "Food Price Policies and Nutrition in Latin America." Tokyo: United Nations University, pp 66–77.

"Annual Report of the Ministry of Health for the Year Ending 31st December 1977." Port of Spain, Trinidad: Ministry of Health.

"Annual Statistical Digest, Trinidad and Tobago, 1980" (1983): No 27, Central Statistical Office, Port of Spain, Trinidad: Ministry of Finance.

Antrobus ACK (1971): Child growth and related factors in a rural community in St. Vincent. J Trop Pediatr 17:187–209.

Ashworth A, Picou D (1974): Nutritional status in Jamaica 1968–73. Paper presented at the Conference on Food and Nutrition Policy, Kingston, Jamaica.

Burke M (1979): Inter-American Investigation of Mortality in Childhood, Report on a household sample. In Burke M, Yorke M, Sande I (eds): PAHO Sci Pub 386, Washington DC: PAHO, pp 1–54.

CFNI (Caribbean Food and Nutrition Institute) (1974): "Strategy and Plan of Action to Combat Gastroenteritis and Malnutrition in Children Under Two Years of Age." Kingston, Jamaica: CFNI.

CFNI (Caribbean Food and Nutrition Institute) (1977): "Nutritional Status of Young Children in the English-Speaking Caribbean" (Revised). CFNI-J-54-77. Kingston, Jamaica: CFNI, pp 1–55.

CFNI (Caribbean Food and Nutrition Institute) (1980): "Country Nutrition Profile." CFNI-J-72-80. Kingston, Jamaica: CFNI, pp 1–11.

Desai P, Miall WE, Standard KL (1968): The social background of malnutrition. Maternal Child Care 4:161.

Desai P, Standard KL, Miall WE (1970): Socio-economic and cultural influences on child growth in rural Jamaica. J Biosoc Sci 2:133–143.

FAO (1981): The uses of energy and protein requirement estimates. Food Nutr Ser 3:45–53.

FAO (1982): "Production Yearbook." Rome: FAO, Vol 35.

Food and Nutrition Bulletin (1981): The uses of energy and protein requirement estimates. Food and Nutr Bull 3:45–53.

Fraser HS (1980): An overview of obesity in the Caribbean, its prevalence, prevention and treatment. Cajanus 13:131–138.

Grenier T, Latham MC (1981): Factors associated with nutritional status among young children in St. Vincent. Ecol Food Nutr 10:135–141.

Gueri M (1982): Childhood malnutrition in the Caribbean. Cajanus 15:76–83.

Guerney JM (1982): Food supply and nutrition in primary health care in the Caribbean. Cajanus 15:221–237.

Jenkins CL (1982): Factors in the aetiology of poor growth in Belize. Cajanus 15:172–184.

Jonsson V (1981): The causes of hunger. Food Nutr Bull 3:1–9.

Klein RE, Arenales P, Delgado H, Engle PL, Guzmán G, Irwin M, Lasky R, Lechtig A, Martorell R, Mejía Pivaral V, Russel P, Yarbrough C (1976): Effects of maternal nutrition on fetal growth and infant development. Bull Pan Am Health Organ 10:301–316.

Le Franc E (1981): Social structure, land use and food availability in the Caribbean. Food Nutr Bull 3:5–11.

Marchione TJ (1980): Factors associated with malnutrition in the children of Western Jamaica. In Jerome N, Kandel R, Pelto G (eds): "Nutritional Anthropology." New York: Redgrave, pp 223–273.

Marchione TJ (1981): Child nutrition and dietary diversity within the family. A view from the Caribbean. Food Nutr Bull 3:10–14.

Marchione TJ, Prior FW (1980): The dynamics of malnutrition in Jamaica. In Greene LS, Johnston FE (eds): "Social and Biological Predictors of Nutritional Status." New York: Academic, pp 201–222.

Mc Glashan ND (1982): Causes of death in ten English-speaking Caribbean countries and territories. Bull Pan Am Health Organ 16:212–223.

Mc Intosh CE (1980): Food price and subsidy policies and nutrition: Experiences in Trinidad and Tobago. In Solimano G, Taylor L: "Food Price Policies and Nutrition in Latin America." Tokyo, United Nations University, pp 78–96.

PAHO (1982): "Health for All by the Year 2000. Plan of Action for the Implementation of Regional Strategies." PAHO Official Document No 179. Washington DC: PAHO.

Puffer RR, Serrano CV (1973): "Patterns of Mortality in Childhood." PAHO Sci Pub 262. Washington DC: PAHO.

Puffer RR, Serrano CV (1975): "Birth Weight, Maternal Age and Birth Order: Three Important Determinants in Infant Mortality." PAHO Sci Pub 294. Washington DC: PAHO.

Sukhatme PV, Basu D (1972): The present situation: Pattern of food production and availability of foods in Asia. In "Proceedings of the First Asian Congress of Nutrition, Hyderabad, India."

Malnutrition: Determinants and Consequences, pages 29–43

Food and Nutrition Problems in Urbanized Latin America: Misdirected Development

Ricardo Uauy, MD, PhD**, Rolando Chateauneuf, and Sergio Valiente,** MD
Instituto de Nutrición y Tecnología de los Alimentos (INTA), University of Chile, Santiago 11, Chile

INTRODUCTION

The last decades have been associated with important demographic changes in Latin America. Urbanization has been the dominant force in this change. Rapid population growth, lower mortality, and urbanization have definite implications for food and nutrition problems. The impact of the rural-urban shift can be perceived in the region. The insufficiencies of most urban centers to accommodate their new settlers and satisfy their basic needs have not detered others from coming. Latin American cities continue to grow. Masses of human beings living under conditions of extreme poverty distributed as rings or large pockets have mushroomed in the periphery of most if not all large cities in Latin America. The expectation of a better life in the city is the motivation that attracts millions of people to the crowded urban centers; the lack of consistent rural development policies is the force that discourages people from staying in the villages and other small agricultural settlements.

Food and nutrition are important components of basic human needs. The marginalized segments of the population of cities in the region have unmet needs for food, housing, health, sanitation, water, employment, recreation, education, and clean air. In some cities, governments impose a further restriction on the self-expression and community participation needs of poor urban dwellers, limiting their search for solutions.

The malnutrition present in the urban centers of Latin America is the result of the inadequacy (deficit or excess) of diets to meet the nutritional needs under the prevailing environmental conditions. Food scarcity and nutritional need cannot be dissociated from the integrum of basic human needs. Malnutrition is not only a problem of food scarcity; it is part of a poverty situation in which most human needs are not appropriately met. Food consumption patterns in the city are largely dependent on food availability and effective demand. In real terms this means food prices and purchasing capacity. Urban centers are not self-sufficient in food. Moreover, the shift in consumption patterns that occurs in the city increases the need for food imports and external dependency. The urban demand for food is sustained by income derived from the industrial, commercial, and service sectors of the economy, which flourish in the city. Yet income maldistribution and unemployment curtail the food-purchasing capacity of many and determine most of the nutritional problems. Formal and nonformal education as well as propaganda will modulate in part the response of the consumer in purchasing food commodities. Food utilization and satisfaction of nutritional needs are determined by overall health, especially the presence of infection and level of environmental sanitation. The decline in breast-feeding practices in the urban areas aggravates further the problems of nutrition and health of the vulnerable infant.

This basic framework will help in the interpretation of nutritional problems of urban Latin America. Although some differences exist between countries, the main variations are within cities and countries. Maldistribution is the key word in this phenomenon. Food, health, education, work, sanitation, housing, and income are not distributed according to need but are heavily determined by the social and economic structures of society at the national and international level. The urban poor are selectively marginalized by the urban marketplace both in their basic demands and as suppliers of labor. Nutritional problems and their consequences are also grossly maldistributed. Protein energy malnutrition, anemia, xerophthalmia, endemic goiter, and rickets—all related to nutrient deficits—coexist with obesity, diabetes, and atherosclerosis in the urban centers of Latin America. This chapter will focus on the available data on the nutritional problems related to food scarcity and excess in urban Latin America.

URBAN GROWTH IN LATIN AMERICA
Characteristics of the Latin American Population

Latin America has exhibited rapid population growth over the last four decades. In 1950 there were 164 million inhabitants, data for 1980 showed 364 million, by year 2000 a figure of 566 million is projected, and for 2025 the expected population is 864 million. This is over five times the 1950 figure. This explosive demographic growth is explained by the progressive widening in the gap between birth and death rates exhibited by most Latin American countries. The fall in birth rate lags considerably behind the observed decline in mortality figures associated with public health and nutrition improvements.

This in turn has delayed the demographic transition and has resulted in faster population growth than that shown by the developed world in the nineteenth century. The Latin American population is growing at an annual rate of 2.47%; this is faster than any other region in the world. Many countries in Central America and the Caribbean will double their population in less than 25 years. Most of this explosive growth is and will be concentrated in the urban centers. Table I compares projected urban and rural growth for Latin America [CELADE, 1981].

Accelerated Urban Growth

There are wide disparities in the definitions of urban centers. Most Latin American countries choose demographic criteria based on the population: ie, more than 1,000, 1,500, 2,000, 5,000, or 20,000 inhabitants. Some countries consider additional characteristics of basic infrastructure such as street plan, commerce, or public services. To avoid problems of definition the United Nations system has suggested that settlements with greater than 20,000 inhabitants be considered urban. All agree with defining as urban those settlements where the predominant economic activity is not agricultural [SIEP/UNESCO, 1982].

Urban growth in Latin America has been fueled by massive rural-urban migration as well as by the gap between birth and death rates in urban centers. As the proportion of urban dwellers increases, migration from rural settlements becomes progressively less important. The demographic transition associated with decreased birth rates eventually contributes to slowing urban growth. For some countries urban growth came late but very rapidly. In Guatemala, El Salvador, Honduras, Nicaragua, Dominican Republic, Haiti, Ecuador, Bolivia, Paraguay, and Costa Rica, urban growth exceeds 4.2%, but their urban dwellers are still less than 50% of the population. For countries such as Colombia, Mexico, Brazil, Peru, Venezuela, and Panama urban growth came late but less rapidly. These countries have 50–70% of their total inhabitants in cities but

TABLE I. Projected Annual Population Growth Rates (%) for Latin America, 1940–2025

Period	Urban	Rural	Urban/rural
1940–1950	5.00	1.50	3.3
1950–1970	5.20	1.50	3.5
1971–1980	3.50	1.08	3.5
1981–1990	3.19	0.81	4.0
1991–2000	2.77	0.59	4.6
2001–2025	2.13	0.39	5.5

Based on information obtained from CELADE (Latin American Demographic Center), 1981.

growth is around 4%. Countries with early urbanization have almost completed their demographic transition and show urban growth rates under 2.5%. Argentina, Chile, and Uruguay have more than 80% of their total population in urban centers. The exception in this group is Cuba, with a 65% urban population. Table II shows annual urban growth rates and projected population figures by year 2000 for Latin American countries categorized according to onset and velocity of urban growth as previously described [CELADE, 1981].

Urban growth in Latin America can thus be accounted for by a net difference between birth and death rates in the city, by rural-urban migration, and by a reclassification of rural centers as urban. For developed countries the latter two explain 60% of urban growth. In contrast, more than 60% of Latin

TABLE II. Latin American Estimated Population in 1983, Urban Growth Patterns, and Projected Figures for 2000

	1983		2000		
Country	Total population (thousands)	% Urban	Annual urban growth rate (%)	Total population (thousands)	% Urban
Argentina	28,033	82.67	1.78	32,861	89.14
Cuba	9,906	64.64	2.15	12,717	74.03
Chile	11,682	81.11	2.44	14,934	89.41
Uruguay	2,935	84.78	1.01	3,448	90.59
Brasil	131,146	64.14	4.22	212,507	78.33
Colombia	27,518	67.64	3.71	42,441	80.81
México	76,085	66.36	4.57	132,244	78.96
Panamá	2,038	54.42	3.79	2,823	67.02
Perú	19,162	65.47	3.97	29,468	77.92
Venezuela	17,258	78.85	4.21	25,705	88.47
Bolivia	6,034	40.19	4.05	9,299	51.40
Costa Rica	2,374	45.85	4.07	3,377	59.30
Ecuador	8,810	44.32	4.24	14,596	54.14
El Salvador	5,232	44.40	4.16	8,708	54.61
Guatemala	7,931	38.43	4.40	12,739	48.54
Haiti	6,258	24.98	4.79	9,860	37.66
Honduras	4,092	40.20	5.54	6,978	55.28
Nicaragua	3,015	54.31	4.78	5,154	68.23
Paraguay	3,476	42.08	4.19	5,273	52.35
República Dominicana	6,402	47.22		9,332	62.71
Latin America	390,850	63.00		495,000	76.00
Less developed countries	990,000	30.00		2,155,000	43.00
Developed countries	864,000	71.00		1,174,000	81.00

Source: Latin American Demographic Center [CELADE, 1982].

American urbanization at present is derived from the net gain derived from high birth rates and low mortality. Urban growth in Latin America accounted for 82.3% of the total population increase during the 1960–1980 period. The projection for 1980–2000 shows that 93.5% of the net population gain will come from the expansion of urban centers [SIEP/UNESCO, 1982].

Metropolization in Latin America

A metropolis is defined as an urban settlement that has more than 100,000 inhabitants. While in 1950 Latin America had only 61 metropolises, by 1960 there were 92; in 1972 the number had grown to 148 and by 1980 there were 229. The progression in time of Latin American urban centers with more than a million inhabitants has been a unique phenomenon. Less than 4% of the population in 1920 lived in these cities; by 1980 this figure had risen to 27.3% (101 million people). Latin America in 1980 had a greater percentage of its population living in cities of over a million people than the developed countries combined (26.6%). The percentage of the Latin American population residing in cities of over 5 million for 1980 was 13.6%. This is second only to North America, which has 18.3% of its people living in large cities, whereas Africa has only 1.6%, Asia 4.1%, Europe 7.7%, and the Soviet Union 2.9% [SIEP/UNESCO, 1982].

Some cities, such as Tijuana in Mexico and Chimbote in Peru, have exhibited annual growth rates in excess of 9%, which means that they have doubled their population in less than 8 years. Most metropolitan cities are growing at a rate greater than 5%, which implies a doubling of population in less than 15 years. For many countries, one-third to one-half of the population lives in the capital city. The high concentration of people beyond what the urban infrastructure is capable of handling and the explosive population growth rates explain the failure of these settlements to satisfy the basic human needs of their inhabitants. Urban slums mushroom in the large metropolises of Latin America. They are called *favelas* in Brazil, *tugurios* in Colombia, *ranchos* in Venezuela, *barriadas* in Peru, *callampas* in Chile, *villas miseria* in Buenos Aires, *cantegriles* in Uruguay, *colonias proletarias* or *chozas* in Mexico, *barriadas brujas* in Panama, and *bidonvilles* in Haiti. The names may vary but the the phenomenon is still the same: gross inadequacies in satisfying all basic needs. Crowded, fragile cardboard houses, two or three families per dwelling, three or four children per bed, contaminated water, pests, parasites, insects, rodents, and waste are part of the failed hope for a better life in the city. The contrast between affluence and poverty; cultural highlights and illiteracy; modern skyscrapers and slums; gluttony and hunger — all are a part of the typical Latin American urban metropolis. Figure 1 shows the evolution of the population for six of the largest cities in Latin America during the second half of this century.

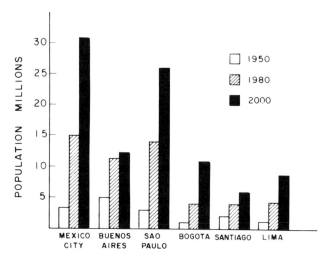

Fig. 1. Past, present, and projected population of the six largest Latin American metropolises. From SIAP/UNESCO [1982], with permission.

IMPACT OF URBANIZATION ON FOOD AND NUTRITION PROBLEMS

In this section we will explore in further detail the impact of urbanization on food and nutritional problems. There are potential benefits and of course significant problems associated with urban life. The dream of a better future in the city is sometimes frustrated and turns into a dreadful nightmare of life in the slum, where unemployment, poor health, malnutrition, and family disruption become a forceful awakening.

Urbanization and Food Availability

The impact of urbanization on food availability in several countries in the region has been directly measured by household consumption surveys and also estimated indirectly from national food availability data, income of various segments of the population, and income elasticities of food commodities. These figures show that for the urban poor there are marked insufficiencies in the availability of cereals, sugar, fruits, meat, milk and dairy products, and fats and oils. Roots and tubers, legumes, vegetables, and eggs are also in inadequate supply but to a lesser degree. A notable exception is the availability of corn, which compensates for the insufficiency of other cereal products in many countries. The Economic Commission for Latin America (ECLA) has estimated for 1980 that 52 million people consume less food than that required to satisfy their needs. The monetary value of this food gap was considered to be US$3,161 million for 1980. Milk products, meat, and cereals make up 62% of the total value. The food gap for the region corresponds to 4.3% of the internal agricultural product of Latin America, US$73,833,000,000 for 1980 [Molina, 1983]. Based on household consumption data available for Brazil, Honduras, Mexico, Peru, Dominican Republic, and Venezuela, a simple correlation analysis between degree of urbanization and the gap in food purchases of the poor expressed as a percentage of the national mean shows a significant negative correlation between food insufficiency and urban population as a percentage of total population. Those countries with less urbanization show higher food gaps. The correlation coefficient is −0.78 (Table III shows data base).

The stable supply of food in urban centers favors adequate consumption. Furthermore, the mean per capita energy availability expressed as percentage of requirements is significantly higher in countries with high urbanization. The intercountry correlation coefficient in this case is 0.53 (n = 20 $P < 0.05$) (Table III shows data base). Moreover, many countries in the region have food fortification programs. Wheat flour is enriched with vitamin B complex, iron, and calcium in 15 countries. Sugar is fortified with retinol in 5 countries. Fluoridation of the water supply is found in 5 countries, and iodization of salt is mandatory in 17 countries of the region. These programs predominantly favor the urban population and are important preventive measures for nutrient-specific deficiencies [UNICEF, 1979]. A large number of countries have national food distribution programs to improve the nutritional status of vulnerable groups. The coverage varies widely but undoubtedly the cities receive the largest proportion of this direct food aid or indirectly benefit through subsidies that favor the urban consumer to the detriment of the agricultural sector, which will often have fixed prices for basic staples.

The data on the satisfaction of energy needs of urban versus rural dwellers varies for different studies and even within a country it may vary between locations. For Brazil as a whole the World Bank estimated a mean per capita energy gap of 119 kcal, distributed as 210 kcal for the urban population and 2 kcal for the rural sector. The figures for Southeast Brazil are −143 kcal for urban and +209 kcal for the rural area [Gray, 1982]. In any case these energy gaps do not match the nutritional status of rural population groups. Furthermore, these results are confounded by inadequacy in the estimation of energy needs, especially of sedentary populations in urban centers, where, indeed, overestimation of requirements is probably the case.

Although city dwellers may be on the average better off than the rural in terms of food availability and satisfaction of needs, the marginalized urban poor are potentially under worse conditions than their rural counterparts. Low income and inadequate commercialization channels condition food purchases of the urban poor. They buy less food and have to pay more for it. The poorest among the urban poor would probably be better off in the rural areas.

TABLE III. Food and Nutrition Status Indicators for Latin America

Country	Population, thousands (1980)	Urban population, % (1980)	Poor population, % (1980)	Income per capita, US dollars (1980)	Food insufficiency, % median income (1980)	Energy availability, % requirement (1980)	Schooling, % (1980)	Illiteracy, % (1980)
Argentina	28,033	82.67	8	1,140	—	127	71	7.4
Cuba	9,905	64.64	—	—	—	118	75	—
Chile	11,682	81.11	16	1,088	—	112	70	11.0
Uruguay	2,955	84.78	—	1,415	19.9	107	54	10.2
Brasil	131,146	64.14	43	956	—	105	58	33.6
Colombia	27,518	67.64	43	831	—	99	55	19.1
Mexico	76,085	66.36	29	1,167	14.5	120	65	25.8
Panamá	2,038	54.42	37	1,150	—	99	77	21.7
Perú	19,162	65.47	49	670	18.6	92	70	27.2
Venezuela	17,258	78.85	24	1,312	16.9	107	58	23.5
Bolivia	6,034	40.19	—	381	—	87	53	37.3
Costa Rica	2,374	45.85	22	996	—	117	59	11.6
Ecuador	8,810	44.32	—	640	—	91	64	25.8
El Salvador	5,232	44.40	—	423	—	94	52	42.9
Guatemala	7,931	38.43	—	558	—	94	35	53.8
Haití	6,258	24.98	—	147	—	83	24	75.3
Honduras	4,092	40.20	64	338	31.8	96	48	40.5
Nicaragua	3,015	54.31	—	350	—	102	47	42.1
Paraguay	3,476	42.08	—	630	—	126	50	19.8
Rep. Dominicana	6,402	47.22	—	558	—	94	60	33.1
Source	CELADE [1981]	CELADE [1981]	Molina [1983]	ECLA [1980]	Molina [1983]	Molina [1983]	ECLA [1980]	ECLA [1980]

Urbanization in the region is associated with important changes in consumption patterns, with an increase in wheat, sugar, oil, and animal protein intake and declines in the more traditional staple foods based on corn, beans, or other legumes and tubers. This change usually brings about an increase in food imports and an increase in outside dependency. Processed foods in the urban centers are promoted by international agribusiness conglomerates and may cause further deterioration in the quality of the diet of the urban poor.

Effects of Accelerated Urbanization on Health and Nutrition

The growth of urban centers has been fueled by a net population increase resulting from lower mortality and stable birth rates. Undoubtedly the health and nutrition of urban dwellers on the average are better than for the rural sector. This can be explained mainly by better access to preventive measures but also by the influence of modern medical care. Immunizations and other health maintenance programs have greater coverage in urban centers. Epidemiologic and nutritional surveillance usually predominantly encompasses the urban population. Nutrition intervention programs such as supplementary feeding, sanitary improvements, food fortification, and malnutrition prevention and recovery centers have a wider coverage in the cities. These programs may target all those in need but their efficiency is greater in the city. Furthermore the urban centers are usually politically more relevant and are easier to reach than the rural areas. Some of these programs may even thrive in spite of doubtful effectiveness as long as they retain urban-based political support.

Simple correlation analysis conducted between countries of the region according to percentage urbanization and multiple health and nutrition indicators shows that the degree of urbanization is positively correlated with rate of measles immunization per child under 5 years ($r = 0.46, P < 0.05$). For Haiti this rate was 0.003 in 1976; for the more urbanized countries it exceeds 1.0 [Horwitz, 1980]. Infant mortality is negatively related to percentage urbanization ($r = -0.32$). Preschool child mortality is also negatively related to percentage urbanization; this correlation is stronger than for infants ($r = -0.69$). The available data for seven countries show a nonsignificant correlation ($r = -0.26$) between percentage urbanization and first-degree malnutrition by a weight-for-age criterion but a significantly negative one with second- and third-degree malnutrition ($r = -0.70$). A statistically significant positive correlation was found between life expectancy and percentage urbanization ($r = 0.51$) for 20 countries of the region [UNICEF, 1979]. The absolute number of inhabitants and percentage urbanization were not significantly correlated. Details of the data base for these intercountry correlations can be found in Table IV. Although these results in no way signify causality, they do suggest that urban life is associated with significant improvements in the food, nutrition, and health status of the population.

TABLE IV. Health and Nutrition Status Indicators for Latin America

Country	Urban population with clean water, % (1977)	Urban population with clean waste disposal, % (1977)	Infant mortality, per 1,000 (1975)	Infant mortality, per 1,000 (1980)	Mortality of 1 to 5-year-olds, per 1,000 (1975–1980)	I-degree malnourished in age group ≤ 5 years, % (1976)	II- and III-degree malnourished in age group ≤ 5 years, % (1976)	Measles immunization per child aged 5 years (1976)	Life expectancy, in years (1975–1980)
Argentina	68	40.0	41	40.8	2.2	36.0	9.3	0.72	69.2
Cuba	60	46.0	24	22.6	0.9	–	–	–	72.8
Chile	79	67.0	62	38.7	1.5	11.9	3.4	1.07	65.7
Uruguay	75	58.0	42	38.2	1.1	–	–	1.84	69.5
Brasil	63	34.0	82	–	–	–	–	0.07	61.8
Colombia	64	65.0	59	46.7	5.6	43.1	19.5	0.26	62.2
Mexico	59	41.0	60	57.0	4.9	–	–	0.50	64.4
Panamá	82	97.0	38	33.0	4.5	–	–	0.65	69.7
Perú	45	50.0	109	37.2	5.9	31.0	13.0	0.91	57.1
Venezuela	81	52.0	45	33.9	2.4	35.3	13.6	0.68	66.2
Bolivia	38	42.2	142	–	–	30.4	21.6	0.11	48.6
Costa Rica	60	42.0	45	22.1	1.3	40.1	12.4	0.34	69.7
Eduador	46	63.0	83	57.5	10.1	–	–	0.29	60.0
El Salvador	55	36.0	79	53.4	6.1	52.3	22.1	1.16	62.2
Guatemala	40	31.0	89	72.3	13.1	47.5	34.9	0.57	57.8
Haití	10	–	121	31.4	6.5	25.9	52.3	0.003	50.7
Honduras	42	48.0	95	21.9	–	43.0	38.0	1.32	57.1
Nicaragua	74	31.0	96	–	2.0	46.0	22.6	0.55	55.2
Paraguay	12	15.0	49	47.1	5.0	27.0	5.0	0.05	64.1
Rep. Dominicana	57	27.0	74	30.8	3.0	42.0	24.0	0.002	60.3
Source	ECLA [1980]	ECLA [1980]	ECLA [1980]	ECLA [1980]	Horwitz [1980]	PAHO [1979]	PAHO [1979]	Horwitz [1980]	ECLA [1980]

Urbanization may also have a negative effect on health and nutrition. Sedentary life styles, increased animal food and energy availability, and the psychological stress of the city influence mortality associated with obesity, atherosclerosis, and diabetes in the more urbanized countries of the region. For Argentina, Chile, Colombia, Jamaica, and Uruguay cardiovascular disease is the leading cause of death among adults living in the urban centers [Valiente, 1983].

Urbanization has often been ranked as a leading factor in the decline in breast-feeding practices observed among women in many countries of the region. Most data show that the prevalence of breast feeding in the cities is less than half of that observed in the rural areas [Mardones, 1980]. This difference is only partly explained by the involvement of women in the labor force and may be an example of the effects of the urban culture, where the penetration of foreign habits is strongest.

Increased chemical and microbiologic contamination in the cities may explain the paradox of increases in communicable enteric disease, such as typhoid fever, paralleling urban growth. Sanitation in the city may often be qualitatively worse than in the rural sector. There is a significant intercountry correlation between clean water supply and percentage urbanization ($r = 0.69$, $P < 0.01$). Within countries, rural dwellers are usually worse off quantitatively than those in urban centers, but the microbiologic threat can be greater in the city. Figure 2 shows typhoid fever morbidity and mortality in Chile from 1930 to 1980. The metropolitan Santiago population comprises 60–70% of the cases. During this period the country has doubled its percentage of urban population and the city has grown close to 10 times. Mortality from typhoid has nevertheless been reduced from 7 to 0.4 per 10^5 for this period [Colegio Médico, 1983]. The failure of the urban infrastructure to accommodate the explosive growth spurt is also evidenced by an increase in death rates from traffic accidents. The chemical pollution for some cities may carry added health hazards in terms of pulmonary disorders and neoplastic disease associated with environmental carcinogens.

Sociocultural Changes in Urban Centers

The city growth attracts people to an "enlightened cultural life." Access to schooling and nonformal education is enhanced by urbanization. The rural population has very limited educational opportunities. The intercountry analysis shows that illiteracy rates are negatively correlated with percentage of urban population ($r = -0.54$) and that the percentage of children under 12 years of age remaining in school is positively correlated with urbanization ($r = 0.62$). Improved educational opportunities also imply better access to health and nutrition knowledge, although this may take a longer time to accomplish, since most formal educational programs do not cover these subjects ade-

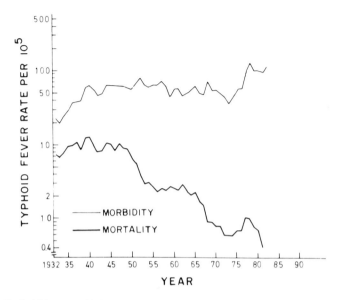

Fig. 2. Typhoid fever morbidity and mortality in Chile per 100,000 inhabitants during the last five decades. From Colegio Médico [1983], with permission.

quately. Nonformal education may fill in many of these gaps in practical knowledge and contribute to the modification of habits [UNICEF, 1979].

The conflict between the urban and rural cultures may take more than a generation to resolve; the conflict is omnipresent in the marginal periurban areas. The new generation raised in the city is not fully integrated and is a source of potential problems that may cause family disruption. Individual families are progressively isolated in the slums and are easy prey to social vices, alcoholism, drugs, child neglect, and prostitution. Disrupted families are many times a factor in the food and nutrition problems found in the cities. The effect of urbanization on breast-feeding practices is a good example of the adverse consequences of the urban culture. Market-oriented propaganda may further aggravate the food and nutrition status of the vulnerable urban poor. Nonessential food items may often displace more nutritious traditional staples and have potentially adverse nutritional consequences.

Political and Economic Change in Urbanized Centers

The rural-urban shift is associated with a transfer of wealth and power from an agriculturally based economic and political system to an industrially oriented urban society with increasing demands for income and power redistribution. Mechanization of agricultural labor and rural population growth have generated a migratory drive to the cities. Development strategies in the region have usually favored industrialization and have created progressive impoverishment of the farmers. The increase and expansion in communication systems have facilitated and precipitated rural-urban migrations. Progress in the cities has been idealized and this image projected and promoted among the rural areas. The city allows more direct access to political participation. Organized labor movements have gained and retained an important share of power under democratic and even authoritarian rulers. Populism, in its attempts to please the masses, has been a political constant in most countries and despite its adverse economic consequences it has usually meant increased social benefits for the urban poor.

Our intercountry analysis based on minimum income required to satisfy basic needs, as suggested by ECLA's definition of poverty, shows a significantly negative correlation (r = -0.66, $P < 0.05$) between percentage urban and percentage poor for ten countries of the region. Argentina, a highly urbanized country, has 8%, while Honduras has 64%, below the poverty line. There is also a high correlation between percentage urban population and mean national income (r = 0.85, $P < 0.001$).

The cost of food represents a large percentage of the income. For the urban poor it may exceed 50% and for some subgroups among the poor it may reach as high as 70% [Valiente et al, 1982]. In many countries inflation poses a serious threat to the food-purchasing capacity of the urban workers. Salaries are always lagging behind inflation. The push for higher wages and the ever increasing demands for better living conditions contribute to higher inflation rates. This spiral has in some countries escaped control, with the predictable final results of loss of purchasing capacity and an overall economic deterioration. On the other hand modest inflation is almost a necessity to satisfy the progressive rise in expectations associated with development. Urban life for the poor is also afflicted by the scourge of unemployment or more frequently subemployment. Urban development strategies have not been able to create enough jobs for the rapidly growing labor force. In times of economic depression, as during the last 3 years, unemployment figures have surged above 15%; for some countries up to 30% of the labor force is underemployed or not employed at all [Chateauneuf, 1983].

Gross inequalities and maldistribution of wealth underlie the social disruption of many urban developing societies. Income distribution has not improved over the last decades and economic growth has predominantly benefited the middle- and higher-income groups. The poor may be relatively poorer today than 10 years ago according to ECLA estimates. Development may in fact aggravate social and economic injustices [Molina, 1983]. This situation is the breeding ground for politicians who offer more than can be realistically provided in order to get elected and attain power. Demagogy is the name of the game. The race for better and more benefits from the state has definite limits; frustration is the final result. Social and political disruption may end up in chaos, revolution, or military intervention. Any of these results will end up restricting individual freedoms and they have different modalities of social control. The city, with its contrasts, inequalities and injustices, is an underlying cause of these phenomena.

CONCLUSIONS

Analysis of the consequences of urbanization on food and nutritional problems reveals that the balance between the positive and negative greatly favors the living conditions that exist in the urban settlements. The results are not as clear if we examine the situation of the marginalized groups in the large metropolis, especially if we project their growth into the future and consider the present failure of the urban infrastructure of most Latin American cities. The demographic trends clearly point in the direction of continued urban growth with a disproportionate increase in the population of large metropolises. The expected result is continued growth in the proportion of urban poor living under subhuman conditions where basic needs, including food, will not be appropriately met. In this setting progress and development mean further social and economic injustices for the poor. In the final analysis, this situation calls for a basic change in development strategies. Actions to redirect development that stresses integrated rural development based on agricultural production rather than promoting industry in the large cities are badly needed. This would increase the job opportunities in the rural or small urban centers and contribute to the development of intermediate cities. The accelerated growth of the large metropolises should be stopped if living conditions of the marginalized urban groups are to be expected to improve. The health, nutrition, education, and other service facilities for the rural or small urban centers should be expanded if we expect to maintain more people in the rural areas and hopefully reverse the rural-urban shift. Large cities should give a high priority to improving the basic infrastructure of the marginalized urban poor rather than investing further in the more developed areas. Although these measures may seem unrealistic, they are only reasonable if we would like cities to fulfill their heritage as centers of civilization for all citizens. As an epilogue we have adapted a portion of the speech given by Mario Moreno "Cantinflas," a famous Latin American comedian, upon receipt of the 1982 FAO World Food Day Award. "I am afraid you will not understand me; you do not understand me but appear as if you did. . . . Just as there are street dogs, there are homeless children longing for love and hungry for a bite. We do not need to go to faraway war places to find them. In our own cities within the reach of our egoism and our indifference neglected children stride ignored by the economically privileged classes.... I do not want to wipe out the rich, I would like to eradicate poverty."

ACKNOWLEDGMENTS

The authors gratefully acknowledge the collaboration of Dr. Sandra Hirsch, who assisted in collecting and processing data, Mr. Oscar Ruiz for his review and valuable suggestions and Ms Genoveva Escobar for secretarial assistance.

REFERENCES

CELADE (Latin American Demographic Center) (1981): Boletín Demográfico No 28, July 28, 1981. Santiago, Chile: CELADE.

Chateauneuf R (1983): "Algunas Consideraciones Sobre la Evolución de la Población de América Latina. FAO Consultación en Urbanización Intensiva y Sus Repercusiones Alimentarias y Nutricionales en América Latina." RLAT 802/Bas-1. Santiago, Chile: FAO.

Colegio Médico (1983): "Algunas Consideraciones Sobre la Salud en Chile, Hoy." Santiago, Chile: Colegio Médico de Chile.

Gray CW (1982): Food Consumption Parameters for Brazil and Their Application to Food Policy." Washington, DC: International Food Policy Research Institute.

ECLA (1980): ECLA (Economic Commission for Latin America) (1980): Sintesis Estadística de América Latina 1960–1980 (versión revisada) Santiago, Chile: CEPAL.

Horwitz A (1980): La Malnutrición en Las Américas. In "VII Reunión del Consejo Directivo de la Asociación Latinoamericana de Academias Nacionales de Medicina." Santiago, Chile: Instituto de Chile, Academia de Medicina.

Mardones SF (1979): History of breast-feeding in Chile. Food Nutr Bull 1:15–22.

Molina S (1983): "El Desarrollo Latinoamericano y la Urbanización: Sus Relaciones con La Pobreza y La Alimentación. FAO Consultación en Urbanización Intensiva y sus Repercusiones Alimentarias y Nutricionales en América Latina." RLAT 802/Exp-1. Santiago, Chile: FAO.

PAHO (1979): Sci Publ No. 381 "Condiciones de Salud del Niño en las Américas." Washington, DC: PAHO.

SIEP/UNESCO (1982): "La Educación en Población y el Proceso de Urbanización. Enlace." Boletín Informativo. Santiago, Chile: SIEP/UNESCO.

UNICEF (1979): "Situación de la Infancia en América Latina y el Caribe." Santiago, Chile: Editorial Universitaria.

Valiente S et al (1982): "Situación de Familias Pobres en el Gran Santiago y Políticas Para Satisfacer Sus Necesidades Básicas: Un Caso de Estudio." E/CEPAL/L.277 Santiago, Chile: CEPAL.

Valiente S (1983): "Problemas Nutricionales Urbanos en Chile. FAO Consultación en Urbanización Intensiva y sus Repercusiones Alimentarias y Nutricionales en América Latina." RLAT 802/Bas-1. Santiago, Chile: FAO.

Malnutrition: Determinants and Consequences, pages 45–58
© *1984 Alan R. Liss, Inc., 150 Fifth Avenue, New York, NY 10011*

Malnutrition in Industrialized North America

Frederick L. Trowbridge, MD

Division of Nutrition, Center for Health Promotion and Education, Centers for Disease Control, Atlanta, Georgia 30333

BACKGROUND

In industrialized North America, as in less industrialized areas of the world, nutritionalists in public health have tended to focus on problems of undernutrition, such as growth stunting in children, iron deficiency anemia, and inadequate nutrient intakes during pregnancy and among the elderly. These problems occur with increased frequency among low-income populations and among specific ethnic and geographically defined groups. Because of the potential impact of these nutrition-related conditions on health, they continue to deserve attention and commitment of resources for prevention and treatment.

Despite the importance of inadequate nutrient intake in some populations, however, nutrition-related illness in industrialized North America has become increasingly related to nutritional excess rather than to nutritional deficiency. The importance of nutritional excess as a public health issue is reflected in the 1990 nutrition objectives for the nation formulated by the U.S. Department of Health and Human Services in 1980 [1]. Most of the objectives are concerned not with nutrient deficiency but with reducing risk factors related to overnutrition or an imbalance of dietary constituents.

An assessment of malnutrition in industrialized North America requires a review of nutritional inadequacies among high-risk groups. However, attention must increasingly be directed towards nutrition-related risk factors such as obesity, high sodium intake, and low dietary fiber, which are linked to the development of chronic conditions such as heart disease, diabetes, and hypertension.

SOURCES OF DATA

The sources of data that are most useful for defining nutritional status in industrialized North America include both sample survey data relating to the general population such as the Health and Nutrition Examination Surveys (HANES) in the United States [2] and the Nutrition Canada Survey [3], and surveys and studies directed at more specific, high-risk populations, such as the Ten-State Nutrition Survey [4]. In addition, nutritional surveillance data have been collected by the Centers for Disease Control (CDC) since the mid-1970s, providing an additional source of data on principally low-income pediatric and prenatal populations attending publicly supported health clinics in the United States. Taken together, data sources like these provide a data base that can be used to characterize general nutritional status as well as the nutritional status of low-income populations.

It is apparent, however, that these data sources have inherent limitations. Surveys such as the HANES provide an overview of nutritional status in the general population but do not provide information specific to regions, states, or subpopulations that may have specific nutritional problems. Studies directed at low-income populations, such as the Ten-State Nutrition Survey, are now 13–15 years old and may be out of date. Surveillance data can provide current information on children and women attending publicly supported clinics, but these data reflect the nutritional status of individuals who choose to attend such clinics and may not reflect the nutritional status of those not served by these facilities. Despite their limitations these data sources can serve to describe an overview of nutritional status and to define some trends over time.

REFERENCE STANDARDS

The selection of appropriate reference standards for assessing malnutrition is critical, since choosing a higher or lower standard can increase or diminish the apparent prevalence of nutritional problems. In regard to growth data the most commonly used standard in the United States is the NCHS-CDC reference population [5]. The fifth percentile of this reference population can serve as a useful although arbitrary cutoff point to define "low" values when comparing the relative growth of different ethnic groups and subpopulations. However, this criterion will be less useful for defining the absolute prevalence of growth stunting in the general population of the United States as measured, for example, by the HANES I survey. Since the reference standard is based, in part, on HANES I data, by definition 5% of children in the HANES I survey will fall below the fifth percentile and will be classified as "low" in terms of growth.

Another issue in regard to growth standards is the appropriateness of NCHS-CDC percentiles for assessing the growth of different ethnic groups. Race-specific differences in growth potential exist, but growth is also affected by environmental factors, including diet as well as infectious disease and other factors. In the developing world, environmental factors are likely to outweigh genetic influences in determining growth attainment [6]. In industrialized countries, however, adverse environmental factors are substantially reduced, and genetic factors may be relatively more influential, complicating the interpretation of ethnic-group growth differences.

The same issues arise in regard to reference standards for defining the prevalence of anemia. There is no firm consensus on the appropriate cutoff points to be used for defining anemia for different age and sex groups. Since hemoglobin and hematocrit levels normally change with age and change differentially in regard to sex, fixed cutoff points can provide only a rough definition of "low" values. A partial solution is to define sex-specific percentile values for hemoglobin and hematocrit for each month of age through puberty — in effect to develop a growth chart for hemoglobin and hematocrit. Percentile distributions of this type have been defined by CDC on the basis of HANES I data [7]. Despite the limitations imposed by small sample size, age- and sex-specific fifth percentile curves from the HANES I data have been used to define "low" values in the hematologic data from CDC surveillance presented in this chapter. In the future, HANES II data may provide a more adequate basis for developing percentile curves for hematologic data.

PROBLEMS RELATING TO NUTRITIONAL DEFICIENCY
Linear Growth Stunting

Retardation in linear growth has been identified in low-income populations in numerous surveys. The Ten-State Nutrition Survey indicated a clear relationship between levels of family income and reduced height growth. In that survey growth stunting was especially prominent among Hispanic populations. More current data from CDC nutritional surveillance of predominantly low-income populations indicate that growth stunting is a continuing concern among Hispanic children. Data for 1982 (Fig. 1) indicate that during infancy height growth is generally similar among ethnic groups, but by 1 to 2 years of age stunting becomes more prevalent among Hispanic and Native American children, a trend that increases in the later preschool years.

The ethnic groups with the highest prevalence of stunting also have the highest prevalence of high weight-for-height values that suggest obesity. As illustrated in Figure 2, beyond infancy, high weight-for-height is most prevalent among Hispanic and especially Native American children. High weight-for-

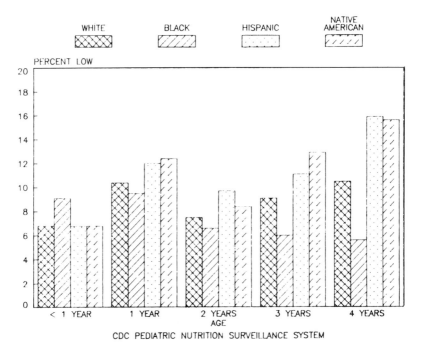

Fig. 1. Prevalence of low height-for-age by age and ethnic group. CDC Nutritional Surveillance, 1982.

height among Native American children may be a precursor to the obesity that is a significant problem among adult Native Americans, and that is associated with a high rate of diabetes. Similar concerns may also apply to Hispanic populations, as reflected in the relatively high weight-for-height values for their children.

The causes of linear growth retardation in these ethnic groups and the extent to which such causes represent nutritional deficiencies are not clear. However, the observation of high weight-for-height values, presumably representing obesity, suggests a qualitative rather than a quantitative nutrient deficiency. The diet of these children appears to supply sufficient energy intake as reflected in high weight-for-height status. However, their diet may fail to supply other nutrients needed for maximal linear growth.

The nutrient deficiencies that contribute to reduced linear growth are not well defined; perhaps marginal deficiencies of high-quality protein, vitamin A, or zinc are contributing factors. Relatively low levels of serum vitamin A and of dietary intake of vitamin A were observed in Mexican-American populations in the Ten-State Nutrition Survey. However, research is needed to pro-

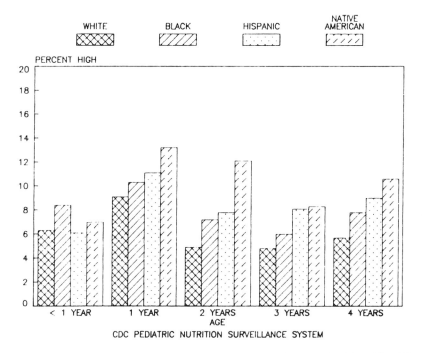

Fig. 2. Prevalence of high weight-for-height by age and ethnic group. CDC Nutritional Surveillance, 1982.

vide conclusive data on the nature of deficiencies contributing to growth stunting.

Overall trends in the prevalence of growth stunting are difficult to define. Nutrition surveillance data suggest a decline in prevalence among children from low-income families using publicly supported health services. As illustrated in Figure 3, a downward trend in prevalence is generally observed from 1976 to 1982 among children less than 2 years of age for all ethnic groups, although for Hispanics and Native Americans the trends appear to have leveled out in recent years. The prevalence of stunting is greatest among black children in this age group.

For children 2–5 years of age, trends over time are not consistent (Fig. 4). However, it is of interest that in this age group black children are the least stunted of the four ethnic groups; the prevalence of stunting approaches the 5% level "expected" to be found below the fifth percentile. Among Hispanic and Native American children, levels of stunting are relatively high and indicate an important public health concern.

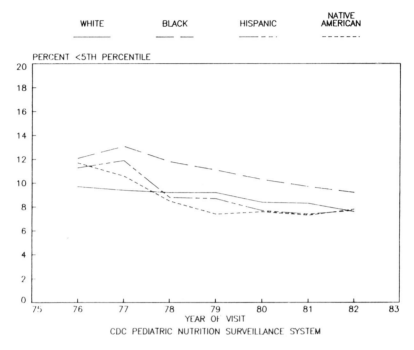

Fig. 3.   Prevalence of low length-for-age among children less than 2 years of age by ethnic group. CDC Nutritional Surveillance, 1976-1982.

Examination of comparable data for high weight-for-height over the same period indicates a general downward trend in prevalence for all ethnic groups among children less than 2 years of age (Fig. 5), which suggests improvement in the prevalence of obesity among infants. Among older preschool children 2-5 years of age, no consistent trends in regard to prevalence are observed (Fig. 6). As previously noted, the prevalence of high weight-for-height values in this age group is consistently greater among Hispanic and especially among Native American children. The extent to which this high weight-for-height represents obesity is not well defined. It may be that genetically determined differences in body proportions affect weight-for-height status [8]. However, high weight-for-height, probably reflecting obesity, must be cited as a continuing concern among Hispanic and Native American children.

Anemia

As for linear growth stunting, anemia has generally been observed to be most common among low-income populations. The Ten-State Nutrition Sur-

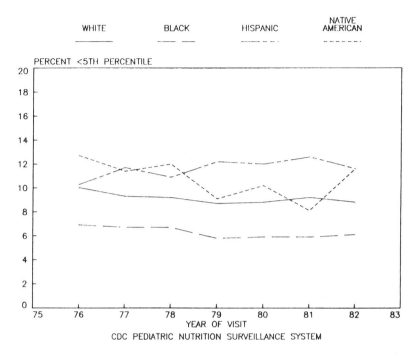

WHITE   BLACK   HISPANIC   NATIVE AMERICAN

Fig. 4.   Prevalence of low height-for-age among children 2–5 years of age by ethnic group. CDC Nutritional Surveillance, 1976–1982.

vey documented a higher prevalence of anemia among low-income groups and especially among black populations. Data from states reporting hemoglobin values to the CDC Pediatric Nutrition Surveillance System indicate that rates of anemia are generally higher among black children than among children of other ethnic groups.

Surveillance data indicate a modest downward trend in the prevalence of low hemoglobin values since 1976 (Fig. 7). These trends are generally shared by white, black, Hispanics, and Native American children. These trends are encouraging, suggesting that prevalence of anemia among low-income children served by publicly supported programs is declining.

Anemia in pregnancy is another issue of conern, particularly in low-income populations. Data from the Collaborative Perinatal Study [8a] show that anemia is more common among black pregnant women than among white women during pregnancy. Approximately 40% of black pregnant women had hemoglobins below 10 gm/dl, compared to approximately 12% of white pregnant women (Fig. 8).

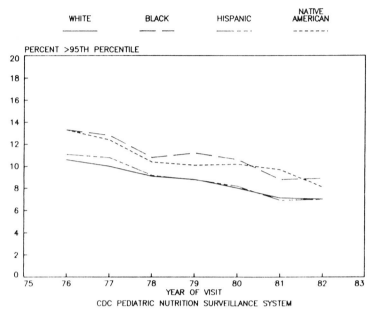

Fig. 5.   Prevalence of high weight-for-height among children less than 2 years of age by ethnic group. CDC Nutritional Surveillance, 1976–1982.

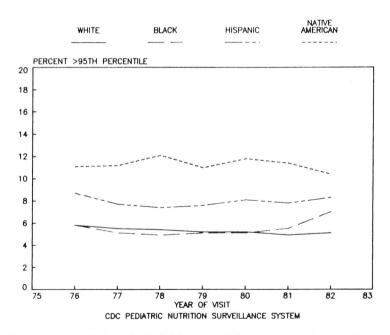

Fig. 6.   Prevalence of high weight-for-height among children 2–5 years of age by ethnic group. CDC Nutritional Surveillance, 1976–1982.

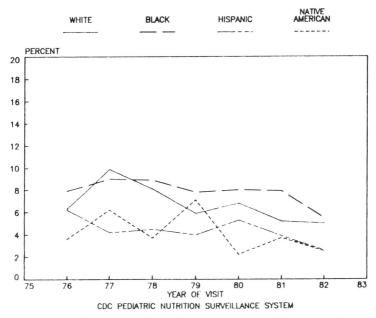

Fig. 7.   Prevalence of low hemoglobin by ethnic group among children 6 months–5 years of age. CDC Nutritional Surveillance, 1976–1982.

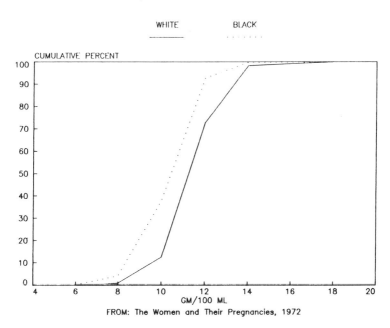

Fig. 8.   Cumulative percent distribution of hemoglobin among pregnant women by ethnic group. Collaborative Perinatal Study. From "The Women and Their Pregnancies" [8a], with permission.

Osteoporosis

Another nutrition-related condition of considerable public health importance in industrialized North America is osteoporosis. Particularly among the elderly, this condition underlies the occurrence of pathologic fractures, which cause significant morbidity and mortality. Fractures of the hip are estimated to end fatally for 15% of the elderly who suffer such injuries, to cause about half of the survivors to be committed to nursing homes, and to cost over US$1 billion annually for health care costs alone [9].

The development of osteoporosis may be affected by nutritional factors, such as calcium, vitamin D, protein, and fiber intake, as well as by physical activity and hormonal factors. A recent review of nutritional problems among elderly persons [10] recommended an increase in calcium intake as a step towards reducing the incidence of osteoporosis.

EXCESS AND IMBALANCE OF NUTRIENT INTAKE

Although problems related to nutrient deficiency are of public health concern, especially among low-income and elderly populations, the larger role of nutritional factors in morbidity and mortality in industrialized North America is related to an excess rather than a deficiency of nutrient intake. Nutritional factors are of etiologic significance in regard to many of the leading causes of mortality in the United States, including heart disease, cancer, cerebral vascular disease, cirrhosis of the liver, and diabetes. While it is difficult to quantify the contribution of nutritional factors to mortality from each of these causes, nutritional factors do play a significant role.

Data sources for assessing the prevalence of nutrition-related conditions such as obesity include the HANES surveys and the Ten-State Nutrition Survey. A more recent source is data from state-based behavioral-risk-factor surveys, collected by means of random-digit-dialing telephone surveys [11]. Since the beginning of 1982, more than 30 states have conducted this type of survey, which includes self-reported height and weight data along with data on nutrition-related behaviors, such as exercise and alcohol consumption.

The evaluation of data from any of these sources raises the same issues regarding standards that arise in evaluating the prevalence of conditions related to nutrient deficiency. Establishing criteria for obesity is particularly complex. The table of "ideal weights" proposed by the Metropolitan Life Insurance Company in 1959 [12] was widely used until the controversial revision of these reference standards in 1980 [13]. Application of the new standards, with their generally higher "ideal weight" levels, would lower the apparent prevalence of obesity.

Whatever the criteria, the prevalence of obesity in most surveys increases from young adulthood into middle age for both men and women and tends to fall off again among those over 65 years of age. Data from the Ten-State Nutrition Survey showed this pattern of increasing obesity in middle age when obesity was defined as a skinfold thickness above the 85th percentile for individuals of the same sex in the age group 20–29 years. Among men in the Ten-State Nutrition Survey obesity was more common in whites, whereas among women obesity was more prevalent in blacks. Data from recent behavioral risk factor surveys in 27 states and Washington, DC [14] in which obesity was defined as 120% of ideal weight-for-height based on the 1959 Metropolitan Life tables [12] indicate a similar pattern of prevalence with age (Fig. 9). These surveys found that more than 30% of middle-aged individuals were obese.

The prevalence of obesity in adults in the United States as well as long-term trends may also be assessed on the basis of data from the National Center for Health Statistics Surveys (Table I). In these data overweight and obesity have been defined as above the 85th percentile of weight-for-height and of skinfold

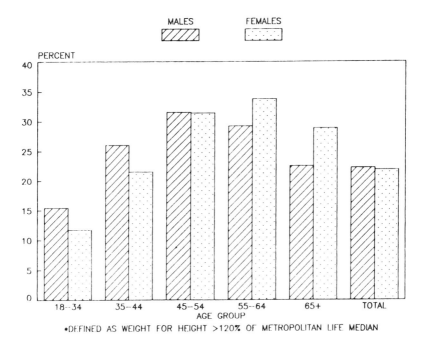

Fig. 9. Prevalence of obesity in adult populations in 27 states and Washington, DC by age and sex. State-based risk factor surveys compiled by CDC, 1982. Obesity defined as weight-for-height > 120% of Metropolitan Life median.

TABLE 1. Age-Adjusted Prevalence of Overweight and Obesity Among Adults Aged 20–74 Years by Race and Sex: United States 1960–1962, 1971–1974 and 1976–1980

Sex/race groups	1960–1962 (HES)		1971–1974 (HANES I)		1976–1980 (HANES II)	
	% Overweight	% Obese	% Overweight	% Obese	% Overweight	% Obese
Men	21.6	17.0	22.7	15.0	22.8	21.9
White	21.9	17.7	22.8	15.0	22.9	21.5
Black	20.2	12.1	24.1	15.6	25.3	25.9
Women	24.7	11.1	25.5	14.1	25.8	23.8
White	22.5	10.4	23.6	12.8	23.9	21.9
Black	41.5	16.7	42.4	26.1	43.5	40.0

Source: National Center for Health Statistics (1983): unpublished data.

thickness, respectively, for individuals of the same sex in the age group 20–29 years in the 1976–1980 (HANES II) survey. It may be observed that the prevalence of overweight has undergone a modest increase in both men and women. Obesity as measured by skinfold thickness has undergone a more marked increase, especially among blacks and particularly among black women, in whom prevalence of obesity rose from 16.7% in 1961–1962 to 40% in 1976–1980.

The increasing prevalence of obesity especially in specific high-risk groups has important implications for the development of chronic illnesses such as diabetes, hypertension, and cardiovascular disease and constitutes a significant public health concern.

TRENDS IN NUTRITIONAL PRACTICES

Although nutritional factors—especially overnutrition—appear to contribute significantly to morbidity and mortality in industrialized North America, there are some encouraging trends. Public awareness of nutritional issues is high, having been stimulated by a great outpouring of books, articles, and coverage in the media, albeit of variable quality and accuracy. Interest in physical conditioning has increased significantly, ranging from group exercise programs to individual activities, such as jogging and cycling. Consumption of foods with reduced calorie and saturated fat content is increasingly popular. Some combination of these behavioral factors may underlie the 33% reduction in mortality from heart disease and the 57% reduction in stroke mortality noted between 1950 and 1978 in adults 25–64 years of age [15]. This downward trend has been increasingly pronounced in the last decade.

In contrast to these encouraging trends, other types of nutrition-related behaviors with potentially negative implications for health are being recognized with increased frequency. Practices such as the consumption of megadose levels of vitamins can result in clinical toxicity. The effects of alternative dietary practices and nutritional abuses during pregnancy are a source of increasing concern [16]. A significant increase in mortality was documented among individuals on severe, prolonged reducing diets based on liquid-protein preparations [17], and the effects of radical reducing diets on health are a continuing concern.

Social pressures to be thin may be among the factors that underlie eating disorders such as anorexia nervosa or bulimia, conditions that are becoming more common [18]. Acute and chronic misuse of alcohol, with possible nutritional as well as other health consequences, is an increasing concern. Overall, although the nature of malnutrition problems may be changing, nutrition-related illness remains an issue of major public health concern.

CONCLUSION

A description of malnutrition in industrialized North America is as complex as the heterogeneous populations and diverse socioeconomic and cultural environments that make up its population. In some populations, deficiency disease remains an important concern and deserves commitment of resources for prevention and treatment. At the same time, the more traditional view of malnutrition as a deficiency disease must be modified to recognize the very substantial contribution of nutritional excess to chronic diseases. It is both an opportunity and a challenge to consider that many of the nutritional factors that contribute to illness in contemporary industrialized North America are factors that can be modified by individual choice. Therefore, fresh efforts must be made to increase awareness of the health effects of behavioral choices, including choices about nutrition-related behaviors such as diet, exercise, and alcohol consumption. More effective ways must be found to modify behavior and nutritional choices in ways that promote both individual and public health.

REFERENCES

1. DHHS (US Department of Health and Human Services, Public Health Service) (1980): "Promoting Health/Preventing Disease. 1990 Objectives for the Nation."
2. DHHS (US Department of Health and Human Services, Public Health Service, National Center for Health Statistics) (1977): Data from the National Health Survey, Series 11.
3. Nutrition Canada (1973): "National Survey. Nutrition, A National Priority: A Report by Nutrition Canada to the Department of National Health and Welfare." Ottawa: Information Canada.
4. DHEW (US Department of Health Education and Welfare, Health Services and Mental Health Administration, CDC) (1971): "Ten-State Nutrition Survey. Historical Development, Demographic Data." HMS 72-8130, 1968–1970.
5. NCHS (National Center for Health Statistics) (1977): "NCHS Growth Curves for Children:

Birth–18 years." United States Vital and Health Statistics, Series 11, No. 165 (DHEW Publication No. PHS 78-1650), November 1977.

6. Habicht JP, Martorell R, Yarbrough C, Malina RM, Klein RE (1974): Height and weight standards for pre-school children: How relevant are ethnic differences in growth potential? Lancet 1:611–614.

7. DHHS (US Department of Health and Human Services, Public Health Service) (1983): "CDC Nutrition Surveillance. Annual Summary 1980." CDC 83-8295:44.

8. Garn SM (1977): The anthropometric assessment of nutritional status. In Smith M (ed): "Proceedings of the Third National Nutrition Workshop for Nutritionists from University-Affiliated Facilities." The Child Development Center, University of Tennessee Center for Health Sciences, Memphis, Tennessee, April 4–9, 1976, pp 3–16.

8a. DHEW (US Department of Health, Education and Welfare) (1972): "The Women and Their Pregnancies, The Collaborative Perinatal Study of the National Institute of Neurological Diseases and Stroke." Niswander KR, Gordon M (eds), Philadelphia, London, Toronto: W.B. Saunders Company.

9. Gallagher JC, Melton LJ, Riggs BL, Bergstralh E (1980): Epidemiology of fractures of the proximal femur in Rochester, Minnesota. Clin Orthop 150:163–171.

10. Heaney RP, Gallagher JC, Johnston CC, et al (1982): Calcium nutrition and bone health in the elderly. Am J Clin Nutr 36:986–1013.

11. DHHS/PHS (US Department of Health and Human Services/Public Health Service) (1983): "CDC Morbidity and Mortality Weekly Report. Behavioral Risk Factor Prevalence Surveys—United States, First Quarter, 1982." 32:141–143.

12. Metropolitan Life Insurance Company (1959): New Weight Standards for Men and Women. Statistical Bulletin 40(1), January–June, 1959.

13. Metropolitan Life Foundation (1983): 1983 Metropolitan Height and Weight Tables. Statistical Bulletin 64(1), January–June, 1983.

14. CDC: Unpublished data.

15. DHHS (US Department of Health and Human Services, Public Health Service, Office of Disease Prevention and Health Promotion) (1982): "Prevention 82. Healthier Adults." Publication No. 82-50157, pp 30–36.

16. NAS (National Academy of Sciences) (1982): "Alternative Dietary Practices and Nutritional Abuses in Pregnancy: Summary Report." Washington DC: National Academy Press.

17. Sours HE, Frattali VP, Brand D, et al (1981): Sudden death associated with very low calorie weight reduction regimens. Am J Clin Nutr 34:453–461.

18. Bruch H (1982): Anorexia nervosa: Therapy and theory. Am J Psychiatry 139(12):1531–1538.

1983 W.O. ATWATER MEMORIAL LECTURE

Malnutrition: Determinants and Consequences, pages 61–81
1984 Alan R. Liss, Inc., 150 Fifth Avenue, New York, NY 10011

Energy in Human Nutrition: Perspectives and Problems

George H. Beaton, PhD
Department of Nutritional Sciences, Faculty of Medicine, University of
Toronto, Toronto, Ontario, Canada M5S 1A8

At the turn of this century W.O. Atwater and his colleagues E.B. Rosa and F.G. Benedict made a monumental contribution to the study of the physiology of energy metabolism and related aspects of human nutrition [Atwater and Rosa, 1897; Atwater and Benedict, 1899]. Having constructed a human calorimeter, they conducted painstaking experiments to establish, with high precision of measurements, that the Law of Conservation of Energy applies to the human as well as animal. This may seem obvious now but it was not obvious at that time. With this observation we had the basic tennet of the nutritional aspects of energy metabolism:

Energy intake = Energy expenditure + Change in energy content of body

Many may argue that in the three-quarters of a century since then we have not progressed much farther —not because we have not learned much more about energy metabolism, its regulations and aberrations, and about the components and costs of energy expenditure, but rather because we have learned so much. While we still accept, and keep returning to, the concept established for the human by Atwater, we continue to be confused and confounded in attempting to appreciate some of the practical implications of this relationship in relation to the definition and description of energy requirements.

For many years the science of nutrition devoted its attention to human needs for the vitamins and minerals and largely neglected the field of energy. In the period since World War II and most particularly in the last decade or so, interest in energy metabolism and energy requirement has mounted very rapidly — and with this rising interest has come controversy and confusion of concepts.

In my presentation I do not intend to attempt to review the now very large field of energy in human nutrition but rather to start with a review of a particular controversy that has arisen in the past decade and illustrate some of the dimensions and issues that arise from this controversy. The ultimate objective is to generate a perspective and perhaps argue for a different approach to interpretation of energy requirements and indeed a different approach to research directed toward the definition of energy requirement. In keeping with the theme of the Congress, these remarks are directed particularly toward issues relevant to the developing countries.

I can think of no better way to begin than with the current controversy about assessment of the magnitude of the current nutrition problem—the problem that is perceived to be dominantly one of inadequate food or energy intake.

ESTIMATION OF THE MAGNITUDE OF THE NUTRITION PROBLEM
Macroanalyses of the Adequacy of Energy Intake

A few years ago I undertook a comparative analysis of two widely known approaches to the gross analysis of the adequacy of food supplies—the approaches adopted by FAO in connection with the Fourth World Food Survey [FAO, 1977] and Agriculture: Toward 2000 [FAO, 1979] and the approach adopted by Reutlinger and Selowsky [1976], later modified by Reutlinger and Alderman [1980]. The motivation for becoming involved was the desire to determine why these two approaches gave such different estimates of the magnitude of the problem. Table I portrays the published estimates. It is informative and germane to consider some of the highlights of that comparative analysis.*

First, it should be clearly understood that neither analysis had access to information on actual intakes. Rather, both were addressing the issue of the apparent adequacy or inadequacy of per capita food supplies collated and reported by FAO as a part of the World Food Survey. Second, it should be recognized that in order to model the distribution of food intakes within the populations, both approaches assumed that income was a major determinant of food demand and food intake. Therefore income distribution was used as a major variable in the derivation of a proxy distribution of intakes. Implicitly these distributions referred to aggregated consumer units; there was no attempt to take into account any inequity of distribution that may have taken place within families nor any attempt to predict which demographic segments of the population were more seriously affected. The income data bases used by

---

*The author is indebted to the staff of FAO for making available data used in comparative calculations in this chapter and to Dr. Reutlinger and his colleagues for carrying out most of the actual calculations.

TABLE I. Comparison of Published Estimates of the Magnitude of the Nutrition Problem

Source	Descriptor used	Data base year	Prevalence (millions)
Fourth World Food Survey [FAO, 1977]	Intakes below critical minimum limit	1969–1971 1972–1974	401 455
Agriculture: Toward 2000 [FAO, 1979]	Intakes below critical minimum limit	1975	414
Reutlinger and Selowsky [1976]	Calorie-deficient diets a) With deficit of less than 250 kcal/day b) With deficit of more than 250 kcal/day	1965	1,130 290 840
Reutlinger and Alderman [1980]	Calorie-deficient diets Intakes below FAO/WHO per capita requirements Intakes below 90% of FAO/WHO per capita requirements	1965 1973 1965 1973	704 808 578 599

Estimates presented do not encompass all developing countries nor do all estimates apply to the same set of countries.

FAO and by Reutlinger and colleagues are from generally similar sources. Thus, in essence the two approaches start from a similar point, yet reach what appear to be very different answers. There are three potential major sources of these differences: 1) approaches taken to modeling the distribution of intakes; 2) approaches taken to statistical analysis; and 3) adopted definition of "energy requirement." Each of these will be discussed in turn.

Modeling the distribution of intake. FAO accepted that the β-distribution would provide a good descriptor of the skewed distribution of intakes in LDC (Less Developed Country) populations. As noted, FAO also accepted that income was a major determinant of the distribution of intakes although it was recognized that the relationship was not linear. The proportion of income allocated to food purchase decreases as income rises.* FAO estimated the parameters of the β-distribution drawing on: per capita food disappearance data, reported variability of income, calculated income elasticity of demand, and judgmental lower and upper limits for the distribution. In practice, further judgmental limits on the calculated parameters were applied. A continuous distribution was derived.

*The relationship between income and intake assumed by *both* FAO and Reutlinger and colleagues was $C = a + b \ln X$, where C is consumption, a is constant, b is the calorie income propensity calculated as the income elasticity of demand times the specified intake level, and X is the income level.

Reutlinger and colleagues chose a different approach. On the basis of Lorenz curves, they first divided the population into income strata. Then, assuming the same relationship between income and intake as did FAO, they estimated the mean intake for each income stratum. As will be indicated under Statistical Approach, they made a further assumption that there was a variability of intake within income strata that was independent of income [Reutlinger and Alderman, 1980]. Setting that aside for the moment, it is possible to ask whether the basic approach to modeling distribution accounts for the difference in final estimates.

The answer is clearly no; modeling of the overall distribution is not a major factor. This is illustrated in Figure 1, where data for four arbitrarily chosen countries have been used to generate the β-distributions of FAO and the income-related distributions of Reutlinger and colleagues. A third plot portrays the effect of using Reutlinger's assumed elasticity of demand in the derivation of the FAO β-distribution. The important features are that all of the distributions exhibit skewing and thus are in keeping with expectation, and that at the low-intake end of the distributions the Reutlinger approach tends to suggest a somewhat lower proportion of the population with very low intakes (see also Table IV).

Statistical approach. The approach adopted by FAO is a variant of that originally developed by Sukhatme [1961, 1966]. In essence, it applies a fixed cutoff point set two standard deviations below the average requirement and estimates the proportion of the population with intakes below this cutoff. The argument is that it is almost certain that at intakes this low "individuals are most probably suffering from some forms of energy deprivation" (very few would be expected to have requirements this low) [FAO, 1977].

Conversely, the approach adopted by Reutlinger and Alderman accepts that both intake and requirement are variable among comparable individuals (a bivariate distribution) although there may be a correlation between intake and requirement. To apply this approach to the stratified income groups, they assumed that within income strata the distributions of intake and of requirement were both Gaussian, that both had coefficients of variation of 15%, and that a correlation of 0.7 existed between intake and requirement. Other assumptions about correlation were tested.* The Reutlinger and Alderman [1980] approach then is a bivariate probability approach applied within income strata and then summed across strata to obtain a population estimate of the prevalence of intakes below actual requirements. Such an approach looks at probability of in-

---

*The approach developed by Reutlinger and Alderman [1980] is analogous to that developed earlier by Lörstad [1971]. He also conducted sensitivity testing. Between these two analyses it is clear that the impact of changing the assumption about correlation depends upon the positions of the two distributions and their relative variances [Corey and Beaton, 1975].

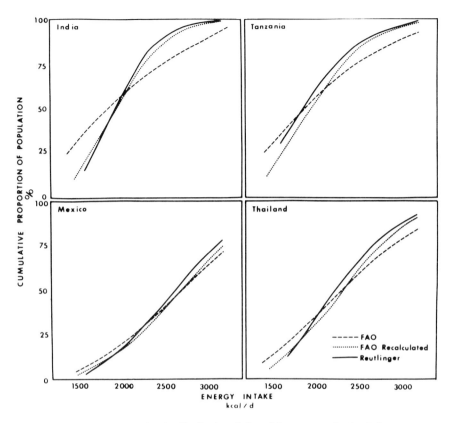

Fig. 1. Comparison of the intake distributions inferred from per capita food disappearance and income distribution data by the approaches of FAO and of Reutlinger and colleagues. The adjusted FAO approach represents to β-distribution of FAO, with application of the income elasticity of demand estimate of Reutlinger and colleagues.

adequacy across the whole of the distribution of intakes rather than at only one tail of the distribution. In theory it is a better approach [Corey and Beaton, 1975], although it requires additional assumptions not needed for the FAO approach.

It is apparent that, at least when mean intake is below mean requirement, the Reutlinger and Alderman approach will give higher estimates of the proportion of people with intakes below their own requirements [Corey and Beaton, 1975]. Is this the major source of difference in the estimates? In Table II, both the FAO and Reutlinger and Alderman approaches have been applied using the same estimate of average requirement, 1.5 BMR (basal metabolic

TABLE II. Apparent Proportion (%) of Population With "Inadequate" Energy Intakes

Country	FAO approach[a]	Reutlinger and Alderman approach[b]		
		"Maintenance requirement"	"Reference requirement"	FAO per capita "requirement"
India	31	41	53	72
Tanzania	31	49	63	77
Mexico	6	14	22	35
Thailand	15	27	32	49

[a]FAO approach is an estimation of proportion of population with intake below 1.2 BMR.
[b]Reutlinger and Alderman approach is a probability estimation based upon bivariate distributions of intake and requirement with assumed mean requirements equal to:

Maintenance requirement = 1.5 BMR
Reference requirement = estimated requirement for moderate activity as published by the FAO/WHO Committee on Energy and Protein Requirements
FAO per capita requirement represents the reference requirement increased by 10% to allow for food wasteage in the household.
Figures are those published by FAO.

rate). The difference in estimated proportion with inadequate intakes that is attributable to statistical approach is clear.

Definition of requirement. Table II illustrates also the third source of difference between the FAO and Reutlinger and colleagues approaches: the definition of requirement adopted in the analysis. As is to be expected, as one raises the estimate of average requirements with a given distribution of intakes, the estimated prevalence of inadequate intakes increases. Presented in Table II under the Reutlinger and Alderman approach is the impact of changing the average requirement estimate from the "Maintenance Requirement" (1.5 BMR) adopted by FAO in the Fourth World Food Survey through the requirement estimate for moderate activity proposed by the FAO/WHO Committee on Energy and Protein Requirements [1973] to the per capita requirement estimate published by FAO in the Fourth World Food Survey [FAO, 1977]. This last estimate was increased by 10% to allow for wastage in the household. (It is argued that per capita food disappearance data are adjusted for wastage to the retail level.) The comparison of published FAO and Reutlinger and Alderman estimates is captured by comparing the first and last columns of Table II.

Clearly, then, the major source of the difference between the estimates published by FAO and by Reutlinger and colleagues lies in the criterion of adequate energy intake (average energy requirement) adopted.*

*Another way of looking at the application of different requirement criteria is that they may be used to obtain estimates of the proportion of population with intakes lying in different ranges of deficit. In a sense this might be seen as a measure of "severity" as well as prevalence [Reutlinger and Selowsky, 1976; Lörstad, 1974].

That both approaches to analysis are sensitive to the criterion of adequacy is demonstrated in Tables III and IV. (Table IV is generated directly from the curves presented in Fig. 1).

Recognize the import of this issue. In essence, FAO has taken the stance that inadequacy of intake means an intake that is too low to meet even maintenance needs — what was suggested to be an estimate of the needs for a very inactive level of existence. Conversely, by adopting the FAO/WHO committee recommendations, Reutlinger and Selowsky and later Reutlinger and Alderman implicitly accepted the notion that inadequate intake was a level of intake that would be insufficient to permit an expected level of activity.

To compare the FAO and Reutlinger approaches is to compare apples and oranges. To criticize one against the other without recognizing the implicit difference in the meanings attached to inadequacy is to miss the major issue. What is it that we wish to estimate? Are we trying to estimate the proportion of people who are likely to be clinically malnourished? Are we trying to estimate the magnitude of any shortfall from developmental goals (defined in terms of "desirable" levels of activity and growth rates)?

ADDITIONAL CRITICISMS AND ALTERNATIVES

During the past decade, and particularly during the past 5 years, there have been major criticisms of these macroanalyses on two valid bases. The first criticism relates to the reliability of the data bases for these analyses — the per capita food disappearance data and the income distribution data. It must be accepted that any use of these data sets can be no better than the inherent quality of the data sets. The second criticism is that aggregate data, even with models of distribution, are no real substitute for disaggregated data: Knowledge of the distribution of intakes at the level of the households or even better at the level of individuals would be preferred [UNU, 1981]. Present approaches depend upon assumptions made about the relationship between income and intake. These assumptions may not hold for all populations or for all segments within populations. As noted earlier, the macroanalyses do not attempt to look at intrahousehold distribution; they make no inference about the age group affected.

Desirable as better data bases may be, they exist for very few countries. At the international level, one is faced with the question of using the information available, recognizing its serious limitations, or not using any information. On this question, of course, opinion is divided!

In a series of single and joint papers, Sukhatme and Margen have introduced a separate issue that has attracted much attention by critics of the Reutlinger and FAO approaches to analysis. It is their contention that the energy requirement of an individual varies over a *wide* range across time [Sukhatme

TABLE III. Comparison of Effects of Changing Estimate of Average Energy Requirements on Predicted Proportion of Population With Intakes Below Actual Requirements (approach of Reutlinger and Alderman)

Country	Assumed average requirement[a]				Reported per capita "intake"[b]
	1.5 BMR	88% Reference	99% Reference	110% Reference	
	Per capita energy requirement (kcal/day)				
India	1858	1768	1990	2210	1970
Tanzania	1873	1856	2088	2320	1958
Mexico	1890	1864	2097	2330	2673
Thailand	1889	1776	1998	2220	2315
	Predicted proportion (%) of persons with intakes below their requirements				
India	41	23	53	72	
Tanzania	49	48	63	77	
Mexico	14	13	22	35	
Thailand	27	20	32	49	

[a]Requirement estimates are adjusted in accordance with the anthropometric and demographic characteristics of the populations. "Per capita requirement" estimates published by FAO are 110% of the reference requirement estimates published by the FAO/WHO Committee on Energy and Protein Requirements, 1973.
[b]Per capita "Intake" is reported per capita food disappearance theoretically adjusted for waste to household purchase level.

TABLE IV. Comparison of Approaches to Derivation of Intake Distributions: Apparent Proportions of Population With Intake Below Fixed Cutoff Points

Approach to derivation of intake distribution	Selected cutoff point[a]		
	1.2 BMR	1.5 BMR	"Moderate activity"
India			
FAO approach	31%	50%	66%
FAO recalculated[b]	12%	41%	70%
Reutlinger and Alderman	11%	43%	76%
Tanzania			
FAO approach	31%	50%	70%
FAO recalculated	17%	45%	76%
Reutlinger and Alderman	23%	52%	80%
Mexico			
FAO approach	6%	16%	33%
FAO recalculated	4%	13%	31%
Reutlinger and Alderman	1%	13%	34%
Thailand			
FAO approach	15%	31%	47%
FAO recalculated	8%	25%	46%
Reutlinger and Alderman	11%	26%	51%

[a]All cutoff points have been adjusted for anthropometric and demographic characteristics of populations.
[b]FAO recalculated is the β-distribution of FAO but using the income elasticity assumption of Reutlinger and Alderman.

and Margen, 1982]. It is argued that this is accomplished through an autoregulatory process of adjustment of the efficiency of metabolism. It does not involve any change in body size or composition or in activity. The implication taken from this is that within this wide range no individual can be deemed to have an inadequate energy intake, since he possesses the inherent ability to adjust metabolic expenditure of energy. The further implication is that there is no "functional cost" associated with this adjustment. Obviously, they argue, if this is correct, current probability approaches, which depend upon the assumption that a particular individual's energy requirement is essentially fixed unless body composition or activity are allowed to change, must be fundamentally incorrect [Sukhatme and Margen, 1982; Sukhatme, 1981; Margen, 1983]. Sukhatme [1981] has suggested that the coefficient of variation (CV) of this range of homeostasis may be 12–15% of average requirement. Thus, he infers that individuals can adapt to intakes as low or as high as -30% to $+30\%$ of average requirement with no disadvantageous effects!

Recognize that this is fundamentally different from the concept of variability of requirement between individuals. That concept of variability has been generally accepted (although not always applied). It is the focus of major discussion in the forthcoming FAO/WHO/UNU report on Energy and Protein Requirements [FAO/WHO/UNU, 1983]. Rather, the essence of the Sukhatme and Margen argument is that the variability of requirement within individuals overwhelms variability between individuals and indeed makes existing concepts of individual variability of requirement seriously misleading.

We would all accept that there are mechanisms, even if poorly understood, that operate to stabilize energy balance over the long run. Descriptions of possible systems have been offered (see, for example, Payne and Dugdale [1977] and Garby [1983]). This is not the real issue. The issue is the proposed extent of this homeostatic adaptability suggested by Sukhatme [1981].

Unfortunately, there are no data sets now existing against which the theorem of Sukhatme and Margen can be either proven or disproven. It would be necessary to collect continuous long-term data sets encompassing a number of parameters of intake, of expenditure, and of body composition.* Until such data sets become available, the proposal is likely to remain a matter of theoretical interest to scientists involved in studies of the homeostasis of energy balance, but an item of major dispute among those wishing to assess the probable adequacy of existing food supplies or future food needs.

At least some economists have decided to wash their hands of the whole argument and to look for other approaches to planning. This may represent a

---

*It is anticipated that a longitudinal data set encompassing some of these parameters will be forthcoming in connection with the USAID-funded Collaborative Research Support Program on Nutrition and Function.

general disillusionment with the contribution that nutritional sciences is seen as making in the field of development planning [Reutlinger, 1983].

Recently Srinivasan [1983] completed a review of the field of assessment of nutritional problems for planning purposes. After having criticized existing approaches, he concluded in his closing passages that since nutritional problems were clearly related to maldistribution of income, there was little to be gained by looking at food intake. A simpler and more meaningful approach would be examination of income distribution or, as a refinement, such parameters as the proportion of income expended on food or the marginal propensity to spend on food. The rationale may be summarized in Srinivasan's own words:

> It is now well understood that whatever be the true extent of undernutrition in developing countries, the causes "are many and closely interrelated, including ecological, sanitary and cultural constraints but the principal cause is *poverty*" [UN, 1975]. Even though not all poor households are undernourished and not all rich households necessarily are well nourished, and as such being poor and undernourished are not the same, it is nevertheless true, as is to be expected, that undernourished households are to be found mostly among the poor. Thus policies toward elimination under-nutrition really have to address the problem of poverty.

In one regard, of course, Srinivasan is in agreement with the approaches of Reutlinger and of FAO. All three accept income and related food expenditure to be the driving force toward inadequate intakes and nutritional problems. Perhaps the most important distinction is that Srinivasan does not attempt to develop cutoff points, predict the magnitude of the problem or, if you wish, define development goals. He is content to point out that poverty is bad and that when you localize poverty you have a point at which to begin appropriate interventions to alleviate poverty and all of the problems that go with it.

In some regards this is not unlike the position taken by Payne and colleagues in recent writings [Dowler et al, 1982]. He too dismisses attempts to judge the adequacy or inadequacy of observed food intake. He too appears convinced that poverty and inadequate economic security are the root problems that must be attacked. He proposes, therefore, that we seek and measure indices that might serve to localize the populations at risk and hence form a basis for focusing programs. He has suggested such indices as birth weight, weight-for-height or weight-for-age, and mortality, and such economic parameters as land tenure. Like Srinivasan, he does not attempt to define criteria of adequacy; rather he is concerned with indices of subpopulations at risk of a range of health problems.

Still another approach is portrayed by the work of Habicht and his colleagues [Habicht et al, 1982]. Interested in the development of criteria to be used in public health programs, in surveillance systems, or in other applications, Habicht et al point out that both the parameter and the interpretational criterion (cutoff point) must be selected to suit the particular purpose. They deal with the problem as one of specificity and sensitivity of classification, using statistical approaches to predict the proportions of type I and type II errors. They argue that if you are selecting individuals for intervention, you should adopt criteria that will predict responsiveness to intervention. In this approach, Habicht et al are examining indices of nutritional status, such as hemoglobin or anthropometric parameters, as predictors of health outcomes. They are not dealing with questions of food and nutrient intake as predictors of nutritional status.

The arguments of Srinivasan, of Payne, and of Habicht all make sense in their particular connotations. Srinivasan and Payne see nutritional problems as an outcome of economic inequities and conclude that the most practical approach to assessment for purpose of economic intervention is to record indices that describe the segment of the population at particular disadvantage. These could be either economic indices or health indices. They are not interested in counting numbers; rather the question is where do foci or clusters of indices suggest a need and opportunity for intervention. Habicht is interested in numbers but again numbers that are relevant to particular types of actions or potential actions. His focus is more toward a "diagnosis" of an individual rather than identification of a population subgroup that is particularly at risk of ill health.

None of these authors are directly addressing nutritional questions. None are addressing adequacy of food supply as a variable conveying risk. None contribute directly to the planner's dilemma: Are food supply and food intake adequate? Is there really a food-related nutrition problem?

A CONSTRUCT OF THE RELATIONSHIP BETWEEN INTAKE AND FUNCTION

Let us return to the original concept of energy balance and the Law of Conservation of Energy that Atwater and his colleagues established as applying to man. This is described simply as:

Utilizable energy intake = Energy expenditure + Change in energy content of the body

No one has challenged the validity of this equation. Somewhere in the past 50 years we seem to have gone through an evolution of interpretation that gradually stated this equation in different ways. I exemplify this below.

Those interested in obesity (and underweight) saw this equation as:

Change in body weight (or body composition) = Energy intake − Energy expenditure

in which expenditure was almost taken as a given, albeit changing with the existing body mass.

Those interested in child growth fell into the same pattern of thinking, expressing the equation as:

$$\frac{\text{Child growth rate}}{\text{(pregnancy weight change)}} = \text{Energy intake} - \text{Maintenance energy expenditure}$$

Granted, it was recognized from the beginning that if physical activity differed, it would affect the position of the balance or magnitude of the numbers. However, the point is that this led us into a pattern of thinking that has potentially serious consequences.

We have come to accept the notion that the ultimate measure of the adequacy of energy intake is an anthropometric index. In adults we think of underweight or overweight, expected weight being adjusted for height. In children we think of parameters such as weight-for-height and weight-for-age or, if the data sets are adequate, growth rate (change in anthropometry over time). We have coined names for these anthropometric departures including "protein energy malnutrition." We have undertaken many studies in children and in adults to look at the association between anthropometric parameters and health outcomes: birth weight and childhood mortality, growth rate or weight-for-age or -height and childhood mortality, obesity and cardiovascular disease, etc. We have then inferred that we have measured relationships between nutrition and outcomes. Perhaps we have. But have we missed other relationships?

In effect we have fallen into a trap of assuming that anthropometry is an adequate proxy for "nutrition" rather than an index of one aspect of nutritional status.

Our current mode of thinking goes along the following line:

$$\frac{\text{Inappropriate}}{\text{energy intake}} \rightarrow \text{Deviant anthropometric status} \rightarrow \text{Functional abnormality}$$

In our analyses we have tended to accept anthropometric status as a proxy for adequacy of food intake in looking at functional outcomes and as a proxy for functional status in looking at the outcome of change in intake (as in program evaluation). In effect, "normalization" of anthropometry (by whatever standard one chooses) has progressively become the goal of nutritional action.

This could be very misleading. Do we really have any sound evidence that body size and composition make up an intermediary variable in the linkages between intake and function? Do we even have clear evidence that deviation in anthropometry will necessarily accompany a deviation in function? I think that the answer to both questions has to be no. We have to accept that a model of the relationships could be as portrayed in Figure 2 without interdependence of the pathways.

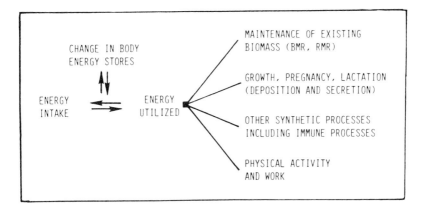

Fig. 2.   Components of the energy balance equation.

In this simplistic model, the point being made is that it is at least conceivable that food intake may relate to activity or to immunologic competence or to other functional outcomes in manner that does not involve intermediary change in anthropometric status. By the same token, it suggests that anthropometric status may differ without implication that other functions are affected. The existing evidence suggests that in the presence of major deviation in anthropometry toward the low side, many of the other functions are compromised. These, of course, are the studies that give rise to the assertion that "severe malnutrition has measurable functional effects." However, evidence exists also that there are effects of intake that do not associate with change in anthropometry.

Again let us step back and look at this for a moment. When we see major deviations from expected body weight, it is reasonable to accept that a nutritional variable is involved. It is fair, then, to describe a child with abnormally low weight-for-height or weight-for-age as probably "undernourished" or "malnourished." It is reasonable also to suggest that when morbidity and mortality associate with this very low weight status, there is an association between malnutrition and disease. I do not challenge this conclusion. Chen et al [1980a, 1981] demonstrated the predictive relationship between depressed anthropometric status in young children and mortality in the ensuing 2 years. Their data "showed that severely malnourished children according to all [anthropometric] indices experienced markedly higher mortality risk whereas normally nourished and mildly and moderately malnourished children all experienced lower but similar risks." In a subsequent note Chen [1982] took issue with the manner in which some had interpreted these findings. He noted that the original intent was to ask whether anthropometric criteria could be used to identify children at risk of mortality, not to define malnutrition. He noted also that although "normal, mild and moderate" malnutrition classifications did not offer differential predictions of mortality, the mortality rates in these children were 30–50 per 1,000 in the 2- to 4-year age group, a rate approximately ten times higher than that seen among more privileged children in rich and poor countries [Chen et al, 1980b]. Chen specifically cautioned against any conclusion that suggested, on the basis of his studies, that "mild and moderate malnutrition," judged by anthropometric indices, could be seen as being without functional consequence. In essence he may be seen as suggesting also that depressed anthropometry is an indicator of a cluster of deprivations, and although serving as a good predictor of risk of mortality it is not necessarily a good descriptor or predictor of the effects of any one of the associated risk factors. Again we face the issue of defining the purpose of any classification, the point made by Habicht et al [1982].

Chandra [1983] has repeatedly made the point that much less severe depressions of anthropometric indices than suggested above are associated with disturbances of components of the immune system, although it is not entirely clear how these relate to either susceptibility to infection or to response to infection. Chen [1982] points out that at least one role of "nutrition" may be in ameliorating the debilitating effects of infection or, phrased another way, facilitating the recovery from infection and fostering "catch-up growth" between periods of infection; this view was expressed also by a UNU Workshop [UNU, 1979]. Martorell et al [1980] make the additional point that food intake is depressed by disease, further confounding the situation.

What about other outcomes of "undernutrition"? Are these necessarily mediated through, or even indicated by, anthropometric status? I think that in the realm of physical activity we have some pretty clear indications that the relationship between intake and activity can be independent of that between intake and anthropometry.

Rutishauser and Whitehead [1972] described a Ugandan child population in which physical growth rates had been maintained at reasonable levels in the face of apparent low food intakes. Further examination of the community suggested that one way in which this had been achieved was by a very low level of activity, play. Chavez and colleagues [Chavez and Martinez, 1972, 1983; Chavez et al, 1972] demonstrated that increased physical movement was an outcome of supplementary feeding in a Mexican community. Anecdotally it has been reported that a common finding in food distribution programs is that the children become a "nuisance," implying perhaps that they exhibit increased and societally atypical patterns of physical activity, even though these same programs may have minimal effect on anthropometric indices [Beaton and Ghassemi, 1982]. Viteri and Torun [1981] reported a series of studies in children strongly suggesting a different and important pattern of relationships.

Physical activity reduction was a response to food intake reduction, a result that is in keeping with the other studies cited. However, physical activity level, independent of food intake, seemed to have an important influence on linear growth. An inference from this is that to maintain a higher level of physical activity that would be associated with good rates of linear growth, a commensurate level of food intake would be required. In this model, intriguingly, physical activity may be an intervening variable between intake and anthropometry!

The sole point of these citations is to establish that we may be seriously misled by a pattern of thinking that places anthropometry in the position of the intervening variable between dietary inadequacy and functional effect — or in accepting too literally the various anthropometric criteria and the designations "normal, mild, moderate, and severe malnutrition" as descriptors of nutritional status rather than at most indicators of one dimension of nutritional status.

If my argument is accepted, then it becomes rather important how we conceptualize the components of Atwater's energy balance equation. I suggest that it might be presented in a manner resembling Figure 3 [Beaton, 1983]. The first important element of this portrayal is the potential independence of the

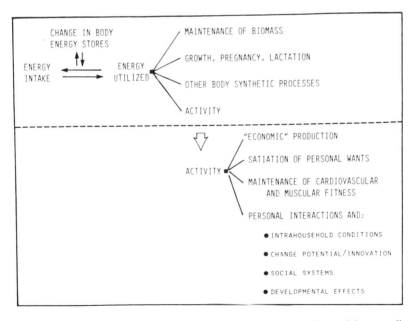

Fig. 3. Some functional implications of the energy balance equation. Some of the expenditure components may be adjusted in keeping with intake adjustment (adaptation). These accommodations may carry functional implications. Based on Beaton [1983].

pathways of relationships. In establishing energy balance, the components could be adjusted independently of one another; observed effects need not be directly associated. This does not eliminate the possibility of interactions between the portrayed components of utilization, as in the activity-growth relationship discussed above. It does mean that measurement of one component does not predict the status of other components. Anthropometry is not a satisfactory proxy for all aspects of energy utilization.

The second important feature of the portrayal is the recognition that if variation in physical activity is a part of the mechanism of adjustment of energy balance, it can lead to other effects. Thus, for example, if it is valid to assume that a child's cognitive development is influenced by its interaction with its physical and human environment, then we can see the possibility of two distinct paths of effect. The child's energy intake and activity are associated; his activity level affects his exploratory behavior and that aspect of environmental interaction. This is a potential direct pathway of effect. The second pathway is indirect. The energy intake of the child's caretaker associates with activity level of the caretaker; in turn this influences the caretaker's response to the child's signals and thus influences the interaction between child and environment. Similar examples might be hypothesized about other aspects of child care, such as sanitation and care during illness.

Although there have been studies of the relationship between intake and functional activity measured as "productivity" in a narrow economic sense, these have tended to suggest that supplementary feeding has little or no operational significance unless the original level of deprivation was severe. Rather, incentives for production seem to have a greater influence (although they entail a need for additional food). This may not imply that there is no functionally significant change in activity with intake but rather that in an equilibrium situation individuals consciously or unconsciously make choices among the activities that will be performed with limited energy intake. There does not appear to have been systematic examination of the levels of "nonwork" activities that associate with changes in intake, nor has there been adequate consideration of the potential significance of these activities, sometimes termed "discretionary activities" [UNU, 1981]. This may change with the newer "household economics."

The inherent issue was recognized in the 1973 FAO/WHO report on energy requirements [FAO/WHO, 1973]. There it was cautioned that while activity was customarily classified in terms of occupations, a major variable might be what people did in their nonoccupational hours. The issue was raised again in a review of that report. Concern was expressed about the dangers of accepting low levels of energy intake that might be achieved by reduction in physical activity [FAO/WHO, 1975]. It was given emphasis in a UNU workshop [UNU, 1981] which urged that there be specific recognition of the importance of "discretionary activity." It will be a part of the forthcoming FAO/WHO/UNU report on energy and protein requirements [FAO/WHO/UNU, 1983].

A RECONCEPTUALIZATION OF "ENERGY REQUIREMENT"?

Where does this leave us? Durnin et al [1973] suggested that these uncertainties meant simply that we cannot describe human energy requirement. Beaton [1982] suggested that we can describe human energy requirements but before we do so we must answer the question "requirement for what?" Today I would suggest that we should reconceptualize what we mean by "energy requirement." Specifically I suggest that we think of this as the *level of energy intake and expenditure at which balance is established.* In itself such a conceptualization makes no assumption about whether food intake restrains expenditure or external influences of society establish expenditure levels that in turn limit intake. Rather, it addresses the overall level and its functional significance.

Consider for a moment what we have learned from recent studies and what constitutes the focus of current debate at the international level. At the level of populations, if we set aside the famine areas and the natural or man-created disasters, it is clear that existing populations are in energy balance. If we accept maintenance of energy balance as a criterion of "requirement," then we must conclude that all populations are currently meeting their energy requirements. There is no need for the calculations of FAO, of Reutlinger, or of the many others. Similarly, there is no need for detailed studies of energy intake and expenditure since under equilibrium conditions they are likely to prove the obvious — energy balance has been achieved! Certainly, within populations, there are individuals who do not manage to maintain long-term energy balance and who die with what we term protein-energy malnutrition or simply starvation. The numbers of such individuals are really rather small in comparison with the estimates of the size of the nutrition problem that I cited earlier. If *this* is the problem that causes us concern, then we would be well advised, as many advocate, to focus upon those individuals with treatment and specific intervention programs.

But are we really prepared to say that these populations are healthy in the sense that the energy flux is at an appropriate level? Let me cite two examples of contrasting situations to make my point.

Critics of the FAO and Reutlinger macroanalytic approaches (eg, Srinivasan [1983]) have cited reported levels of energy intake in North America as an example of the erroneous conclusions that are to be drawn from examination of intake in relation to FAO/WHO requirement estimates. Reported intakes are below the FAO/WHO [1973] or FAO/WHO/UNU [1983] requirement estimates and even below intakes reported for some developing countries. Yet few would say that these populations, with their high prevalence of obesity, are undernourished. This would seem to be a sound criticism in our present mode of thinking about requirement. However, would not most agree that these populations are indeed underactive and that this underactivity carries an associated risk to health? The FAO/WHO/UNU [1983] report makes that precise suggestion. By the thinking of that committee, indeed the North American population has established energy equilibrium at a level below that required for good health and hence good function.

For my second example, I draw upon recent studies of pregnant and lactating women conducted in Gambia. Many others could be cited. In Gambia it is apparent that women can exist on very low intakes of food and can produce viable infants and nourish these infants adequately at the breast such that at 3 months of age their weights are reasonable albeit a bit low by British standards [Prentice et al, 1981; Prentice, 1983]. At one season of the year, food intake was reduced still further and depression of birth weight was seen; however, in the subsequent time period when food intake improved these infants were nursed at a level that permitted a higher growth rate. There was no evidence of a progressive loss of maternal weight across successive pregnancies. The provision of supplemental food did not appear to influence either the mother's or infant's anthropometry [Whitehead, 1983]. It seems reasonable to conclude that the women maintained long-term energy balance. There was no suggestion that this was achieved by a reduction in participation in agricultural work. While one may challenge the estimates of food intake since there was not a validation by estimation of energy expenditure (a requirement for all such studies suggested by James and Shetty [1982]), it is difficult to challenge the conclusion that these women achieved energy balance on intakes well below current requirement estimates [Beaton, 1983]. Again we are faced with a position that published requirement estimates seem too high.

How, then, do we interpret the comment of Prentice [1983]? After concluding that "people in developing countries are more efficient than those in developed countries," he went on to suggest that "although it may be possible to survive on much lower intakes than considered possible hitherto, such dietary conditions are almost certainly not compatible with optimum quality of life." Speaking of the same women, Whitehead [1983] reported that "the first reason given by pregnant and lactating mothers for the popularity of the supplement was that it gave them 'power' for work." On another occasion, Whitehead (personal communication, 1981) reported that the supplemented women "sang while they worked." Are these suggestions of effects of food intake on affective behavior? Are they hints that there are other effects, lying in the social domain, that we have failed to measure in our studies? Can we really say that in these women the level of intake that is sufficient to maintain energy balance really marks energy requirement?

CONCLUSION

This, then, is the core issue that surfaces in a comparative examination of the approaches of FAO and of Reutlinger and colleagues to estimation of the magnitude of the nutrition problem. It is a core issue that must be faced in many of the other approaches now being suggested for defining the problem of designing interventions. It is much more than an issue of defining and applying estimates of energy requirements.

If we once accept that the issue we face is the definition of the level of intake *and* expenditure at which energy balance should be established and the sequelae of shortfalls from that level (the sequelae of achieving energy balance at lower levels of intake and expenditure), then we will have moved to a completely different dimension of thinking. We will realize that the answers lie not in the laboratory of the physiologist, though clearly he must contribute. Rather, the issues we now face combine the domains of biological and psychosocial sciences and only a collaborative approach to the development of understanding will suffice in the future.

It is this new perspective of energy balance and its functional dimensions that has driven the design of the USAID-funded Collaborative Research Support Program on Nutrition and Function (Nutrition CRSP). The research challenges are major; new approaches and methodologies and, perhaps more important, new combinations of approaches and methodologies are required. However great the challenges, the question must be addressed: We must ask about the functional significance of the marginal changes in the position of the energy balance.

What is at risk? What is the import of an improved understanding? I suggest that at least one thing that is at risk is the definition of our goals for development!

Depending upon how we choose to interpret and extend the Atwater energy balance equation, we are likely to conclude either that there are major problems in relation to meeting energy requirements in virtually all countries, developed and developing, or that there are relatively few people who do not meet their energy needs.

ACKNOWLEDGMENTS

The comparative study of the approaches of FAO and of Reutlinger and colleagues to the estimation of the prevalence of inadequate intakes was supported financially by the Food and Agriculture Organization of the United Nations and was conducted with the full collaboration of the World Bank. In large part, the evolution of the concept of the functional significance of the position at which energy balance is established has been the direct result of the author's involvement in the preliminary discussion and later design of the Collaborative Research Support Program on Nutrition and Function (Nutrition CRSP), administratively based in the University of California at Berkeley and involving several US institutions and collaborating national institutions in Egypt, Kenya, and Mexico. The author acknowledges both personal financial support from this project (US Agency for International Development grant DAN-1309-G-SS-1070-00) and the influence of the wide base of individuals involved in the early development phases of the project and more particularly the influence of the collaborating Principal Investigators and of Dr. Doris Calloway, Program Administrator, in the detailed design and implementation phases.

REFERENCES

Atwater WO, Benedict FG (1899): "Experiments on the Metabolism of Matter and Energy in the Human Body." Bull US Dept Agric 69.

Atwater WO, Rosa EB (1897): Report Storrs Agric Exp Station, p 212.

Beaton GH (1982): "Some thoughts on the definition of the world nutrition problem." Paper presented at the Eighth Session of the UN Administrative Committee on Coordination-Subcommittee on Nutrition, Bangkok, Thailand (unpublished).

Beaton GH (1983): Adaptation to, and accommodation of, long term low energy intake. In "Proceedings of the Conference on Energy Intake and Activity, Bellagio, Italy" (in press).

Beaton GH, Ghassemi H (1982): Supplementary feeding programs for young children in developing countries. Am J Clin Nutr 35:864–916.

Chandra RK (1983): Nutrition, immunity, and infection: Present knowledge and future directions. Lancet 1:688–691.

Chavez A, Martinez C (1972): Nutrition and development of children from poor rural areas. Study No. 5. Nutrition and behavioural development. Nutr Rep Int 11:477–491.

Chavez A, Martinez C (1983): Behavioural measurements of activity in children and its relation to food intake in a poor community. In "Proceedings of the Conference on Energy Intake and Activity, Bellagio, Italy" (in press).

Chavez A, Martinez C, Bourges H (1972): Nutrition and development of infants from poor rural areas. Study No. 2. Nutrition and behavioural development. Nutr Rep Int 5:139–144.

Chen LC (1982): Malnutrition and mortality. Nutr Found India Bull, October, pp 1–5.

Chen LC, Chowdhury AKMA, Hufman SL (1980a): Anthropometric assessment of energy-protein malnutrition and subsequent risk of mortality among preschool aged children. Am J Clin Nutr 33:1836–1845.

Chen LC, Rahman M, Sardar AM (1980b): Epidemiology and causes of death among children in a rural area of Bangladesh. Int J Epidemiol 9:25–33.

Chen LC, Chowdhury AKMA, Hufman SL (1981): The use of anthropometry for nutritional surveillance in mortality control programs. Am J Clin Nutr 34:2596–2599.

Corey P, Beaton GH (1975): Safe protein-calorie ratios in diets: Reply to Drs Sukhatme and Payne. Am J Clin Nutr 28:1195–1199.

Dowler FA, Payne PR, Seo Y, Thomson AM, Wheeler EF (1982): Nutritional status indicators—interpretation and policy making role. Food Policy 7:99–112.

Durnin JVGA, Edholm OG, Miller DS, Waterlow JC (1973): How much food does man require? Nature 242:418.

FAO (1977): "The Fourth World Food Survey." FAO Nutr Rep Ser, No. 10; FAO Statistics Ser, No. 11.

FAO (1979): "Agriculture: Toward 2000." FAO Conf Rep C79/24.

FAO/WHO (1973): "Report of a Joint FAO/WHO Ad Hoc Expert Committee on Energy and Protein Requirements." FAO Nutr Meet Rep Ser, No. 52; WHO Tech Rep Ser, No. 522.

FAO/WHO (1975): Energy and protein requirements: Recommendations by a joint FAO/WHO informal gathering of experts. Food Nutr 1(2):11–19.

Garby L (1983): Energy balance and obesity. In "Proceedings of the International Workshop on Genetic Factors in Nutrition, Teotihuacan, Mexico, 1982."

Habicht J-P, Meyers LD, Brownie C (1982): Indicators for identifying and counting the improperly nourished. Am J Clin Nutr 35:1241–1254.

James P, Shetty PS (1982): Metabolic adaptation and energy requirements in developing countries. Human Nutr Clin Nutr 36C:331–336.

Lörstad MH (1971): Recommended intakes and their relation to nutrient deficiency. FAO Nutr Newsl 9(1):18–31.

Lörstad MH (1974): On estimating incidence of undernutrition. FAO Nutr Newsl 12(1):1–11.

Margen S (1983): Autoregulatory processes to maintain energy balance in the individual. In "Proceedings of the Conference on Energy Intake and Activity, Bellagio, Italy" (in press).

Martorell R, Yarbrough C, Yarbrough S, Klein RE (1980): The impact of ordinary illnesses on the dietary intakes of malnourished children. Am J Clin Nutr 33:345–350.

Payne PR, Dugdale AE (1977): A model for the prediction of energy balance and body weight. Ann Hum Biol 4:525.

Prentice AM (1983): Adaptation to long term low energy intake. In "Proceedings of the Conference on Energy Intake and Activity, Bellagio, Italy" (in press).

Prentice AM, Whitehead RG, Roberts SB, Paul AA (1981): Long term energy balance in childbearing Gambian women. Am J Clin Nutr 34:2790–2799.

Reutlinger S (1983): Policy implications of research on energy intake and activity level. In "Proceedings of the Conference on Energy Intake and Activity, Bellagio, Italy" (in press).

Reutlinger S, Alderman H (1980): "The Prevalence of Calorie Deficient Diets in Developing Countries." World Bank Staff Working Paper, No. 374.

Reutlinger S, Selowsky M (1976): "Malnutrition and Poverty. Magnitude and Policy Options." World Bank Staff Working Paper, No. 23.

Rutishauser IHE, Whitehead RG (1972): Energy intakes and expenditure in 1–3 year old Ugandan children living in a rural environment. Br J Nutr 28:145–197.

Srinivasan TN (1983): "Malnutrition in developing countries: The state of knowledge of the extent of its prevalence, its causes, and its consequences." Unpublished distributed paper.

Sukhatme PV (1961): The world's hunger and future needs in food supplies. J Roy Statist Soc 124:463–585.

Sukhatme PV (1966): The world's food supplies. J Roy Statist Soc 129:222–243.

Sukhatme PV (1981): Relationship between malnutrition and poverty. First National Conference on Social Sciences, New Delhi. Unpublished paper.

Sukhatme, PV, Margen S (1982): Autoregulatory homeostatic nature of energy balance. Am J Clin Nutr 35:355–365.

UN (1975): Extracts from papers of the World Food Conference. UNU Food Nutr Bull 1(1): 23–26.

UNU (1979): "Protein Energy Requirements Under Conditions Prevailing in Developing Countries: Current Knowledge and Research Needs." UNU World Hunger Program WHTR-1/UNUP-18.

UNU (1981): The uses of energy and protein requirement estimates. Report of a workshop. UNU Food Nutr Bull 3:45–53.

Viteri FE, Torun B (1981): Nutrition, physical activity and growth. In Ritzen M et al (eds): "The Biology of Human Growth." New York: Raven, pp 265–273.

Whitehead RG (ed) (1983): "Maternal Diet, Breast Feeding Capacity and Lactational Infertility." UNU Food Nutr Bull, Suppl 6.

THE MATERNAL/INFANT DYAD

—

Malnutrition: Determinants and Consequences, pages 85–100
© 1984 Alan R. Liss, Inc., 150 Fifth Avenue, New York, NY 10011

Physiology of Lactation: An Integrative Perspective

J.E. Chappell, BASc, and M.T. Clandinin, PhD

Department of Nutritional Sciences, Faculty of Medicine, University of
Toronto, Toronto, Ontario, Canada M5S 1A8

INTRODUCTION

From a nutritional viewpoint, understanding of hormonal influences over
transfer of nutrients from mother to infant is fundamental to appreciation of
mechanisms that provide an essential milk nutrient content. This composition
is thought to approximate the need for these nutrients by the infant for tissue
development. Partitioning and transfer of nutrients is regulated by the endocrine system of the mother, and is subjected to the influence of exogenous factors, such as maternal diet and the essential interactive stimulus of the suckling
infant. Moreover, recent findings appear to indicate that the cascade of hormonal events that become internalized within the secretory cells of the mammary gland may in themselves be of physiologic significance in the developing
neonate.

Our present understanding of the physiology of human lactation is based
largely on principles drawn from animal experiments, tissue explants, and human studies of varying acute physiologic states. Extrapolation of controlling
mechanisms from these sources must be viewed with some reservation. A complex series of coordinated and perhaps synergistic hormonal events results in
development of the mammary gland preparatory to lactation. During the peri-
partum period, shifts in levels of maternal hormones derived from placental,
uterine, and gonadal tissues combined with increasing prolactin (PRL) levels
are associated with proliferation of receptor-mediated functions in the mammary gland.

In addition, the events of lactation should not be considered as solely limited to activities in mammary tissues, for indeed homeorrhetic controls encompass direct and indirect functions and responses of extramammary tissues. Relationships between maternal nutrient intake and the composition of lactation

have been extensively studied. However, underlying mechanisms for these alterations in milk composition have not been defined and may result from interaction with a limited maternal postprandial endocrine response.

Many investigators now recognize that by analysis of breast fluid and milk the intracellular messengers can be successfully identified, thus depicting prior cellular events. Furthermore, perceptive examination of transitional or altered, yet naturally existing, states of lactation may improve current knowledge of underlying hormonal relationships responsible for milk composition. This chapter will examine aspects of human lactation with an emphasis placed on how controls over lactogenesis may be assessed in man.

MAMMARY GLAND DEVELOPMENT

There is great variation in both the general appearance and the pattern of development of mammary glands among species; however, the transitions in function, resulting in copious secretory activity, are broadly similar. The fine control of this cycle from quiescence through regression is not well understood. At present, a major portion of current knowledge concerning anatomic changes in the breast preparatory to lactation is inferred from animals subjected to hypophysectomy, oophorectomy, or adrenalectomy followed by hormone replacement therapy [Lyons, 1958; Cowie et al, 1969] or is derived from cell culture studies, in which complete control of hormonal enrivonment is feasible [Topper, 1970; Borst, 1980]. Interpretation across species is an obvious concern. The significance of potential compounding influences, such as prior "priming," administration of pharmacologic doses of semipure hormones, and stromal/lymph contamination of cell cultures must be examined [Rivira, 1976].

In this chapter, the conventional division of the lactation process into specific stages should not imply a rigid format of events or influences. The phenomenon of "witch's milk" from the newborn infant illustrates the overwhelming hormonal impact on an anatomically "fetal" gland [Buehring, 1982]. Compositional analysis of this secretion may disclose the impact of minimal structural differentiation on the synthetic process [Wiersbitzky and Weyrauch, 1970]. Structural differentiation of the mammary gland is mediated within a hormonal environment. Primary steps of the dynamic process include, sequentially, development of the lobuloalveolar structure, emergence of characteristic secretory activity, hypertrophy of active secretory cells, and finally, usually at weaning, cessation of synthetic activity followed by disappearance of lobuloalveolar structure [Delouis et al, 1980].

Resting Phase

Prior to onset of puberty the mammary gland is composed of primary ducts with minimal branching and terminal budding, multilayered epithelial cells, and narrow lumina. Ultrastructural examination of a parallel stage in mouse mammary development indicates limited ultrastructural development of cytoplasmic and subcellular organelles [Hollman, 1974]. Hormonal changes associated with puberty induce limited cell proliferation and differentiation such that by the end of adolescence a characteristic ductular-alveolar structure exists [Vorherr, 1978]. In analogy with changes in the endometrium, breast tissue also sustains cyclic fluctuations in growth, subsequent to periodic release of hormones by ovarian and hypothalamic tissues. Breast fluid, present in 50% of caucasian women, may reflect accumulation of secretory material subsequent to the ebb and flow of hormonal stimuli. Currently, cancer researchers are examining this secretion to detect potential early markers inherent in breast cancer development [Wynder and Hill, 1977; Petrakis et al, 1981]. Examination of nutrient and hormonal patterns of breast fluid may also generate insight into the fundamental biology of the nonlactating mammary gland.

Relactation (nonpuerperant lactation associated with infant adoption) offers further opportunity to examine some of the controls surrounding mammary gland function. In this regard, Kleinman et al [1980] recently reported that, while total milk protein concentration from nonbiologic mothers decreased with time in a pattern analogous to that of postpartum lactation, the level of secretory IgA, α-lactalbumin, and albumin was significantly lower when appropriate comparison was made with the level of these components in postpartum lactations. This transitional-mature profile for milk protein concentration during relactation suggests that the hormonal environment of pregnancy is essential for secretion of colostrum. Furthermore, Kleinman and coworkers [1980] reported that a woman who stimulated her breasts prior to delivery did not produce the protein pattern characteristic of colostrum until the immediate postpartum period. Analysis of alterations in milk nutrient profile might serve to identify possible reasons for variable success rates of relactation [Bose et al, 1981].

Antepartum Phase

Pregnancy initiates a process of extensive transformation in the mammary gland subsequent to increase in plasma estrogen (E) and progesterone (PG) levels. While specific hormones are mammogenic, it is difficult to associate individual hormones with each step in the cascade of events. Rudimentary branching and budding develop by sprouting of the terminal portion of the duct system (now tertiary) and by true alveolar elaboration. In animal models duct growth is influenced by estrogen, adrenal steroids, and growth hormone, whereas lobuloalvcolar growth is induced by PG and PRL [Friesen et al, 1973]. This intensified expansion gradually displaces much of the surrounding and previously predominant adipose and connective tissues. By 3–4 weeks of gestation, glandular development, which includes increased mammary blood flow and increased interstitial water and electrolyte levels, exceeds the respective changes occurring during the menstrual cycle [Vorherr, 1979]. The major anatomic process to occur in the breast during pregnancy is multiplication of epithelial cells and formation of the characteristic lobuloalveolar structure. Insulin may be permissive at this stage, PRL being the functioning mitogen (reviewed by Forsyth [1971]). This architectural change involves transition of a two-cell layer of alveolar epithelium into a monolayer secretory unit in combination with dichotomic ductular proliferation, whereas the cytoplasm remains poorly organized with small mitochondria and nucleoli [Vorherr, 1979]. It is also thought that hydrocortisone, insulin, and PRL result in cytologic and functional differentiation of epithelial cells (reviewed by Topper [1970]). Hydrocortisone induces increased rough endoplasmic reticulum and increased lateral paranuclear Golgi apparatus, which are essential for protein synthesis and secretion. PRL synergistically with insulin induces synthesis of new RNA, which eventually culminates in milk synthesis. Placental lactogen, growth hormone, thyroxine, and other hormones have been observed from animal experiments to be involved at this stage; however, their role in human mammary gland development remains speculative.

The hormonal stimuli concomitant with advancing pregnancy facilitate progressive yet controlled development of this exocrine gland. The concept of mammary gland immaturity prior to a full-term gestational period should perhaps be re-evaluated, given reports of milk-like secretions following spontaneous or therapeutic abortions, at as early as 16 weeks gestation [Smith et al, 1972; Yue et al, 1974]. The nutrient and hormonal composition of these secretions may mirror the architecture and synthetic potential present at this phase of gestation. Observations by Atkinson et al [1978] indicate not only that mothers delivering at 26 weeks of gestation can secrete milk, but also that the total milk nitrogen content is significantly higher from mothers delivering premature infants of 26–33 weeks gestational age than from women delivering full-term infants. This and other reports have sparked renewed interest in the appropriateness of human milk for the high-risk premature infant [Gross et al, 1981; Lemons et al, 1982; Chappell and Clandinin, 1982]. There is little evidence to suggest that this milk secretion has a teleologic origin; however, it does raise the consideration of an underlying hormonal relationship responsible for this observation on milk composition. Controversy or variance in results reported to date [Sann et al, 1981; Anderson et al, 1983] may also be better understood if "preterm milk" is examined as an event secondary to an altered or interrupted hormonal status.

During the second half of gestation, high placental-luteal hormone levels are believed to inhibit proliferation of mammary PRL receptors and thus prepartum lactation [Djiane and Durand, 1977]. As circulating PG/E levels are lower at 30 weeks than at 38–40 weeks of gestation [Parker et al, 1979; Buster et al, 1979; Goh et al, 1982], it may be inferred that women delivering premature infants initiate lactation with lower circulating PG/E levels and thus a potentially relatively greater number of mammary PRL receptors. It is conceivable that this difference in receptor number may result in higher rates of mammary synthesis (eg, lipogenesis) reported for mothers of preterm infants [Guerrini et al, 1981]. This concept is further supported by increased levels in preterm milk of medium-chain fatty acids synthesized de novo [Chappell and Clandinin, 1982; Bitman et al, 1983] and by the relationship between medium-chain fatty acid synthesis and increasing PRL levels in mouse mammary gland explants [Borst, 1980].

Anderson [submitted] has proposed that differences found between "preterm" milk and "full-term" milk are subsequent to an immature mammary system, which permits paracellular transport [Peaker, 1976] to continue unabated following parturition. Since evidence for paracellular transport in human lactation [Hartmann and Kulski, 1978; Hartmann and Prosser, 1982] is associated with hormonal changes, this argument may also be seen as an extension of a hormonal mechanism rather than its antithesis. However, the existence and pattern of transitional "preterm" milk constituents [Anderson et al, 1981; Lemons et al, 1982] does not lend support to the proposal.

Extensive differentiation required to support varied metabolic and neuroendocrine activities of lactation must therefore be operative as early as midgestation. Increased secretion of PRL, adrenal corticotropic hormone, E, thyroid-stimulating hormone, and human chorionic somatotropin has been implicated in the complex transition from mammotropic to lactogenic stimuli. Increasing numbers and subcellular positioning of mitochondria, Golgi apparatus, and endoplasmic reticulum result in accumulation of lipid droplets and granule-laden vacuoles in the apical region of the alveolar cells. Intracellular degradation is apparently less important than in the preceding phase; however, dense bodies and multivesicular bodies are still present.

Initiation

Signals involved in parturition may also be those associated with initiation of lactation [Liggins et al, 1977]. While attempts have been made to stimulate blood-borne and/or neuroendocrine signals thought to be responsible, the actual sequence of events is not well understood. Parturition is associated with marked hormonal shifts, but these may not be the pivotal factor, as many mammary cellular changes occur in advance of parturition. It should also be noted that lactogenesis or initiation of milk secretion is a different process from that maintaining established milk production (reviewed by Tucker [1979]). Before parturition in the mouse, mammary secretory activity is intense, resulting in an increase in number and size of fat globules [Hollman, 1974]. The lumen, while still narrow, is filled with protein granules, occasional lipid droplets, and colostrum corpuscles. Immediately preceding parturition, the lumen becomes markedly distended with newly formed lipid droplets, whereas degradation bodies are no longer observed. These shifts in synthetic capacity parallel noticeable changes in number of mitochondria, positioning of rough endoplasmic reticulum, and development of Golgi vacuoles. Hormonal mediation of these events is similar to prior stages of development, but now induces a heightened response due to precipitous decrease in concentrations of placental and luteal hormones [Kuhn, 1969; Nicholas and Hartmann, 1981]. In primates the increase of E concentration mediates intraovarian release of prostaglandin $F_{2\alpha}$ [Sotrel et al, 1981]. This luteolytic agent may alter luteinizing hormone/chorionic gonadotropin receptor, resulting in decreased PG secretion. In addition, removal of placental secretions results in a dramatic decrease in both systemic and local inhibition [Turkington and Hill, 1969]. For the goat, elevated mammary gland prostaglandin $F_{2\alpha}$ synthesis during late pregnancy also accounts for a portion of local inhibition of mammary secretion [Walker and Peaker, 1980]. Extensive metabolism to DHK-prostaglandin $F_{2\alpha}$ or release into the lumen at parturition may insure a mechanism to free secretory cells from down-regulation. It is noteworthy that various prostaglandins are present in human milk [Reid et al, 1980; Lucas and Mitchell, 1980; Chappell et al, 1983]. It is not known whether milk prostanoids reflect specific exogenous release or endogenous mediation of hormonal stimuli. In this "essential" endocrine milieu the presence of PRL converts "presecretory" alveolar epithelium to active milk-synthesizing and milk-releasing cells (reviewed by del Pozo and Brownell [1979] and Shiu and Friesen [1980]). In addition it is known that in animals decline in sex steroids and chorionic somatotropin fosters a hypothalamic decrease of PRL inhibiting factor such that a further increase in transmembranal secretion of PRL occurs from pituitary lactotrophs. The pattern of initially high colostrum concentrations of PRL [Healy et al, 1980], cortisol, insulin, growth hormone, and thyroid-stimulating hormone [Kulski and Hartmann, 1981a; 1983] followed by marked decreases over the first few days of lactation suggests a multiphasic requirement for "triggering" lactation. Similar lactation outcomes following caesarian and normal deliveries [Kulski et al, 1981a], in spite of different plasma PRL surges [Rigg and Yen, 1977], indicate that other "priming" influences cannot be overlooked. For example, in the goat and cow, low concentrations of ionized calcium may be crucial for normal epithelial integrity at the onset of lactation [Neville and Peaker, 1981].

One of the most dramatic events following removal of "blocking activity" is increased synthesis of α-lactalbumin and subsequently lactose [Turkington and Hill, 1969; Kulski et al, 1977]. During pregnancy α-lactalbumin is present in plasma and these levels stabilize at 26 weeks until term [Martin et al, 1980]. The presence of this protein in plasma may reflect paracellular leaking; however, the absence of fat droplets suggests that liberation of protein granules is subsequent to a physiologic process. Plasma and milk levels of α-lactalbumin increase markedly following labor and remain elevated in both lactating and nonlactating women during the first few postpartum days. This transition in secretory activity is not suckling-dependent [Kulski and Hartmann, 1981b]. Subsequent increase in milk lactose content has been demonstrated by many researchers [Brew, 1969].

Milk Synthesis and Secretion

Net increase in enzyme activity has been viewed by many to signal the phase transition from colostrum to milk [Tucker, 1979] and occurs between 32 and 40 hr after delivery [Kulski and Hartmann, 1981b]. Operating within a hormonal complex, PRL by way of its receptor induces the synthetic apparatus resulting in the characteristic milk profile [Skarda et al, 1982]. Many PRL operants have been identified [Shiu and Friesen, 1980]. Prolactin receptors are enriched in plasma membrane and appear to be high-affinity lipoprotein complexes [Shiu et al, 1973]. Receptor content in cat and rat mammary glands is induced following parturition [Djiane and Durand, 1977] concomitantly with the surge in PRL release. Immunochemical studies imply that PRL may be internalized within the secretory cell [Nolin and Witorsch, 1976]. Molecular events subsequent to hormone/receptor interaction remain hypothetical. In the mouse, phospholipase activation is involved, implicating a secondary messenger [Rillema and Wild, 1977]. The resultant release of arachidonic acid from membrane phosphatidylcholine may trigger release of prostaglandins (B_2, E_2, and $F_{2\alpha}$). The action of PRL, potentiated by hydrocortisone, in milk protein secretion may be mediated by these prostaglandins [Rillema, 1975]. α-Lactalbumin and casein are synthesized on the rough endoplasmic reticulum and then are moved to the Golgi body for vesicular incorporation. These vesicles migrate to the luminal surface, where a process of reverse pinocytosis occurs, resulting in escape of vesicle contents into the lumen [Hollman, 1974].

Lactose synthesis is catalyzed by galactosyltransferase [Ebner and McKenzie, 1972] attached to the Golgi apparatus and by a second component, α-lactalbumin, which controls the substrate specificity of the enzyme complex. T_3 potentiates induction of lactose synthesis by PRL in mice [Vonderhaar, 1977]. Lactose is formed in the lumen of the Golgi apparatus and draws water with it as lactose is secreted (reviewed by Jenness [1974] and Peaker [1976]). While this process is heightened at parturition, the observation of lactose in the urine of pregnant women as early as 8 weeks of gestation indicates that synthesis does occur in a majority of women throughout pregnancy [Flynn and Harper, 1953; SA Atkinson, personal communication].

Endocrine control of mammary gland lipid metabolism is not well understood. In mice PRL stimulates fatty acid synthesis in the presence of insulin and hydrocortisone. Furthermore, it is known that lipoprotein lipase activity in rat mammary gland is increased by a prostaglandin-mediated PRL influence, thereby facilitating uptake of exogenous fatty acids for triglyceride synthesis [Spooner et al, 1977]. Esterification of fatty acids takes place on the endoplasmic reticulum. The triglycerides produced form small droplets that markedly increase in size as they approach the cell apex (reviewed by Patton [1976]). These droplets become enveloped in apical membrane and are released by apocrine secretion (reviewed by Smith and Abraham [1975]).

PRL also has been implicated in maintaining low milk sodium concentrations by promoting alveolar retention [Bern and Nicoll, 1968]. Na$^+$,K$^+$-ATPase activity may be the focus of this PRL influence (reviewed by Falconer [1980]). When PRL is administered to sex steroid-primed virgin mice, the number of IgA-bearing plasma cells increases dramatically in the mammary gland [Weisz-Carrington et al, 1978]). The mechanism appears to be specific for IgA-bearing cells. PRL is also involved in active elaboration of secretory IgA, in the "initiated" mammary gland.

Maintenance of Lactation (Galactophoresis)

Mechanical stimuli associated with maintenance of established lactogenesis involves hypophyseal release of both oxytocin and PRL. Milk formed is secreted continuously and retained in alveoli and small ducts in the gland until the neuroendocrine milk ejection reflex occurs [Cobo et al, 1967]. Suckling stimulates nerve endings in the areola and nipple to induce release of oxytocin, which results in contraction of myoepithelial cells surrounding the alveoli and duct system moving milk towards the terminal ducts and sinuses [Lincoln and Paisley, 1982]. Physical removal of the "let-down" milk by the infant is a continuing stimulus for further milk synthesis.

During this later stage of lactation when copious secretions are produced, the nonsuckling levels of PRL decline. Following suckling, a surge in PRL release results in a severalfold transitory increase in circulating plasma PRL levels [Tyson et al, 1972; Grosvenor et al, 1979]. While the role of metabolic hormones in human milk production is not well understood, this shift in plasma PRL levels associated with the maintenance of lactation has been interpreted to signal a diminishing role for PRL. This shift in PRL level occurs in the absence of elevated PG levels or other potential inhibitors of the PRL effect. Thus, without data on PRL receptor numbers, turnover, or sensitivity, the role of PRL cannot be interpreted solely on the basis of its circulating levels.

Administration of Br-ergocryptine, a known inhibitor of PRL release, results in suppression of lactation [Brun del Re et al, 1973; del Pozo and Brownell, 1979]. Thus human pharmacologic data appear to support the concept that PRL exerts its lactogenic effect at both the initiation and maintenance stages of lactation. In addition, studies of nonpuerperal lactation subsequent to abnormal PRL metabolism [Chang, 1978] may further develop our understanding of prolactin dynamics. In this regard, Kulski et al [1981b] suggest that lactation in nonpregnant, nonparturient women may provide "a model for studying hormonal control of lactation in the absence of the complicating factors of a fetus, inhibitory hormones and infant suckling."

The pivotal role of the infant in sustaining lactation has become increasingly obvious, especially in Western countries where women have recently followed advice such as rigid feeding regimen and supplementary feedings. Lactation failure, while complex in origin, is rarely associated with a maternal defect [Lawrence, 1980]. Recently, Davies [1979] has documented two breast-feeding styles linked with failure to thrive in breast-fed infants; the "fretful underfed" and the "contented underfed" baby. Failure to remove milk from the breast decreases milk synthesis and subsequent secretion because milk-dilated alveoli obstruct mammary blood flow in addition to the combined effect of declining oxytocin and PRL pulse due to subnormal intensity of stimulation. Stress and anxiety place the maternal-infant dyad at even greater risk of failure. While both functional and emotional support are widely recognized as essential factors inherent in successful lactation, further recognition of the hurdles impeding successful breast feeding is also essential.

The total "hormonal milieu" is implicit in maintenance of lactation. Characteristic changes in nutrients present in milk that are concomitant with ovulation during lactation have been interpreted as representing the existence of paracellular transport [Hartmann and Prosser, 1981]. However, Prosser and Hartmann [in press] in recent examination of these shifts found that while milk sodium and chloride levels were elevated with an associated decrease in lactose and potassium, the protein and glucose content was not increased as would be expected. If a direct paracellular route for transfer exists at this time the concentration gradient shift should result in increased glucose and protein levels. Therefore, these authors conclude that decreased milk glucose concentrations may signal a period of limited availability of substrate for energy and synthetic processes. These nutrient shifts occur 5–6 days before and after ovulation; thus, it has been speculated that endocrine controls resulting in gradual change in hormone levels associated with ovulation also induce compositional transitions in milk lactated. In support of this concept, short-term cyclic changes also occur in salivary glucose levels with ovulation in both lactating and nonlactating women [Prosser and Hartmann, in press]. Since these acute salivary changes also occurred in nonlactating women, these authors suggest that hormones controlling ovulation overide those influencing lactation. Cyclic changes in basal metabolic rate [Soloman et al, 1982] and energy intake [Dalvit, 1981] also fluctuate together during the menstrual cycle. Thus it might be hypothesized that metabolic adaptation associated with lactation cannot respond to the further energy demands of menses without a resultant transitory decrease in substrate availability for milk synthesis.

EXTRA-MAMMARY GLAND DEVELOPMENT

Striking maternal adaptations occur during pregnancy so as to enable mammary gland development. There is an increase of 30–50% in the size of the pituitary, primarily owing to hypertrophy of PRL cells as a consequence of sex steroid levels [Vorherr, 1979]. Synthesis of PRL increases some 10-fold to 20-fold over normal levels, resulting in increased plasma PRL levels as gestation advances [Tyson et al, 1972]. Together, these hormonally controlled transitions in microanatomy of secretory cells in the breast and pituitary exemplify critical tissue interdependence and synergism. From animal model studies it is also apparent that during lactation fundamental shifts occur in metabolism between tissues. For example, it is known that during lactation the weight and length of the rat small intestine increases and that dipeptidase and glucose-6-phosphate dehydrogenase activity increases [Williamson, 1980]. These synchronized events imply a higher order of endocrine regulation in support of the dominant physiological process, lactation [Bauman and Currie, 1980]. This hemeorrhetic regulation implies a coordination of metabolism of body tissues so as to facilitate a priority development [Bauman et al, 1982].

PRL may be a key component responsible for flow or partitioning of nutrients and reciprocal compensatory nutrient utilization by competing tissues [Bauman and Currie, 1980; Benito et al, 1982]. Several researchers have proposed that PRL directs lipid metabolism in adipose tissue and liver in a manner that distributes nutrients to the mammary gland [Zinder et al, 1974; Aqius et al, 1979]. PRL may inhibit directly or indirectly [Spooner et al, 1977] the synthesis of adipose tissue lipoprotein lipase while conversely stimulating mammary gland lipoprotein lipase activity. This metabolic adaptation may be augmented by pregnancy-stimulated and lactation-suppressed anabolic effects of insulin/receptor interactions [Flint et al, 1979]. In rat liver, lactation is associated with increased glucose utilization, lipogenesis, and fatty acid esterification, whereas ketogenesis and triglyceride secretion are decreased [Williamson, 1980]. Furthermore, it has been proposed that protein and mineral metabolism are also directed to support lactation, indicating that lactation is not solely a mammary gland phenomenon [Bauman and Currie, 1980].

Perhaps this "buffering" capacity of body tissues permits an overall uniformity of human milk composition. Indeed, a direct diet-to-milk nutrient interaction has usually been observed when nutritional "status" is such that the coordination process or intake is no longer within a range compatible with adaptation [Deodhar et al, 1964]. For example, low B_{12} levels in milk have been reported only following a prolonged vegan diet [Higginbottom et al, 1978] or in the presence of maternal pernicious anemia [Johnson and Roloff, 1982]. While there are exceptions to this hypothesis [Forsum and Lonnerdal, 1980; Deodhar et al, 1964], the overwhelming similarities across socioeconomic and food selection patterns reinforce the teleologic basis of human milk for the developing newborn (reviewed by Jelliffe and Jelliffe [1978] and Atkinson [1979]). Perhaps by reexamining either the proportion of variance in milk composition attributable to diet [Vuori et al, 1982] or milks of abnormal composition from apparently normal subcellular development [Asnes et al, 1982], we may further delineate the controlling mechanisms involved. Dietary fat alters the structure and function of plasma membranes [Neelands and Clandinin, 1983]. Modulation of secretory cell membrane structure and function by diet is also likely, but it has not been examined as a factor relating diet to mammary gland functions.

Hormonal controls differ among species. This genetic difference in controlling mechanisms is believed to be responsible for marked species differences in milk nutrient content. For humans further examination of the relationship between endocrine controls and expression of subcellular functions in the epithelial cell is essential to understanding the basis of the nutrient content of milk.

SUMMARY

In general it can be concluded that as the endocrine balance affects morphologic and biosynthetic changes occurring in mammary secretory cells, it might be expected that factors interfering with this endocrine balance will alter the composition of milk produced. Considerable study remains to be accomplished to define these factors and their influence on human milk composition.

Principles established primarily through animal model research have provided the framework for understanding of the process of human lactation. Further development of this unique area of research should include assessment of human milk for markers of subcellular function and control. While numerous reports exist regarding the presence of hormones (reviewed by Koldovsky [1980]) and secondary messengers in human milk, confounding factors such as hormone receptors and artifactual procedures cannot be overlooked [Chappell et al, submitted; Gala et al, 1975].

Furthermore, the hormones of maternal origin present in human milk may have the potential for short- and long-term effects on neuroendocrine activity in neonates [Angelucci et al, 1983; Strbak et al, 1978]. The hypothesis that maternal endocrine status influences neonatal endocrine function through the vehicle of suckled milk is a fascinating relationship between mother and her developing neonate that merits further exploration.

TEACHING AID

This paper is available as a separate text adapted for use with accompanying visual aids. Inquiries should be sent to Dr. M.T. Clandinin at the University of Toronto.

REFERENCES

Anderson DM, Williams FH, Merkatz RB, Schulman PK, Kerr DS, Pittard WB (1983): Length of gestation and nutritional composition of human milk. Am J Clin Nutr 37:810–814.

Anderson GH (submitted for publication): The effect of prematurity on milk composition and physiological basis.

Anderson GH, Atkinson SA, Bryan MH (1981): Energy and macronutrient content of human milk during early lactation from mothers giving birth prematurely and at term. Am J Clin Nutr 34:258–265.

Angelucci L, Patacchioli FR, Chierichetti C, Laureti S (1983): Perinatal mother-offspring pituitary adrenal interrelationship in rats: Corticosterone in milk may affect adult life. Endocrinol Exp 17:191–205.

Aqius L, Robinson AM, Girard JR, Williamson DH (1979): Alterations in the rate of lipogenesis in vivo in maternal liver and adipose tissue on premature weanling of lactating rats: A possible regulatory role of prolactin. Biochem J 180:689–692.

Asnes RS, Wisotsky DH, Migel PF, Seigle RL, Levy J (1982): The dietary chloride deficiency syndrome occurring in a breast-fed infant. J Pediatr 100:923–924.

Atkinson SA (1979): Factors affecting human milk composition. Can Dietet Assoc J 40: 213–222.

Atkinson SA, Bryan MH, Anderson GH (1978): Human Milk: Difference in nitrogen concentration in milk from mothers of term and preterm infants. J Pediatr 93:67–69.

Bauman DE, Currie WB (1980): Partitioning of nutrients during pregnancy and lactation: A review of mechanisms involving homeostasis and homeorrhesis. J Diary Sci 63:1514–1529.

Bauman DE, Eisemann JH, Currie WB (1982): Hormonal effects on partitioning of nutrients for tissue growth: Role of growth hormone and prolactin. Fed Proc 41:2538–2544.

Benito M, Lorenzo M, Medina JM (1982): The role of prolactin in the regulation of hepatic lipogenesis in vivo during late gestation in the rat. Horm Metab Res 14:614–615.

Bern HA, Nicoll CS (1968): The comparative endocrinology of prolactin. Recent Prog Horm Res 24:681–713.

Bitman J, Wood DL, Hamosh M, Hamosh P, Mehta NR (1983): Comparison of the lipid composition of breast milk from mothers of term and preterm infants. Am J Clin Nutr 38:300–312.

Borst DW (1980): Hormonal regulation of medium chain fatty acid synthesis by mouse mammary gland explants. Lipids 15:913–917.

Bose CL, D'Ercole J, Lester AG, Hunter RS, Barret JR (1981): Relactation by mothers of sick and premature infants. Pediatrics 67:565–569.

Brew K (1969): Secretion of α-lactalbumin into milk and its relevance to the organization and control of lactose synthetase. Nature 222:671–672.

Brun del Re R, del Pozo E, de Grandi P, Friesen H, Hinselmann M, Wyss H (1973): Prolactin inhibition and suppression of puerperal lactation by a Br-ergocryptine (CB 154). Obstet Gynecol 41:884–890.

Buehring GC (1982): Witch's milk: Potential for neonatal diagnosis. Pediatr Res 16:460–462.

Buster JE, Chang RJ, Preston DL, Elashoff RM, Cousins LM, Abraham GE, Hobel CJ, Marshall JR (1979): Interrelationships of circulating maternal steroid concentrations in the third trimester pregnancies. I. C_{21} steroids: Progesterone, 16α-hydroxyprogesterone, 17α-hydroxyprogesterone, 20α-dehydro-progesterone, Δ^5-pregnenolone sulfate, and 17-hydroxyΔ^5-pregnenolone. J Clin Endocrinol Metab 48:133–138.

Chang RJ (1978): Normal and abnormal prolactin metabolism. Clin Obstet Gynecol 21:125–137.

Chappell JE, Clandinin MT (1982): Comparative fatty acid content of human milk. Fed Proc 41:A473.

Chappell JE, Clandinin MT, Barber GJ, Armstrong DT (1983): Prostanoid content of human milk: Relationship to milk fatty acid content. Endocrinol Exp 17:351–358.

Chappell JE, Ruse J, Clandinin MT (submitted for publication): Is there a prolactin receptor in human milk?

Cobo E, DeBernal MM, Gaitan E, Quintero CA (1967): Neurohypophyseal hormone release in the human. II. Experimental study during lactation. Am J Obstet Gynecol 97:519–529.

Cowie AT, Hartmann PE, Turvey A (1969): The maintenance of lactation in the rabbit after hypophysectomy. J Endocrinol 43:651–662.

Dalvit SP (1981): The effect of menstrual cycle on patterns of food intake. Am J Clin Nutr 34: 1811–1815.

Davies DP (1979): Is inadequate breast feeding an important cause of failure to thrive? Lancet 1:541–542.

Delouis C, Djiane J, Houdebine LM, Terqui M (1980): Relation between hormones and mammary gland function. J Dairy Sci 63:1492–1513.

del Pozo E, Brownell J (1979): Prolactin I. Mechanisms of control, peripheral actions and modification by drugs. Hormone Res 10:143–174.

Deodhar AD, Rajalakshmi R, Ramakrishnar CV (1964): Studies on human lactation. Part III. Effects of dietary supplementation on vitamin contents of breast milk. Acta Paediatr 53: 42–48.

Djiane J, Durand P (1977): Prolactin-progesterone antagonism in self-regulation of prolactin receptors in the mammary gland. Nature 266:641–643.

Ebner KE, McKenzie LM (1972): α-Lactalbumin and galactosyltransferase in rat serum and their relationship to milk secretion. Biochem Biophys Res Comm 49:1624–1630.

Falconer IR (1980): Aspects of the biochemistry, physiology and endocrinology of lactation. Aust J Biol Sci 33:71–84.

Flint DJ, Sinnett-Smith PA, Clegg RA, Vernon RG (1979): Role of insulin receptors in the changing metabolism of adipose tissue during pregnancy and lactation in the rat. Biochem J 182:421–427.

Flynn FV, Harper C (1953): Lactosuria and glycosuria in pregnancy and the puerperium. Lancet 2:698–704.

Forsum E, Lonnerdal B (1980): Effect of protein intake on protein and nitrogen composition of breast milk. Am J Clin Nutr 33:1809–1813.

Forsyth IA (1971): Reviews of the progress of dairy science. Section A. Physiology. Organ culture techniques and the study of hormone effects on the mammary gland. J Dairy Res 3: 419–444.

Friesen HG, Fournier P, Desjardins P (1973): Pituitary prolactin in pregnancy and normal and abnormal lactation. Clin Obstet Gynecol 16:25–45.

Gala RR, Singhakowinta A, Brennan MJ (1975): Studies on prolactin in human serum, urine and milk. Hormone Res 6:310–320.

Goh HH, Lim LS, Wong PC, Ratnam SS (1982): Plasma oestriol in pregnancies complicated by diabetes mellitus. Aust J Exp Biol Med Sci 60:529–540.

Gross SJ, Geller J, Tomarelli RM (1981) Composition of breast milk from mothers of preterm infants. Pediatrics 68:490–493.

Grosvenor CE, Mena F, Whitworth NS (1979): The secretion rate of prolactin in the rat during suckling and its metabolic clearance rate after increasing intervals of nonsuckling. Endocrinology 104:372–376.

Guerrini P, Bosi G, Chierici R, Fabbri A (1981): Human milk: Relationship of fat content with gestational age. Early Hum Dev 5:187–194.

Hartmann PE, Kulski JK (1978): Changes in the composition of the mammary secretion of women after abrupt termination of breast feeding. J Physiol 275:1–11.

Hartmann PE, Prosser CG (1982): Acute changes in the composition of milk during the ovulatory menstrual cycle in lactating women. J Physiol 324:21–30.

Healy DL, Rattigan S, Hartmann PE, Herington AC, Burger HG (1980): Prolactin in human milk: Correlation with lactose, total protein, and α-lactalbumin levels. Am J Physiol 238 (Endocrinol Metab 1):E83–E86.

Higginbottom MC, Sweetman L, Nyhan WL (1978): A syndrome of methylmalonic aciduria, homocystinuria, megaloblastic anemia and neurologic abnormalities in a vitamin B_{12} deficient breast fed infant of a strict vegetarian. N Engl J Med 299:317–323.

Hollmann KH (1974): Cytology and fine structure of the mammary gland. In Larson BL (ed):

"Lactation: A Comprehensive Treatise." New York: Academic, pp 3–95.

Jelliffe DB, Jelliffe EFP (1978): The volume and composition of human milk in poorly nourished communities. A review. Am J Clin Nutr 31:492–515.

Jenness R (1974): Biosynthesis and composition of milk. J Invest Dermatol 63:109–118.

Johnson PR, Roloff JS (1982): Vitamin B_{12} deficiency in an infant strictly breast-fed by a mother with latent pernicious anemia. J Pediatr 100:917–919.

Kleinman R, Jacobson L, Hormann E, Walker WA (1980): Protein values of milk samples from mothers without biological pregnancies. J Pediatr 97:612–615.

Koldovsky O (1980): Hormones in milk. Life Sci 26:1833–1836.

Kuhn NJ (1969): Progesterone withdrawal as the lactogenic trigger in the rat. J Endocrinol 44: 39–54.

Kulski JK, Hartmann PE (1981a): Changes in the concentration of cortisol in milk during different stages of human lactation. Aust J Exp Biol Med Sci 59:769–778.

Kulski JK, Hartmann PE (1981b): Changes in human milk composition during the initiation of lactation. Aust J Exp Biol Med Sci 59:101–114.

Kulski JK, Hartmann PE (1983): Milk insulin, growth hormone and thyroid stimulating hormone: Relationship to changes in milk lactose, glucose and protein during lactogenesis in women. Endocrinol Exp 17:317–326.

Kulski JK, Smith M, Hartmann PE (1977): Perinatal concentrations of progesterone, lactose and α-lactalbumin in the mammary secretion of women. J Endocrinol 74:509–510.

Kulski JK, Smith M, Hartmann PE (1981a): Normal and caesarian section delivery and the initiation of lactation in women. Aust J Exp Biol Med Sci 59:405–412.

Kulski JK, Hartmann PE, Saint WJ, Giles PF, Gutteridge DH (1981b): Changes in the milk of nonpuerperal women. Am J Obstet Gynecol 139:597–604.

Lawrence RA (1980): Management of the mother-infant nursing couple. In Lawrence RA (ed): "Breastfeeding, a Guide for the Medical Profession." St. Louis: C.V. Mosby, pp 109–134.

Lemons JA, Moye L, Hall D, Simmons M (1982): Difference in the composition of preterm and term human milk during early lactation. Pediatr Res 16:113–117.

Liggins GC, Forster CS, Grieves SA, Schwartz AL (1977): Control of parturition in man. Biol Reprod 16:39–56.

Lincoln DW, Paisley AC (1982): Neuroendocrine control of milk ejection. J Reprod Fertil 65: 571–586.

Lucas A, Mitchell MD (1980): Prostaglandins in human milk. Arch Dis Child 55:950–952.

Lyons WR (1958): Hormonal synergism in mammary growth. Proc Soc B 149:303–325.

Martin RH, Glass MR, Chapman C, Wilson GD, Woods KL (1980): Human α-lactalbumin and hormonal factors in pregnancy and lactation. Clin Endocrinol 13:223–230.

Neelands PJ, Clandinin MT (1983): Diet fat influences liver plasma-membrane lipid composition and glucagon-stimulated adenylate cyclase activity. Biochem J 212:573–583.

Neville MC, Peaker M (1981): Ionized calcium in milk and the integrity of the mammary epithelium in the goat. J Physiol 313:561–570.

Nicholas KR, Hartmann PE (1981): Progressive changes in plasma progesterone, prolactin and corticosteroid levels during late pregnancy and the initiation of lactose synthesis in the rat. Aust J Biol Sci 34:445–454.

Nolin JM, Witorsch RJ (1976): Detection of endogenous immunoreactive prolactin in rat mammary epithelial cells during lactation. Endocrinology 99:949–958.

Parker CR, Everett RB, Quirk JG, Whalley PJ, Gant NF (1979): Hormone production during pregnancy in the primigravid patient: I. Plasma levels of progesterone and 5α-pregnane-3,20-dione throughout pregnancy of normal women and women who developed pregnancy-induced hypertension. Am J Obstet Gynecol 135:778–782.

Patton S (1976): Structure and function of mammary epithelium. In Patton S, Jensen RG (eds):

"Biomedical Aspects of Lactation." New York: Pergamon, pp 22-51.

Peaker M (1976): Lactation: Some cardiovascular and metabolic consequences, and the mechanisms of lactose and ion secretion into milk. In Wolstenholme G (ed): "Breastfeeding and the Mother." Ciba Foundation Symposium, No. 45, Amsterdam: Elsevier-Excerpta Medica-North Holland, pp 87-101.

Petrakis NL, Gruenke LD, Craig JC (1981): Cholesterol and cholesterol epoxides in nipple aspirates of human breast fluid. Cancer Res 41:2563-2566.

Prosser CG, Hartmann PE (in press): Saliva asnd breast milk composition during the menstrual cycle of women. Aust J Exp Biol Med Sci.

Reid B, Smith H, Friedman Z (1980): Prostaglandins in human milk. Pediatrics 66:870-872.

Rigg LA, Yen SSC (1977): Multiphasic prolactin secretion during parturition in human subjects. Am J Obstet Gynecol 128:215-218.

Rillema JA (1975): Possible role of prostaglandin $F_{2\alpha}$ in mediating effect of prolactin on RNA synthesis in mammary gland explants of mice. Nature 253:466-467.

Rillema JA, Wild EA (1977): Prolactin activation of phospholipase A activity in membrane preparations from mammary glands. Endocrinology 100:1219-1222.

Rivira EM (1976): Hormonal control of cellular events during lactogenesis: Some unresolved problems. In Josimovich JB (ed): "Lactogenic Hormones, Fetal Nutrition, and Lactation." New York: Wiley, pp 279-295.

Sann L, Bienvenu F, Lahet C, Bienvenu J, Benthenod M (1981): Comparison of the composition of breast milk from mothers of term and preterm infants. Acta Paediatr Scand 70:115-116.

Shiu RPC, Kelly PA, Friesen HG (1973): Radioreceptor assay for prolactin and other lactogenic hormones. Science 180:968-971.

Shiu RPC, Friesen HG (1980): Mechanism of action of prolactin in the control of mammary gland function. Annu Rev Physiol 42:83-96.

Skarda J, Urbanova E, Houdebini LM, Delouis C, Bilek J (1982): Effects of insulin, cortisol and prolactin on lipid, protein and casein synthesis in goat mammary tissue in organ culture. Reprod Nutr Dev 22:379-386.

Smith ID, Shearman RP, Korda AR (1972): Lactation following therapeutic abortion with prostaglandin $F_{2\alpha}$. Nature 240:411-412.

Smith S, Abraham S (1975): The composition and biosynthesis of milk fat. Adv Lipid Res 13:195-239.

Solomon SJ, Kurzer MS, Calloway DH (1982): Menstrual cycle and metabolic rate in women. Am J Clin Nutr 36:611-616.

Sotrel G, Helvacioglu A, Dowers S, Scommegna A, Auletta FJ (1981): Mechanism of luteolysis: Effect of estradiol and prostaglandin $F_{2\alpha}$ on corpus luteum luteinizing hormone/human chorionic gonadotropin receptors and cyclic nucleotides in the rhesus monkey. Am J Obstet Gynecol 139:134-140.

Spooner PM, Garrison MM, Scow RO (1977): Regulation of mammary and adipose tissue lipoprotein lipase and blood triacylglycerol in rats during late pregnancy. Effect of prostaglandins. J Clin Invest 60:702-708.

Strbak V, Macho L, Skultetyova M, Michalickova J (1978): Thyroid activity in early weaned and suckling infants and their lactating mothers. Endocrinol Exp 12:103-107.

Topper YJ (1970): Multiple hormone interactions in the development of mammary gland in vitro. Recent Prog Horm Res 26:287-302.

Tucker HA (1979): Endocrinology of lactation. Semin Perinatol 3:199-223.

Turkington RW, Hill RL (1969): Lactose synthetase: Progesterone inhibition of the induction of α-lactalbumin. Science 163:1458-1460.

Tyson JE, Hwang P, Guyda H, Friesen HG (1972): Studies of prolactin secretion in human pregnancy. Am J Obstet Gynecol 113:14–20.

Vonderhaar BK (1977): Studies on the mechanism by which thyroid hormones enhance α-lactalbumin activity in explants from mouse mammary glands. Endocrinology 100:1423–1431.

Vorherr H (1978) Human lactation and breast feeding. In Larson BL (ed): "Lactation: A Comprehensive Treatise." New York: Academic, pp 181–280.

Vorherr H (1978): Hormonal and biochemical changes of pituitary and breast during pregnancy. Semin Perinatol 3:193–198.

Vuori E, Kiuru K, Makinen SM, Vayrynen P, Kara R, Kuitunen P (1982): Maternal diet and fatty acid pattern of breast milk. Acta Paediatr Scand 71:959–963.

Walker FMM, Peaker M (1980): Local production of prostaglandins in relation to mammary function at the onset of lactation in the goat. J Physiol 309:65–79.

Weirsbitzky S, Weyrauch P-Ch (1970): Die Serumproteine des Brurstdrusensekretes bie menschichen Neugeborenen. Acta Biol Med Germ 24:911.

Weisz-Carrington P, Roux ME, McWilliams M, Phillips-Quagliata JM, Lamm ME (1978): Hormonal induction of the secretory immune system in the mammary gland. Proc Natl Acad Sci USA 75:2928–2932.

Williamson DH (1980): Integration of metabolism in tissues of the lactating rat. FEBS Lett 117: K93–K105.

Wynder EL, Hill P (1977): Prolactin, oestrogen, and lipids in breast fluid. Lancet 2:840–842.

Yue DK, Smith ID, Turtle JR, Shearman RP (1974): Effect of prostaglandin $F_{2\alpha}$ on the secretion of human prolactin. Prostaglandins 8:387–395.

Zinder O, Hamosh M, Clary Fleck TRC, Scow RO (1974): Effect of prolactin on lipoprotein lipase in mammary gland and adipose tissue of rats. Am J Physiol 226:744–748.

Malnutrition: Determinants and Consequences, pages 101–109
© 1984 Alan R. Liss, Inc., 150 Fifth Avenue, New York, NY 10011

Effects of Nutritional Status on Pregnancy and Lactation

Lindsay H. Allen, PhD, RD

Department of Nutritional Sciences, University of Connecticut, Storrs, Connecticut 06268

INTRODUCTION

There is no longer doubt that maternal nutritional status prior to and during pregnancy and lactation affects pregnancy and lactation outcome. Most of the work in this area has focused on the effects of protein-energy malnutrition (PEM) on the size of the infant at birth, and milk volume and composition. This chapter will also address the importance of considering 1) functional measures of pregnancy outcome and the effects of malnutrition on maternal nutritional status, 2) the efficiency of maternal energy utilization, and 3) the effects of mineral and vitamin deficiencies on pregnancy outcome and milk composition.

PROTEIN-ENERGY MALNUTRITION AND PREGNANCY OUTCOME

The reported energy intakes of pregnant and lactating women in the developing world are approximately 20–30% lower than those of women in industrialized societies [Whitehead, 1983]. Supplementation of undernourished pregnant women with sources of energy alone has usually been found as beneficial as supplementation with protein [Naismith, 1981], and high protein intakes may even induce premature delivery [Rush et al, 1980].

Undernutrition during the growing years of women delays menarche [Bongaarts, 1980], but there is little information about its effect on pelvic growth or the development of the female reproductive organs. Maternal growth stunting and low prepregnancy weight-for-height are both associated with a lower pregnancy weight gain and a lower infant birth weight. It has been suggested that maternal nutritional status prior to pregnancy is as important a predictor of birth weight as nutrition during pregnancy [Habicht et al, 1973].

The established and possible effects of maternal undernutrition during pregnancy are shown in Table I. Pregnancy weight gain is clearly lower in malnourished women, and dietary supplementation produces some improvement in this parameter [Chavez et al, 1981; Rush et al, 1980]. When nondietary factors [such as maternal height, weight-for-height, parity, and smoking) are controlled statistically or by subject selection criteria, maternal energy intake explains only 20% of the variance in weight gain and birth weight in the United States [Picone et al, 1982a]. It therefore appears that individual variability in the efficiency of energy utilization for weight gain may play an important role in total pregnancy gain, even in well-nourished women. Environmental factors that probably impair the efficiency of maternal energy utilization during pregnancy include cigarette smoking and psychologic stress [Picone et al, 1982b]; the extent to which the latter is important in developing countries remains to be determined. Maternal weight gain is strongly associated with birth weight, although adequate gain is more important in women with a low prepregnancy weight-for-height, and less important for overweight women [Naeye, 1979].

Placental cell size and number are both reduced in marginal malnutrition. In malnourished animals, a smaller blood volume expansion may explain the slower placental transfer of nutrients, but this has yet to be studied in malnourished women [Rosso, 1981].

The effect of undernutrition on maternal nutritional status has been insufficiently studied. If energy intake is inadequate, less maternal fat will be stored during pregnancy, and maternal fat reserves may be used to buffer the consequences of dietary inadequacy on birth weight. The consequence of depleted fat reserves is likely to be greatest during lactation, when these stores are used to support milk production if energy intake is inadequate [Paul et al, 1979; Schutz et al, 1980]. Little is known about whether undernutrition during pregnancy compromises other aspects of maternal function, such as immunocompetence, disease resistance, physical activity (activities performed and/or quality of performance), and mental well-being.

Established detrimental effects of maternal malnutrition on the condition of the neonate at birth include low birth weight and a reduced ponderal index [Miller and Hassanein, 1973]. Gestational age is slightly shorter [Delgado et al, 1982]. The Brazelton Neonatal Assessment Scale has been used to demonstrate impairment of neurobehavioral performance of the neonate in low-weight-gain pregnant women in the United States [Picone et al, 1982b] and Guatemala [Brazelton et al, 1977]. The most obvious behavioral changes are in visual habituation, auditory and visual orientation, regulation of state, motor performance, and reflexes. Visual habituation of the neonate was improved by maternal pregnancy supplementation in Colombia [Vuori et al, 1979]. An intriguing possibility is that infants with these behavioral changes are more difficult and unresponsive, and less able to interact with their environment and

TABLE I. Effects of Inadequate Maternal Nutritional Status on
Pregnancy Outcome

Maternal effects	
Established:	↓ Pregnancy weight gain
	↓ Placental weight and cell number
Possible:	↓ Blood volume expansion
	↑ Maternal morbidity
	↑ Maternal ketonuria
	↓ Physical activity
Neonatal effects	
Established:	↓ Birth weight
	↓ Head circumference
	↓ Ponderal index
	↑ Morbidity/mortality
	Retarded neurobehavioral development
Possible:	↓ Mother-infant interaction
	↓ Immunologic competence
	↓ Activity

caretakers. Thus, the potential harmful effects of suboptimal infant care-taking and inadequate milk supply should both be considered as factors in the slower growth rate and increased morbidity of infants born to low-weight-gain women.

The reasons for the increased morbidity and mortality of infants born to malnourished women have not been studied systematically. In addition to poorer environmental conditions, possible biologic explanations include maternal ketonuria during pregnancy [Naeye, 1979] and impaired transfer of immunologic factors from maternal milk [Miranda et al, 1983].

In an analysis of the effects of the Dutch famine on pregnancy outcome, maternal food intake, and weight gain in the third trimester accounted for all of the effects of famine on maternal weight, infant size, and placental weight [Stein and Susser, 1973]. However, maternal weight gain in the second trimester, when neuronal cell division is most rapid, accounted for almost all of the effects of maternal weight gain on infant neurobehavioral performance in a US study [Picone et al, 1982b]. This observation emphasizes the importance of including functional measures of pregnancy outcome, and it has obvious implications for the timing of intervention programs.

MINERAL AND VITAMIN DEFICIENCIES AND PREGNANCY OUTCOME

The US recommended dietary allowance (RDA) for energy is increased by only 15% during pregnancy, but the recommended increment of minerals and vitamins is proportionately greater than this. Deficiencies of minerals and vitamins are likely to occur if maternal food intake is inadequate.

Iron deficiency anemia is one of the most commonly encountered problems in pregnant women; the incidence has been reported to be 22% in Latin America [Cook et al, 1971] and 88% in India [Baker, 1981]. Anemia is associated with a shortened length of gestation, low birth weight, and a greater incidence of medical abnormalities [Garn et al, 1981]. In developed nations, megaloblastic anemia due to folate deficiency occurs in a significant number of pregnant women. In Wales, women who consumed poor diets during pregnancy had low serum and red blood cell folate levels, and produced infants with a higher incidence of neural tube defects. Supplements of 360 μg of folic acid daily, before and during early pregnancy, lowered the risk of recurrence of neural tube defects in later pregnancies [Smithells et al, 1981].

An interesting hypothesis has emerged concerning the role of calcium deficiency in the etiology of eclampsia. If the per capita calcium intake of a country is above approximately 800 mg/day, eclampsia occurs infrequently, regardless of the general health and nutritional status of the population [Villar et al, 1983]. Calcium supplements of 1-2 gm/day prevent the rise in blood pressure that usually occurs in late gestation in healthy women [Belizan et al, 1983]. Trials of the effectiveness of calcium supplementation in countries with a high incidence of toxemia are needed.

The zinc intake of pregnant women, even in the United States, averages only 12 mg/day, compared to the RDA of 20 mg/day. In most women, serum zinc levels fall during pregnancy. Of concern is the fact that low maternal serum zinc levels early in pregnancy may be associated with prematurity, malformations, abnormal delivery, and prolonged pregnancy [Jameson, 1976]. A supplement of 45 mg zinc per day greatly improved the chances of a normal pregnancy outcome in such women. In contrast, Hambidge et al [1983] claim that a fall in serum zinc is a normal occurrence during pregnancy and is not prevented by supplements of 15 mg/day. Of additional concern is that dietary iron-to-zinc ratios greater than 2:1 strongly inhibit zinc absorption [Solomons and Jacob, 1981]. This ratio is often exceeded in prenatal supplements, and high iron intakes were associated with low plasma zinc levels in one study of pregnant women in the United Stats [Hambidge et al, 1983]. Little is known about the importance of zinc deficiency during pregnancy in developing countries, but both intake and availability are expected to be low.

Vitamin B$_6$ is a vitamin often consumed in low amounts by pregnant women. Those with low intakes in the United States gave birth to infants with low Apgar scores, and they had low milk B$_6$ levels at 3 days postpartum. This situation was exacerbated if the woman had taken oral contraceptive agents for more than 30 months prior to pregnancy, and it could be improved by raising B$_6$ intake to 6 mg/day with supplements of the vitamin [Roepke and Kirksey, 1979].

Thus, recent work suggests that marginal deficiencies of a number of minerals and vitamins may influence pregnancy outcome even in developed countries. Further studies are needed to confirm these findings and to extend them to developing countries.

EFFECTS OF NUTRITIONAL STATUS ON LACTATION

Considering the large amounts of nutrients secreted in breast milk over the course of lactation, the volume and composition of milk appear to be remarkably conserved in malnourished lactating women. In well-nourished women, milk volume is 650–800 gm/day through the first 4 months of lactation, whereas the output of malnourished mothers is closer to 500–700 gm/day during the first 6 months, falling to 450–600 gm/day during the second 6 months and to 300–500 gm/day during the second year [Jelliffe and Jelliffe, 1978; Whitehead et al, 1983]. It has been suggested that maternal protein deficit may be more important than energy deficit in determining milk output [Hennart and Vis, 1980], but data from The Gambia show a very close correlation between energy intake and breast milk production [Prentice, 1980]. Surprisingly, attempts to increase milk output by maternal supplementation have met with limited success [Whitehead et al, 1983].

Except in cases of extreme maternal undernutrition, the concentrations of protein and lactose are unaffected in breast milk [Jelliffe and Jelliffe, 1978; Lonnerdal et al, 1976]. Fat concentration may be slightly reduced [Prentice et al, 1980]. Milk fat composition generally resembles that of the mother's diet, but if maternal fat stores are used during energy deficiency, the pattern of milk fatty acids is closer to that of her subcutaneous fat [Hambreus, 1980]. A reduced content of lysine and methionine was reported in the milk of malnourished Indian women [Lindblad and Rahimtoola, 1974], and of lysine and tryptophan in Guatemalan women consuming large quantities of maize [Wurtman and Fernstrom, 1979].

Little is known of the changes in mineral content of milk that result from maternal malnutrition. Calcium is the only nutrient occasionally reported as excreted in lower amounts, but if dietary intakes are inadequate, calcium is probably mobilized from maternal bone [Slater and Thomas, 1982].

Current maternal intake of water-soluble vitamins affects their concentration in milk more directly than does maternal vitamin status [Sneed et al, 1981]. Maternal supplementation rapidly increases the levels in milk [Deodhar et al, 1964] whereas an improvement in maternal status may take longer to occur [Bates et al, 1981; Metz, 1980; Sneed et al, 1981]. In The Gambia, seasonal fluctuations of most water-soluble vitamins occurred in milk, and riboflavin concentration was consistently low [Whitehead et al, 1983]. Fat-soluble vitamins probably show similar, but less dramatic, associations with maternal intake, but few data are available.

The reduced morbidity and mortality of breast-fed infants has commonly been attributed to reduced ingestion of pathogenic organisms in breast milk compared to home-prepared formulas. However, a considerable amount of infant immunity to disease can probably be attributed to antimicrobial substances transferred in colostrum and breast milk. Miranda et al [1983] showed recently that the secretion of these substances was reduced in the milk of malnourished Colombian women. In colostrum, malnutrition was associated with reductions in albumin, complement C3, and immunoglobulins IgA and IgG; at 2 weeks postpartum IgG and albumin were lower, and albumin and lysozyme were reduced at 4 weeks. By 8 weeks all differences had disappeared. Whether this occurs in other populations remains to be tested.

MATERNAL ADAPTATIONS TO MALNUTRITION IN PREGNANCY AND LACTATION

In theory, the magnitude of reported differences between the energy intakes of pregnant and lactating women in developing and industrialized countries would predict more devastating effects on maternal nutritional status, and on pregnancy outcome and milk production, than actually occur. There is, therefore, much interest in whether and how such women in developing countries "adapt" to the energy deficit.

If energy restriction occurs during pregnancy, less or no maternal fat is deposited, so that weight gain is lower. Gains of only 0.5 kg/month have been reported when energy intake was 1,350–1,450 kcal/day [Prentice, 1980], but gains of 1.6 kg/month (equivalent to those reported in developed countries) occurred with intakes of only 1,600–1,700 kcal/day in Gambia [Prentice, 1980]. In well-nourished women, weight loss during lactation is 0.6–1.0 kg/month [Manning-Dalton and Allen, 1983]. When low energy intakes and high energy demands for activity coincide, a similar rate of loss occurs, ie, 0.4–1.0 kg/month [Schutz et al, 1980; Prentice et al, 1980]. Gambian women actually gained weight during early lactation at the rate of 0.4 kg/month while consuming only 1,600–1,750 kcal/day [Whitehead et al, 1983]. Thus, in the above studies, and in those of others [Durnin, 1980; Rajalakshimi, 1980], the weight loss of malnourished lactating women is less than expected.

Explanations for these apparent "adaptations" to energy deficit include a reduction in maternal energy expenditure [Durnin, 1980], although data on this are practically nonexistent [Schutz et al, 1980]. In Gambia, 93% of a 720 kcal/day supplement fed to lactating women was not used for milk production or changes in weight gain. While increased physical activity seems a likely explanation of the missing calories, this was not measured. Basal metabolic rates

(BMR) of undernourished individuals in developing countries have been reported as slightly low, or normal, probably because lean body mass is relatively unaffected by malnutrition. Comparative data on BMR in pregnant and lactating ill- and well-nourished women in the same population are not available. Nonshivering and dietary-induced thermogenesis are reduced during pregnancy and particularly during lactation in mice [Trayhurn et al, 1982], but the relevance of this to the human situation is unknown.

Observed hormonal changes in undernourished pregnant women include low levels of insulin, T_3, and estradiol; in lactation levels of prolactin are higher, and then fall with energy supplementation [Delgado et al, 1983]. Such changes would be expected to alter the efficiency of maternal energy utilization, but the evidence neither for this nor for a change in maternal energy expenditure for physical activity is available. Until data to the contrary are obtained, we should assume that inadequate food intake impairs the quality of life of pregnant and lactating women.

REFERENCES

Baker SJ (1981): Nutritional anemias. Trop Asia Clin Hematol 10:843–871.

Bates C, Prentice AM, Paul AA, Sutcliffe BM, Watkinson M, Whitehead RG (1981): Riboflavin status in Gambian pregnant and lactating women and its implications for recommended dietary allowances. Am J Clin Nutr 34:928–935.

Belizan JM, Villar J, Zalazar A, Rogas L, Chan D, Bryce GF (1983): Preliminary evidence on the effect of calcium supplementation on blood pressure in normal pregnant women. Am J Obstet Gynecol 146:175–180.

Bongaarts J (1980): Does malnutrition affect fecundity? Science 208:564–569.

Brazelton TB, Tronick E, Lechtig A, Lasky RE, Klein R (1977): The behavior of nutritionally deprived Guatemalan infants. Dev Med Child Neurol 19:364–372.

Chavez A, Martinez C, Schlaepfer L (1981): Health effects of supplementary feeding programs. In Selvey N, White PL (eds): "Nutrition in the 1980's. Constraints on our Knowledge." New York: Alan R Liss, pp 129–139.

Cook JD, Alvarado J, Burnisky A, Jamra M, Labardini J, Layrisse M, Linares J, Loria A, Maspes V, Restrepo A, Reynafarje C, Sanchez-Medal L, Velez H, Viteri F (1971): Nutritional deficiency in Latin America: A collaborative study. Blood 38:591–603.

Delgado H, Martorell R, Brineman E, Klein RE (1982): Nutrition and length of gestation. Nutr Res 2:117–126.

Delgado H, McNeilly AS, Hartmann PE (1983): Non-nutritional factors affecting milk production. In Whitehead RG (ed): "Maternal Diet, Breast-Feeding Capacity, and Lactational Infertility." Tokyo: United Nations University, pp 54–62.

Deodhar AD, Rajalakshimi R, Ramakrinshnan CV (1964): Effects of vitamin supplementation on vitamin contents of breast milk. Acta Paediatr 53:42–47.

Durnin JVGA (1980): Food consumption and energy balance during pregnancy and lactation in New Guinea. In Aebi H, Whitehead RG (eds): "Maternal Nutrition During Pregnancy and Lactation." Berne: Hans Huber, pp 86–95.

Garn SM, Keating MT, Falkner F (1981): Hematological status and pregnancy outcomes. Am J Clin Nutr 34:115–117.

Habicht J-P, Yarbrough C, Lechtig A, Klein RE (1973): Relationships of birthweight, maternal nutrition and infant mortality. Nutr Rep Int 7:533–546.

Hambidge KM, Krebs NF, Jacobs MA, Favier A, Guyette MS, Ikle DN (1983): Zinc nutritional status during pregnancy: A longitudinal study. Am J Clin Nutr 37:429–442.

Hambreus L (1980): Maternal diet and milk composition. In Aebi H, Whitehead RG (eds): "Maternal Nutrition During Pregnancy and Lactation." Berne: Hans Huber, pp 233–244.

Hennart P, Vis HL (1980): Breast feeding and post partum amenorrhea in central Africa. I. Milk production in rural areas. J Trop Paediatr 26:177–183.

Jameson S (1976): Effects of zinc deficiency in human reproduction. Acta Med Scand 593 (Suppl):5–23.

Jelliffe DB, Jelliffe EFP (1978): The volume and composition of human milk in poorly nourished communities. A review. Am J Clin Nutr 31:492–515.

Linblad BS, Rahimtoola RJ (1974): A pilot study of the quality of human milk in a lower socioeconomic group in Karachi, Pakistan. Acta Pediatr Scand 63:125–128.

Lonnerdal B, Forsum E, Gebre-Medhin M, Hambreus L (1976): Breast milk composition in Ethiopian and Swedish mothers. II. Lactose, nitrogen and protein content. Am J Clin Nutr 29:1134–1141.

Manning-Dalton C, Allen LH (1983): The effects of lactation on energy and protein consumption, postpartum weight change and body composition of well-nourished North American Women. Nutr Res 3:293–308.

Metz J (1980): Folate deficiency conditioned by lactation. Am J Clin Nutr 23:843–847.

Miller HL, Hassanein K (1973): Fetal malnutrition in white newborn infants: maternal factors. Pediatrics 52:502–512.

Miranda R et al (1983): Effect of maternal nutritional status on immunological substances in human colostrum and milk. Am J Clin Nutr 37:632–640.

Naeye RL (1979): Weight gain and the outcome of pregnancy. Am J Obstet Gynecol 135:3–9.

Naismith DJ (1981): Diet during pregnancy — a rationale for prescription. In Dobbing J (ed): "Maternal Nutrition During Pregnancy — Eating For Two?" London: Academic, pp 21–40.

Paul AA, Muller EM, Whitehead RG (1979): The quantitative effects of maternal dietary energy intake on pregnancy and lactation in rural Gambian women. Trans R Soc Trop Med Hyg 73:686–692.

Picone TA, Allen LH, Schramm MM, Olsen PN (1982a): Pregnancy outcome in North American women. I. Effects of diet, cigarette smoking, and psychological stress on maternal weight gain. Am J Clin Nutr 36:1205–1213.

Picone TA, Allen LH, Olsen PN, Ferris ME (1982b): Pregnancy outcome in North American women. II. Effects of diet, cigarette smoking, stress and weight gain on neonatal physical and behavioral characteristics. Am J Clin Nutr 36:1214–1224.

Prentice AM (1980): Variations in maternal dietary energy intake, birthweight and breast-milk output in The Gambia. In Aebi H, Whitehead RG (eds): "Maternal Nutrition During Pregnancy and Lactation." Berne: Hans Huber, pp 167–183.

Prentice AM, Whitehead RG, Roberts SB, Paul AA, Watkinson M, Prentice A, Watkinson AA (1980): Dietary supplementation of Gambian nursing mothers and lactational performance. Lancet 2:886–888.

Rajalakshimi R (1980): Gestation and lactation performance in relation to the plane of maternal nutrition. In Aebi H, Whitehead RG (eds): "Maternal Nutrition During Pregnancy and Lactation." Berne: Hans Huber, pp 184–202.

Roepke JLB, Kirksey A (1979): Vitamin B_6 nutriture during pregnancy and lactation. I. Vitamin B_6 intake, levels of the vitamin in biological fluids, and the condition of the infant at birth. Am J Clin Nutr 32:2249–2256.

Rosso P (1981): Nutrition and maternal-fetal exchange. Am J Clin Nutr 34(Suppl 4):744–755.

Rush D, Stein Z, Susser M (1980): A randomized controlled trial of prenatal nutritional supplementation in New York City. Pediatrics 65:683–697.

Schutz Y, Lechtig A, Bradfield RB (1980): Energy expenditures and food intakes of lactating women in Guatemala. Am J Clin Nutr 33:892–902.

Slater P, Thomas MR (1982): Calcium and phosphorus status of lactating adolescents and their infants. Fed Proc 41:472.

Smithells RW, Sheppard S, Schorah CJ, Seller MJ, Nevin NC, Harris R, Read AP, Fielding DW (1981): Apparent prevention of neural tube defects by periconceptional vitamin supplementation. Arch Dis Child 56:911–918.

Sneed S, Zane C, Thomas MR (1981): The effects of ascorbic acid, vitamin B_6, vitamin B_{12}, and folic acid supplementation on the breast milk and maternal nutritional status of low socioeconomic lactating women. Am J Clin Nutr 34:1338–1346.

Solomons NW, Jacob RA (1981): Studies on the bioavailability of zinc in humans: Effects of heme and nonheme iron on the absorption of zinc. Am J Clin Nutr 34:475–482.

Stein Z, Susser M (1975): The Dutch famine, 1944–1945, and the reproductive process. I. Effects on six indices at birth. Pediatr Res 9:70–76.

Trayhurn P, Douglas JB, McGuckin MM (1982): Brown adipose tissue thermogenesis is "suppressed" during lactation in mice. Nature 298:59–60.

Villar J, Belizan JM, Fischer PJ (1983): Epidemiologic observations on the relationship between calcium intake and eclampsia. Int J Gynaecol Obstet (in press).

Vuori L, Christiansen N, Clement J, Mora JO, Wagner M, Herrera MG (1979): Nutritional supplementation and the outcome of pregnancy II. Visual habituation at 15 days. Am J Clin Nutr 32:463–469.

Whitehead RG (1983): Measured dietary intakes of lactating women in different countries of the world. In Whitehead RG (ed): "Maternal Diet, Breast-Feeding Capacity, and Lactational Infertility." Tokyo: United Nations University, pp 12–23.

Whitehead RG, Vis HL, Hartmann PE (1983): Effect of diet on maternal health and lactational performance. In Whitehead RG (ed): "Maternal Diet, Breast-Feeding Capacity, and Lactational Infertility." Tokyo: United Nations University, pp 24–53.

Wurtman JJ, Fernstrom JD (1979): Free amino acid, protein and fat contents of breast milk from Guatemalan mothers consuming a corn-based diet. Early Hum Dev 3:67–77.

Malnutrition: Determinants and Consequences, pages 111–122
© 1984 Alan R. Liss, Inc., 150 Fifth Avenue, New York, NY 10011

The Composition of Human Milk

Mary Frances Picciano, PhD
Department of Foods and Nutrition, Division of Nutritional Sciences, College of Agriculture, University of Illinois, Urbana, Illinois 61801

INTRODUCTION

The human infant is exceedingly vulnerable to nutritional insult owing to its developmental immaturity and rapid rate of growth. Any alteration in the supply of nutrients during this critical period of the life cycle has profound immediate and possible long-term consequences. Requirements for normal growth in infancy have not been established to any degree of certainty. In fact, several researchers have challenged current international dietary recommendations for energy and protein, urging a reassessment [Butte et al, 1983; Whitehead et al, 1982]. Their position is based on recent data of typical patterns of intake of exclusively breast-fed infants exhibiting normal growth. Thus, the composition of human milk represents our key to understanding infant nutritional requirements and to the formulation of appropriate substitutes when human milk is not provided.

Several comprehensive reviews have recently been published on the nutritional [Gaull et al, 1982; Nichols and Nichols, 1981] and immunologic [Hanson and Söderström, 1981; Ogra and Dayton, 1980] characteristics of human milk. This review highlights and supplements previous accounts and is intended to focus on important recent advances in our knowledge of human milk constituents and their significance in infant nutrition.

The study of human milk composition is fraught with difficulty. Human milk exhibits wide biologic variance even when collected under controlled, defined conditions and subjected to modern, reliable, and ultrasensitive techniques of analyses. The greatest source of variance in the measurement of a constituent in human milk is among women. Yet, variations are large even within the same woman [Picciano, 1981]. Ultimately, it is the quantity of a particular nutrient provided via human milk as related to growth and metabolic response of the nursing infant that is of interest. The quantity of human milk provided under normal conditions is also highly variable. It is exceedingly important to establish normal ranges for human milk constituents and intakes of thriving nursing infants. Deviations from these norms have all too recently been related to significant morbidity in both the formula-fed [Holliday, 1980] and the breast-fed infant [Ernst et al, 1981].

ENERGY-YIELDING CONSTITUENTS

The protein content of human milk as traditionally measured was overestimated by approximately 20%. Conventional methods of protein measurement consist of determining total nitrogen and assuming that it is primarily of protein origin and represents approximately 16% of protein structure. When these assumptions hold true, grams of total nitrogen multiplied by the factor 6.25 (100/16) yield a reasonable estimate of protein content. However, human milk contains 15–25% nonprotein nitrogen, a significant portion of which remains unidentified. Determination of the true protein concentration from amino acid analysis has indicated that mature human milk contained 0.8–0.9 gm/100 ml [Lönnerdal et al, 1976]. Current World Health Organization/Food and Agriculture Organization [1973] recommendations for protein intakes during infancy are not based on this new information and accordingly are inflated.

Protein and/or energy malnutrition during lactation has long been known to cause a suppression of milk output. Jelliffe and Jelliffe [1978] indicated that milk production may be reduced by as much as 40% under severe conditions. However, the concentration of energy-yielding nutrients in milk was believed to be little influenced by their relative amounts in the maternal diet. Results of a number of modern studies employing highly sensitive and specific techniques have provided evidence to the contrary. Miranda et al [1983] observed a two-thirds reduction in protein content of colostrum from malnourished Colombian mothers and a concomitant diminution of the immunologic milk factors: C4 complement and immunoglobulins A and G. In well-nourished Swedish women, a positive effect of dietary protein level (20% vs 8% energy from protein) on total nitrogen, true protein, and nonprotein nitrogen contents of mature human milk as well as 24-hour milk output was demonstrated [Forsum and Lönnerdal, 1980]. There have also been reports of very low concentrations of protein and altered free and total amino acid nitrogen profiles in milk of women in India [Deb and Cama, 1962], Pakistan [Lindblad and Rahimtoola, 1974], and Guatemala [Wurtman and Fernstrom, 1979]. These alterations in the nitrogen fraction of human milk may have nutritional and immunologic significance to the nursing infant. Among infants colonized with *Vibrio cho-*

lerae, those who developed the disease had consumed human milk containing significantly lower levels of IgA antibodies to cholera than were present in milk consumed by infants without symptoms [Glass et al, 1983]. However, when dietary amino acid nitrogen is low, other forms of nitrogen may assume importance. Human milk contains a broad spectrum of nucleotides [Janas and Picciano, 1982] and their supplementation to low-protein diets of weanling rats markedly improved growth rate [György, 1971]. A mitogen that stimulated DNA synthesis and induced division of cells grown in culture has also been identified in colostrum, transitional, and mature human milk [Tapper et al, 1979].

Lipids compose the major energy-yielding fraction of human milk and are 97–98% triglycerides. They are by far the most variable constituents in human milk (2–10%) and it is exceedingly difficult to obtain representative samples for analysis without interfering with the lactation process. The characteristic features of human milk lipids are reviewed elsewhere [Jensen et al, 1980]. Briefly, maternal diet has a profound influence on the composition of human milk lipids; the impact on total lipid production is less certain. Within limits, maternal intakes of fatty acids and phytosterol are reflected in the composition of human milk and, in turn, the plasma of nursing infants [Mellies et al, 1978, 1979a,b]. In contrast, human milk cholesterol content bears no relationship to the maternal diet but a 16-fold elevation is noted in milk of women with familial hypercholesterolemia.

Milk triglyceride digestion in the nursing neonate is achieved by a triad of enzymes, one of which is present in human milk [Jensen et al, 1982]. The first is lingual lipase, which initiates hydrolysis in the stomach; the second is bile-salt-stimulated lipase (BSSL), which is indigenous to human milk and works in concert with the third enzyme, pancreatic lipase in the duodenum. Human milk also contains serum-stimulated lipoprotein lipase, a bile-salt-stimulated esterase activity, possibly the same as BSSL; and perhaps, a nonactivated or spontaneous lipolytic activity associated with neonatal jaundice. These latter enzymes are not quantitatively important in fat digestion but have been implicated in several aspects of lipid metabolism in the nursing neonate.

The disaccharide lactose, which averages 7.0 gm/100 ml, is second only to water as a major constituent of human milk. Among species, concentrations of lactose and α-lactalbumin are positively correlated, as the synthesis of this sugar is achieved by coupled reaction of galactosyltransferase with α-lactalbumin. Human milk lactose concentrations are remarkably similar among women; however, recent reports suggest that in face of severe maternal malnutrition, its synthesis is depressed [Edozien et al, 1976; Shinwell and Gorodescher, 1982]. A stimulating effect of lactose on net absorption of calcium, magnesium, and manganese has recently been demonstrated in infants [Ziegler and Fomon, 1983]. Minor quantities of other carbohydrates and their complexes have been identified in human milk. The nitrogen-containing sugars and oligosaccharides have received the most attention because of their growth-promoting properties on several species of bifid flora in the intestine of infants. *Bifidobacterium bifidum* is the principal species in the intestinal flora of breast-fed infants (72%) and the growth-promoting factor(s) is/are absent in cow, sheep, pig, and horse milks as well as infant formula [Beerens et al, 1980]. The predominance of *B. bifidum* is believed responsible for the observed suppression of *Escherichia coli*, *Bacteroides*, and *Clostridium* in the intestine of breast-fed infants, rendering them resistant to gastroenteritis.

A usual constituent of human milk is α-amylase and substantial activity (1,000–5,000 units/liter) is evident even after 6 months of lactation [Jones et al, 1982]. Human milk α-amylase may be of benefit to the nursing infant consuming complex carbohydrates, since pancreatic amylase, while synthesized, is not released into the duodenum until 4–6 months of age.

VITAMINS

The vitamin content of human milk is affected by a number of factors, the nutritional status of the mother being the most important. In general, when maternal vitamin intakes are low, human milk levels are low and respond to supplementation; when they are high, milk vitamin levels approach a plateau and are less responsive to supplementation.

Fat-Soluble Vitamins

The vitamin A in human milk, principally retinyl esters, decreases with advancing lactation from 2,000 to 300–600 μg/liter and is little influenced by maternal intake unless massive quantities are ingested and then the effect is only transient [Tarjan, 1965]. Concentrations of plasma vitamin A and retinol-binding proteins are elevated in early lactation and parallel the decline in milk vitamin A content [Cumming and Briggs, 1983].

The quantity of vitamin D and its metabolites in human milk corresponds to 26 IU/liter [Hollis et al, 1982]. These sterols are present in the nonlipid fraction of milk at 1.5–6% of their concentration in maternal plasma and are secreted attached to plasma and/or cytosol vitamin D binding proteins. Increasing the maternal intake of vitamin D does not appear to appreciably increase the level in milk. However, supraphysiologic daily doses of 40,000 IU for 10 days to seven lactating women increased milk content from nondetectable levels to 120–440 IU/liter [Polskin et al, 1945]. The fact that breast-fed infants on occasion develop rickets — particularly those nursed by mothers, such as strict vegetarians and commune residents, who restrict their intake of vitamin D-rich foods — suggests that maternal plasma levels of this vitamin can fall to critically low levels and limit its transfer to milk. The Committee on Nutrition/

American Academy of Pediatrics [1978] recommends vitamin D supplementation (400 IU) for the breast-fed infant. Results of recent clinical studies are equivocal concerning whether human milk feeding provides sufficient vitamin D for infant bone mineralization [Greer et al, 1982a; Roberts et al, 1981].

Analysis of human milk for vitamin K indicates a concentration of 15 μg/liter, which apparently does not increase with maternal supplementation even when maternal intake is low [Deodhar et al, 1964]. This quantity of vitamin K is insufficient to prevent neonatal hemorrhagic disease and a supplement is indicated for newborn breast-fed infants to achieve normal prothrombin time [O'Connor et al, 1983].

Approximately 83% of the total vitamin E in human milk is α-tocopherol; β-, γ-, and δ-tocopherols are also present in small quantities [Kobayashi et al, 1975]. Concentrations of tocopherols that are high in colostrum (8 mg/liter) decline and stabilize in mature human milk (2–3 mg/liter). High dietary intake of sunflower seed oil rich in vitamin E is reported to cause an increase in vitamin E content of mature milk by 30% [Kramer et al, 1965].

Water-Soluble Vitamins

Mean vitamin C content of mature human milk is 5–6 mg/100 ml and daily intakes of 100 mg are needed to achieve this plateau in milk concentration. There is a corresponding drop of vitamin C levels in milk with maternal intakes less than this amount. It is interesting that milk level is 8–10 times the level in maternal plasma [Bates et al, 1983].

Thiamin concentration is low in colostrum (20 μg/liter) and increases 7–10-fold in mature milk. In contrast, riboflavin content, which is largely a reflection of the maternal diet, is high in early milk and declines to 310 μg/liter as lactation proceeds. After the initial rise in niacin concentration from colostrum (0.75 mg/liter) to mature human milk (2 mg/liter), actual levels are largely dependent on maternal intake and may be as high as 6 mg/liter [Pratt, 1951].

Vitamin B_6 content is low in colostrum and varies between 50 and 250 μg/liter in mature milk. Levels of vitamin B_6 in mature milk are 10 times higher than in maternal serum, are directly related to maternal intake, and are drastically reduced in mothers with a history of oral contraceptive use greater than 30 months prior to conception [Roepke and Kirksey, 1981]. In order to increase milk vitamin B_6 content of previous oral contraceptive users and reverse neurologic symptoms of deficiency in their infants, supplements of 20 mg/day were required, eight times the recommended amount for lactating women [Roepke and Kirksey, 1981].

Vitamin B_{12} and folate in milk are secreted bound to whey proteins, which are usually present in excess. Heat processing drastically reduces milk excess binding capacities for these vitamins. It has been demonstrated in vitro that milk and isolated binding proteins for vitamin B_{12} and folate will inhibit the growth of organisms requiring these vitamins until they become saturated. A similar role in vivo has been proposed but unconfirmed [Cole et al, 1983].

The accepted normal range for the vitamin B_{12} concentration of mature human milk is 0.1–1.5 μg/liter. Average content in the milk of women receiving a vitamin B_{12} containing supplement was 1.0 μg/liter compared to 0.6 μg/liter for those unsupplemented [Thomas et al, 1980]. There are a number of recent reports of vitamin B_{12} deficiency in infants nursed by mothers who were strict vegetarians or generally malnourished or who had latent pernicious anemia secondary to hypothyroidism [Johnson and Roloff, 1982]. Milk concentrations of vitamin B_{12} that deficient infants received were between 0.05 and 0.075 μg/liter.

Improved methods of analysis have shown that folacin content of human milk is much higher than previously reported. Average values for mature human milk of well-nourished Japanese and American women are between 50 and 100 μg/liter [Tamura et al, 1980; Smith et al, 1983]. The folacin in human milk bears no relation to maternal serum concentration and increases with the progression of lactation even as maternal serum and red cell levels decrease. Considerable portions of milk folacin consist of methyl derivatives with at least four glutamic acid residues [Brown and Picciano, 1984].

MINERALS

Unlike their organic counterparts, the concentrations of inorganic constituents in human milk do not correlate well with the amounts in the maternal diet nor maternal serum. Recent studies have emphasized the high bioavailability of human milk minerals as well as their interrelationships with other nutrients that impact on their absorption, metabolism, and excretion.

Major Minerals

Milk concentrations of calcium, phosphorus, and magnesium do not correspond to their respective values in maternal serum; however Greer and associates [1982b] noted a weak but significant positive correlation between maternal intake of calcium and milk concentration. In this longitudinal investigation, a significant decline was observed in human milk phosphorus from 147 mg/liter at 3 weeks of lactation to 107 mg/liter at 26 weeks. Corresponding values for human milk calcium and magnesium contents at those times were 259–248 and 290–330 mg/liter, respectively. Infant serum phosphorus concentrations were correlated with milk levels and showed a similar decline as lactation progressed. At the same time, infant serum calcium and magnesium concentrations increased. It has been speculated that increased serum calcium and magnesium values, possibly secondary to decreased milk phosphorus content, are important in remodeling of bone in infancy.

An electrical potential gradient in the secretory cell determines the electrolyte concentrations in milk. The synthesis of lactose in the Golgi apparatus osmotically draws water, and the passage of water establishes the potential difference necessary to maintain the low milk electrolyte concentrations. Average amounts of sodium, potassium, and chloride in mature human milk of 7, 15, and 12 mEq/liter are approximately 66, 31, and 36% of their respective levels in colostrum [Macy, 1949]. A number of recent reports have indicated 5- to 40-fold increases in the content of sodium and occasionally chloride in human milk that are associated with maternal emotional stress, cystic fibrosis, mastitis, and diminished milk production, as well as dehydration and malnutrition of infants. Naylor [1982] provides evidence that lack of or inadequate suckling is responsible. Under such circumstances, maternal prolactin production is impaired, which causes a reduction in lactose production and an elevation in the sodium concentration of milk. Moreover, adequate suckling reversed this process. There is a recent case report of chloride deficiency in an infant nursed by a mother whose milk chloride was approximately one-sixth the normal value [Asnes et al, 1982]. Levels of other electrolytes were well within the normal range and the mother had successfully nursed five previous children.

Trace Minerals

Neonates are in negative balance for copper, iron, and zinc even though human milk contents are highest immediately following parturition [Cavell and Widdowson, 1964]. Levels of copper and iron decline rapidly and apparently stabilize in mature mammary secretions at 0.3 mg/liter for both elements, whereas zinc levels continue to decline. Colostrum contains an average of 4 mg/liter of zinc; at 6 months, the values are 1.1 mg/liter and at 1 year, 0.5 mg/liter [Kirksey et al, 1979]. There is no evidence that maternal diet has an influence on milk concentrations of these elements [Vuori et al, 1980; Moser and Reynolds, 1983]. Serum level of copper in nursing infants is more related to concentration of ceruloplasmin, which is low at birth, than to milk content. The serum iron concentration of human milk-fed infants likewise parallels transferrin synthesis, whereas zinc concentration is comparable to that of adults and does not exhibit a development pattern. Liver stores accumulated primarily during the last trimester of pregnancy exert a strong influence on infant copper, iron, and zinc status [Widdowson et al, 1974].

Superior bioavailability of human milk iron and zinc has been clearly demonstrated; however, bioavailability of copper is unknown. The mechanism of iron absorption from human milk and the factors responsible are not completely understood. Under similar conditions, iron from human milk is absorbed five times as efficiently as a similar amount from cow milk [Saarinen et al, 1977]. Consumption of strained pears with human milk reduces the absorption rate of iron by 75% [Oski and Landaw, 1980]. The majority of the iron in human milk is associated with the lipid fraction [Fransson and Lönnerdal,

1980]. It has been proposed that lactoferrin, an iron-binding protein of bacteriostatic significance, accounts for the high bioavailability. However, heat treatment that destroys lactoferrin does not alter the iron absorption rate [McMillan et al, 1977]. Inosine and its metabolites have been shown to enhance iron absorption in rats. Human milk content of inosine as its nucleotide increases two-fold from 2 weeks to 3 months of lactation, the time when infant stores of iron are at or near depletion [Janas and Picciano, 1982]. The rise in plasma zinc concentration is used as an index of zinc absorption. Consumption of 25 mg of zinc with human milk resulted in a significantly higher plasma response than with cow milk [Casey et al, 1981]. Both citric acid [Fransson and Lönnerdal, 1982] and picolinic acid [Evans and Johnson, 1980] contents of human milk have been suggested as responsible agents, but plasma response was unaltered by their addition to cow milk. Both zinc and copper in human milk are associated with proteins and low-molecular-weight constituents [Lönnerdal et al, 1982].

Improved methods of analysis now allow the quantification of manganese and selenium in human milk and in minute biologic samples available from pediatric subjects. Application of these techniques has permitted investigations into the significance of these trace minerals in infant nutrition. Recent reports indicate that manganese concentration in human milk is lower than that in cow milk (3–8 μg/liter and 25 μg/liter, respectively). Manganese level declines in mature milk from 6 μg/liter at 1 month of lactation to 3 μg/liter at 3 and 6 months. Unlike copper, iron, and zinc contents, human milk manganese levels may be influenced by maternal diet [Vuori et al, 1980]. Infant serum concentration of manganese is linearly correlated (r = 0.64) with human milk content [Stastny et al, 1984]. Since the human fetal liver does not accumulate manganese, there is concern whether the infant obtains adequate quantities to meet its growing needs, especially since the neonate is in negative balance and the absorption rate is reportedly poor for this mineral [Widdowson et al, 1972]. Chan and associates [1982] have reported differences between human milk and infant formula in number and type of ligands binding manganese, which may affect bioavailability. Human milk selenium concentrations are high at the initiation of lactation (41 μg/liter), which levels are associated with the protein fraction. Mean values in mature milk display a geographic distribution (7–33 μg/liter), suggesting that maternal diet may exert an influence [Smith et al, 1982]. Breast-fed infants maintain higher serum selenium concentrations than formula-fed cohorts, a fact that can be partially attributed to the high concentration of selenium in human milk. The molecular form of selenium in human milk and bioavailability relative to other milks used in infant nutrition are not known.

CONCLUSIONS

Enormous strides have been made in the development of accurate and reliable techniques of analysis and in their application to studies of factors involved in either the quality or quantity of milk secreted by women. There is an acute need for expansion of modern investigations and repetition of many early investigations. Recent investigations have provided evidence not only that human milk possesses many unique characteristics but that maternal and environmental influences are stronger than previously recognized and appreciated. The fact that more complete data are available for the composition of cow milk indicates that research has not kept pace with available technology. For example, there is no published information on the content of molybdenum, an essential component of several enzymes, in human milk. A complete body of knowledge does not exist to serve as a basis for dietary recommendations to insure optimal nutrition for the nursing dyad. The success of lactation is measured in terms of infant performance, and too often the cost and consequence to the woman are ignored. When breast feeding is contraindicated for whatever reason, modern and reliable data on human milk constituents and their significance to the infant are also essential in the preparation of formulas, especially those not based on cow milk. The adequacy of such preparations cannot always be predicted from compositional analysis alone and must be evaluated with specific nutritional indices as well as traditional anthropometric measures.

REFERENCES

Asnes RS, Wisotsky DH, Migel PF, Seigle RL, Levy J (1982): The dietary chloride deficiency occurring in a breast-fed infant. J Pediatr 100:923–924.

Bates CJ, Prentice AM, Prentice A, Lamb WH, Whitehead RG (1983): The effect of vitamin C supplementation on lactating women in Keneba, a West African rural community. Int J Vitam Nutr Res 53:68–76.

Beerens H, Romond C, Neut C (1980): Influence of breast-feeding on the bifid flora of the newborn intestine. Am J Clin Nutr 33:2434–2439.

Brown CM, Picciano MF (1984): Characterization of the folate content of human milk (submitted for publication).

Butte NF, Garza C, O'Brian Smith E, Nichols BL (1983): Protein/energy intake and growth of 45 exclusively breast-fed infants. Am J Clin Nutr 37:697.

Casey CE, Walravens PA, Hambidge MK (1981): Availability of zinc: Loading tests with human milk, cow's milk and infant formulas. Pediatrics 68:394–396.

Cavell PA, Widdowson EM (1964): Intakes and excretions of iron, copper and zinc in the neonatal period. Arch Dis Child 39:496–501.

Chan W-Y, Bates JM, Rennert OM (1982): Comparative studies of manganese binding in human breast milk, bovine milk and infant formula. J Nutr 112:642–651.

Cole CB, Scott KJ, Henschel MJ, Coates ME, Ford JE, Fuller R (1983): Trace-nutrient-binding proteins in milk and the growth of bacteria in the gut of infant rabbits. Br J Nutr 49:231-240.

Committee on Nutrition/American Academy of Pediatrics (1978): Breast-feeding. Pediatrics 62:591-601.

Cumming FJ, Briggs MH (1983): Changes in plasma vitamin A in lactating and non-lactating oral contraceptive users. Br J Obstet Gynecol 90:73-77.

Deb AK, Cama HR (1962): Studies on human lactation. Dietary nitrogen utilization during lactation and distribution of nitrogen in mother's milk. Br J Nutr 16:65-73.

Deodhar AD, Rajakakshmi R, Romakrishnan CV (1964): Studies on human lactation. III. Effect of dietary vitamin supplementation on vitamin content of breast milk. Acta Paediatr Scand 53:42-48.

Edozien JC, Rahim Khan MA, Waslien CI (1976): Human protein deficiency: Results of a Nigerian village study. J Nutr 106:312-328.

Ernst JA, Wynn RJ, Schreiner RL (1981): Starvation with hypernatremic dehydration in two breast-fed infants. J Am Diet Assoc 79:126-130.

Evans GW, Johnson PE (1980): Characterization and quantification of a zinc binding ligand in human milk. Pediatr Res 14:876-880.

Forsum E, Lönnerdal B (1980): Effect of protein intake on protein and nitrogen composition of breast milk. Am J Clin Nutr 33:1809-1813.

Fransson GB, Lönnerdal B (1980): Iron in human milk. J Pediatr 96:380-384.

Fransson GB, Lönnerdal B (1982): Zinc, copper, calcium and magnesium in human milk. J Pediatr 101:504-508.

Gaull GE, Jensen RG, Rassen DK, Malloy MH (1982): Human milk as food. Adv Perinat Med 2:47-120.

Glass RI, Svennerholm A-M, Stoll BJ, Khan MR, Hossain KMB, Huq MI, Holmgren J (1983): Protection against cholera in breast-fed children by antibodies in breast milk. N Engl J Med 308:1389-1392.

Greer FR, Searcy JE, Levin RS, Steechen JJ, Steichen-Asche PS, Tsang RC (1982a): Bone mineral content and serum 25-hydroxy vitamin D concentrations in breast-fed infants with and without supplemental vitamin D: One year follow-up. J Pediatr 100:919-922.

Greer FR, Tsang RC, Levin RS, Searcy JE, Wu R, Steichen JJ (1982b): Increasing serum calcium and magnesium concentrations in breast-fed infants: Longitudinal studies of minerals in human milk and in sera of nursing mothers and their infants. J Pediatr 100:59-64.

Hanson LO, Söderström T (1981): Human milk: Defense against infection. In Tsang RC, Nichols BL (eds): "Nutrition and Child Health, Perspectives for the 1980s." New York: Alan R Liss, pp 147-160.

Holliday ZMA (1980): Alkalosis in infancy and commercial formulas. Pediatrics 65:639-642.

Hollis BW, Ross BA, Lambert PW (1982): Vitamin D compounds in human and bovine milk. Adv Nutr Res 4:59-75.

Janas LM, Picciano MF (1982): The nucleotide profile of human milk. Pediatr Res 16:659-662.

Gyorgy P (1971): Biochemical aspects of human milk. Am J Clin Nutr 24:970-975.

Jelliffee DB, Jelliffee EEP (1978): The volume and composition of human milk in poorly nourished communities. Am J Clin Nutr 31:492-515.

Jensen RG, Clark RM, Ferris AM (1980): Composition of the lipids in human milk: A review. Lipids 15:345-355.

Jensen RG, Clark RM, deLong FA, Hamosh M, Liao TH, Mehta WR (1982): The lipolytic triad: Human lingual, breast milk and pancreatic lipases: Physiological implications of their characteristics in digestion of dietary fats. J Pediatr Gastro Nutr 1:243-255.

Jones JB, Mehta WR, Hamosh M (1982): Alpha amylase in preterm human milk. J Pediatr Gastro Nutr 1:43-48.

Kirksey A, Ernst JA, Roepke JL, Tsia TI (1979): Influence of mineral intake and use of oral contraceptives before pregnancy on the mineral content of human colostrum and of more mature milk. Am J Clin Nutr 32:30-39.

Kobayashi H, Kanno C, Yamawuchi K, Tsugo T (1975): Identification of alpha-, beta-, gamma- and delta-tocopherols and their contents in human milk. Biochim Biophys Acta 380: 282-290.

Kramer M, Szoke K, Lindner K, Tarjon R (1965): The effect of different factors on the composition of human milk and its variations. III. Effect of dietary fats on the lipid composition of human milk. Nutr Dieta 7:71-79.

Lindblad BS, Rahimtoola RJ (1974): A pilot study of the quality of human milk in a lower socioeconomic group in Karachi, Pakistan. Acta Paediatr Scand 63:125-128.

Lönnerdal B, Forsum E, Hambraes L (1976): Protein content of human milk. 1. A transversal study of Swedish normal material. Nutr Rep Int 13:125-134.

Lönnerdal B, Hoffman BS, Hurley LS (1982): Zinc and copper binding proteins in human milk. Am J Clin Nutr 36:1170-1176.

Macy IG (1949): Composition of human colostrum and milk. Am J Dis Child 78:589-603.

McMillan JA, Oski FA, Lourie G, Tomarelli RM, Landaw SA (1977): Iron absorption from human milk, simulated human milk and proprietary formula. Pediatrics 60:896-900.

Mellies MJ, Ishikawa TT, Gartside P, Burton K, MacGee J, Allen K, Steiner PM, Brady D, Glueck CJ (1978): Effect of varying maternal dietary cholesterol and phytosterol in lactating women and their infants. Am J Clin Nutr 31:1347-1354.

Mellies MJ, Burton K, Laisen R, Fixler D, Glueck CJ (1979a): Cholesterol, phytosterols, and polyunsaturated/saturated fatty acid ratios during the first 12 months of lactation. Am J Clin Nutr 32:2383-2389.

Mellies MJ, Ishikawa TT, Gartside P, Burton K, MacGee J, Allen K, Steiner PM, Brady D, Glueck CJ (1979b): Effects of varying maternal dietary fatty acids in lactating women and their infants. Am J Clin Nutr 32:299-303.

Miranda R, Saravia NG, Ackerman R, Murphy N, Berman S, McMurray DN (1983): Effect of maternal nutritional status on immunological substances in human colostrum and milk. Am J Clin Nutr 37:632-640.

Moser PB, Reynolds RD (1983): Dietary zinc intake and zinc concentrations of plasma, erythrocytes, and breast milk in antepartum and postpartum lactating and nonlactating women: A longitudinal study. Am J Clin Nutr 38:101-108.

Naylor AJ (1982): Elevated sodium concentration in human milk: Its clinical significance. In "Human Milk Banking." Paris: International Institute of Refrigeration, pp 79-84.

Nichols BL, Nichols VN (1981): Human milk: Nutritional resource. In Tsang RC, Nichols BL (eds): "Nutrition and Child Health, Perspectives for the 1980s." New York: Alan R Liss, pp 109-146.

O'Connor ME, Livingstone SD, Hannah J, Wilkins D (1983): Vitamin K deficiency and breast-feeding. Am J Dis Child 137:601-602.

Ogra PL, Dayton DH (1980): "Immunology of Breast Milk." New York: Raven Press.

Oski FA, Landaw SA (1980): Inhibition of iron absorption from human milk by baby food. Am J Dis Child 134:459-460.

Picciano MF (1981): The volume and composition of human milk. In Bond JT, Filer LJ, Leveille GA, Thomson A, Weil WB (eds): "Infant and Child Feeding." New York: Academic, pp 47-61.

Polskin LJ, Kramer B, Sobel HE (1945): Secretion of vitamin D in milk of women fed fish liver oil. J Nutr 30:451-466.

Pratt JP, Hamil BM, Mayer EZ, Kaucher M, Roderick C, Coryell MN, Miller S, Williams HH, Macy IG (1951): Metabolism of women during the reproductive cycle. XVI. The effect of multi-vitamin supplements on the secretion of B-vitamins in human milk. J Nutr 44:141–157.

Roberts CC, Chan G, Folland D, Rayburn C, Jackson R (1981): Adequate bone mineralization in breast-fed infants. J Pediatr 99:192–196.

Roepke JLB, Kirksey A (1981): Effects of vitamin B_6 supplementation during pregnancy on the vitamin B_6 nutriture of previous long-term oral contraceptive users and nonusers. Fed Proc 40.

Saarinen UM, Siimes MA, Dallman PR (1977): Iron absorption in infants: High bioavailability of breast milk iron as indicated by the extrinsic tag method of iron absorption and by concentration of serum ferritin. J Pediatr 91:36–39.

Shinwell ED, Gorodescher R (1982): Total vegetarian diets and infant nutrition. Pediatrics 70: 582–586.

Smith AM, Picciano MF, Milner JA (1982): Selenium intakes and status of breast and formula-fed infants. Am J Clin Nutr 35:521–526.

Smith AM, Picciano MF, Deering RH (1983): Maternal folate status, human milk folate content and their relationship to infant folate status. J Pediatr Gastro Nutr (in press).

Stastny D, Vogel RS, Picciano MF (1984): Manganese intakes and status of human milk-fed and formula-fed infants. Am J Clin Nutr (in press).

Tamura T, Yoshimura Y, Arakawa T (1980): Human milk folate and folate status in lactating mothers and their infants. Am J Clin Nutr 33:193–197.

Tapper D, Klagsburn M, Neumann J (1979): The identification and clinical implications of human breast milk mitogen. J Pediatr Surg 14:803–807.

Tarjan R, Kramer M, Szoke K, Lindner K, Szawas T, Dworschak E (1965): The effect of different factors on the composition of human milk. II. The composition of human milk during lactation. Nutr Dieta 7:136–154.

Thomas MR, Sneed SM, Wei C, Nael PA, Wilson M, Sprinkle EE (1980): The effects of vitamin C, vitamin B_6, vitamin B_{12}, folic acid, riboflavin, and thiamin on the breast milk and maternal status of well-nourished women at 6 months postpartum. Am J Clin Nutr 33:2151–2156.

Vuori E, Makenen SM, Kara R, Knitanen P (1980): The effects of the dietary intakes of copper, iron, manganese and zinc on the trace element content of human milk. Am J Clin Nutr 33: 227–231.

Whitehead RG, Paul AA, Cole TJ (1982): How much breast milk do babies need? Acta Paediatr Scand Suppl 299:43–50.

Widdowson EM, Chan H, Harrison GE, Milner RBG (1972): Accumulation of copper, zinc, manganese, chromium and cobalt in the human liver before birth. Biol Neonate 20:360–367.

Widdowson EM, Dauncey J, Shaw JCL (1974): Trace elements in fetal and early postnatal development. Proc Nutr Soc 33:275–284.

World Health Organization/Food and Agriculture Organization (1973): Energy and protein requirements. World Health Organization Tech Rep Ser, No 522; Food and Agricultural Organization Meetings Rep Ser, No 52.

Wurtman JJ, Fernstrom JD (1979): Free amino acid, protein and fat contents of breast milk from Guatemalan mothers consuming a corn-based diet. Early Hum Dev 3:67–77.

Ziegler EE, Fomon SJ (1983): Lactose enhances mineral absorption in infancy. J Pediatr Gastro Nutr 2:288–294.

Malnutrition: Determinants and Consequences, pages 123–138
© 1984 Alan R. Liss, Inc., 150 Fifth Avenue, New York, NY 10011

Promotion of Breast Feeding, Health, and Survival of Infants Through Hospital and Field Interventions

Leonardo Mata, ScD, Juan J. Carvajal, MD, María E. García, RN,
Patricia Sáenz, MD, María A. Allen, MD, José R. Aráya, MD, and
María E. Rodríguez, BS
Instituto de Investigaciones en Salud (INISA), Universidad de Costa Rica, San
Pedro, Costa Rica (L.M., J.J.C., M.E.G., P.S.) and Hospital San Juan de Dios,
Caja Costarricense de Seguro Social, San José, Costa Rica (M.A.A.,
J.R.A., M.E.R.)

Most authorities agree that the decline in the rate and duration of breast feeding in urban areas in many developing countries has been the result of urbanization and influences of Western culture. Two sequalae have been the transition from extended to nuclear families and the exposure of young mothers to influences affecting their attitudes and working patterns [Jelliffe and Jelliffe, 1978; Elliott and Fitzsimons, 1976]. Experimental studies have demonstrated that early mother-infant stimulation has a marked promoting effect on breast-feeding and bonding. It has become quite obvious that man is not so different from certain animal species in the kind of mechanisms leading to successful nursing and infant-rearing behavior [Bowlby, 1969; Klaus and Kennell, 1976].

A similar decline in breast feeding is also becoming apparent in rural areas, partly owing to a profusion of advertisements of infant formulas and partly to "Westernization" of ways of life [Jelliffe and Jelliffe, 1978; Greiner et al, 1979]. It was not obvious to many, however, that many failures to breast-feed in urban and rural areas have an origin in the inadequacies of medical support during pregnancy and particularly during childbirth and its aftermath [Jelliffe and Jelliffe, 1978]. Such inadequacies have proliferated as institutionalized delivery increases and is expanded to rural populations throughout developing countries. To illustrate, only 50% of births were attended in maternity centers and clinics in Costa Rica in 1960, but in 1970 the rate rose to 71% and in 1980 to 91% [Mata, 1983]. The increment in hospital delivery has not necessarily been accompanied by practices to promote early mother-infant stimulation, bonding, and nursing. Strict separation of mothers and infants after delivery, and feeding neonates with artificial formulas are common practices in the developing world.

This report summarizes observations recorded during 1976–1982 in the population of newborns delivered in the San Juan de Dios Hospital, one of the largest and most prestigious Costa Rican institutions [Mata et al, 1982a, 1983]. Observations were extended to neonates of one particular mountainous rural region, Puriscal, who were born during the period September 1979–September 1980 primarily in the San Juan de Dios Hospital [Mata et al, 1981; Mata, 1982]. The early neonatal morbidity and mortality were calculated across the 7-year period for the 61,478 live births during the observation period. Furthermore, possible effects of hospital practice were evaluated in terms of differentials in rate and duration of breast feeding, health, and growth among Puriscal neonates born from September 1979 to September 1980. Since this effort was part of a long-term prospective observation on nutrition, health, and growth of mothers and infants in a typical rural area, field interventions were also evaluated accordingly.

PROCEDURE
Population

Observations were made of 61,478 live newborns during the period 1976–1982 in the San Juan de Dios Hospital. These newborns belonged to a large sector of the metropolitan population of Costa Rica and to several counties of the southern mountainous rural area that includes Puriscal [Mata, 1982]. The Puriscal region extends to the Pacific Coast and it comprises about 800 square kilometers and approximately 26,000 inhabitants in localities of very sparsely distributed rural population [Mata, 1982]. The region is in rapid transition; most children have access to schools and health services, and about 70% of homes have an indoor piped water supply. The population subsists mainly on agricultural products and sales of food crops, complemented with cash crops such as tobacco; many hold white-collar jobs. The population is predominantly Spanish and, to a lesser extent, Spanish-Amerindian descent; they live in eight district centers and in 146 localities dispersed in valleys and hills. Localities are "rural dispersed" if they have fewer than 500 people, or "rural concentrated" if they have 500–2,000 people. The social development of Puriscal, as in most of rural Costa Rica, is significantly higher than that of traditional Mexico or Guatemala. However, ruralism in Puriscal is more marked than in these countries, and travel between houses may require several hours of walking in the field; some houses may be more than 2 kilometers from the nearest school [Mata, 1982]. Most Puriscal deliveries occur in the San Juan de Dios

Hospital. Adequate coordination between INISA headquarters and the hospitals and clinics allowed the staff of INISA's Field Station to know about most Puriscal deliveries.

Interventions in the Hospital

From 1976 until August 1977, mothers and newborns were completely separated after delivery and during the period of internment. Furthermore, preterm and high-risk neonates were fed glucose solution and infant formulas. Mothers and infants were reunited at the time of discharge, generally 1–3 days after delivery, or after a longer stay due to maternal infection or cesarean birth. Preterm and high-risk neonates remained separated for weeks. In September 1977, a series of innovations were initiated by two of the authors (M.A.A. and J.R.A.; Table I [Mata et al, 1982a, 1983]).

TABLE I. Interventions in the Gynecology and Obstetrics Service, San Juan de Dios Hospital, 1977–1980

Intervention	Date of onset	Description	Approximate percentage of population exposed
A. Mother-infant separation; formula-feeding	1969–1976	a. Brief visual contact at delivery; total separation during hospitalization b. Infants fed glucose solution and milk formulas	100%
B. Rooming-in[a]	September 1977	a. Infants stayed with mothers for about 8 hr per day; infants separated at night	66% (in 1977) 95% (in 1978 +)
C. Colostrum; promotion of breast feeding	January 1978	a. Human colostrum and milk given to preterm and high-risk neonates b. Education of nurses and mothers in feeding practices	50% (mid-1978) 95% (in 1979 +)
D. Early stimulation	July 1979	a. Skin-to-skin contact b. Suction of nipple shortly after birth c. Physical contact of mothers and preterm and high-risk neonates	50% (end 1979) 75% (in 1980 +)

[a]Interventions have been maintained to the present.

Complete and partial rooming-in, initiated in September 1977, consisted of leaving all healthy infants with their mothers during the day. Infants born at night stayed apart from their mothers until a neonatologist examined them the following morning; if neonates were found to be normal, they were given to their mothers during the day. Preterm, high-risk, and other ill neonates (about 5% of the total) were separated from their mothers and kept in an adjoining ward under supervision by neonatologists.

A colostrum feeding program for all neonates, initiated in 1978, was favored by a *milk bank* established in December 1977–January 1978, adjacent to the rooming-in area. Mothers and staff became enthusiastic about the breast pumps. Since most women do not undergo nipple massage before delivery, the pumps helped nipple formation and stimulated lactation [Mata et al, 1983]. Donation of colostrum and milk was carried out before or after mothers breast-fed their own infants. However, emphasis was on suckling of colostrum by the infant itself, and this often occurred on the delivery table after July 1979, when *early mother-infant stimulation* was started, or soon after rooming-in was effected. The program encouraged the nursing of hospitalized infants by their own mothers. For ill neonates who had hyaline membrane disease, congenital abnormalities, birth trauma, infections, or other pathology, pooled fresh colostrum and milk were given in amounts of about 5 ml/kg body weight per day. The pool was collected in sterile plastic bottles, kept under refrigeration, and used not later than 18 hr after collection. Colostrum was administered by tube or bottle as early as 4 hr after birth and generally at 8 hr, but some very ill infants received colostrum at a later date. Healthy neonates (about 95% of the total population) suckled colostrum from their own mothers.

Early mother-infant stimulation was started in 1979, covering about one-half of the mother-infant pairs by the end of the year. Most newborns were given naked to their mothers in the delivery room, although in many instances infants were given clothed. Eye-to-eye contact, and stimulation of the infant's mouth and maternal nipple were emphasized by nurses in the delivery room, although this was not universally practiced. The program has not been wholly successful owing to the firmly established tradition of mother-infant separation immediately after delivery, lack of knowledge about the importance of mother-infant interaction, and alleged limitations of space and time by the nursing staff. In 1979 a professional provided assistance in breast-feeding techniques, focusing mainly on the Puriscal mothers. Rooming-in and other interventions have been very successful; the hospital environment has improved and a relaxed and optimistic atmosphere prevails in the rooming-in wards [Mata et al, 1983]. Interventions remained once they were developed and an additive effect was expected. Other lasting improvements were effected in the hospital by the medical staff. These consisted of an increase in the number of pediatricians, improved diagnostic and therapeutic procedures, and enlarged physical facilities. The possible effect of these changes on neonatal morbidity and mortality could not be quantified during the observation period (1977–1982). A significant improvement in fetal growth was documented in the country as a whole as the prevalence of low birth weight fell from 9.2% to 7.5% in the period 1970–1975 [Mata et al, 1978]. However, no significant further improvement in fetal growth has been recorded after 1975 (unpublished data).

Analyses of Hospital Data

The complete hospital records for the period 1976–1982 were examined by three pediatricians who accurately determined the number of deliveries, characteristics of newborns, and morbidity and mortality during internment. Neonates with illness or defects were transferred at increasing rates, especially after 1979, to the neighboring National Children's Hospital. Care was taken to record the outcome, including deaths, of neonates that were transferred.

The following classifications and definitions were used: *Infection* (acute) comprised diarrhea, sepsis, bronchopneumonia, and meningitis. *Diarrhea* was defined as an increased frequency of watery stools and/or the presence of blood and mucus in the stools; diarrhea could occur in the first 48 hr after birth, but most cases appeared after 48 hr; all cases occurring during internment were considered in the tabulation. *Sepsis* was a state accompanied by pallor, impaired sucking, hypothermia, hypotension, shock, hepatosplenomegaly, and altered platelet and leukocyte profile; most cases were diagnosed in the first 48 hr. *Bronchopneumonia* was characterized by respiratory distress and was confirmed by chest radiography; almost all bronchopneumonia occurred in the first week of life; neonates with aspiration pneumonia were excluded. *Meningitis* was accompanied by pallor, weak sucking, hypothermia, hypotension, tense fontanel with separation of sutures, convulsions, and a pathognomonic cerebrospinal fluid profile; meningitis was diagnosed during the first week of life; deaths also were observed in the first week. *Hyaline membrane disease* (HMD) was a state of lung immaturity generally beginning at birth with intercostal retraction, nasal flarings, hypoventilation, and expiratory grunting; diagnosis was generally by chest radiography; death due to HMD occurred in the first 48 hr of life; doubtful cases without chest plate were excluded from the analysis. Early morbidity and mortality rates were expressed as cases or deaths observed in the first week of life, per 1,000 live births, the denominator being either all live births or only live births after less than 38 weeks of gestation.

Breast feeding in the hospital was defined as successful suckling several times during internment such as to make it unnecessary to administer infant formula. Incidence of breast feeding was expressed as percentage. *Abandon-*

ment of the newborn was the act of giving the child away, generally in the hospital or upon discharge. Infants abandoned were classified as *well*, meaning healthy with adequate gestation and birth weight, or *ill*, meaning that they were preterm, had low birth weight, defects, infections, or other pathology. Rates of abandonment were computed per 10,000 live births.

Interventions in the Field

Several interventions were effected by INISA with the aim of influencing mothers and infants in Puriscal. Because Puriscal women were hard to reach in their widely dispersed homes, most mothers were interviewed while in the hospital. Information collected in precoded forms included antenatal and pregnancy data, delivery characteristics, and description of the newborn and its condition. Upon discharge, mother-infant dyads were monitored from the base of operations, INISA's Field Station in Santiago de Puriscal. Coordination with health workers from the Ministry of Health for coverage of the highly scattered population was required. Rural motor vehicles, motorcycles, and horses were used, but surveillance included foot travel in each instance.

The first yearly cohort comprised 605 infants, distributed in three subcohorts according to the type and intensity of intervention and prospective observation [Mata et al, 1983]. All mother-infant pairs were similarly treated in the hospital (see Table I), but those of the rural dispersed districts of Grifo Alto, Barbacoas, and Candelarita (subcohort 1.1) were visited within the first 10 days postpartum by a field worker, and by the physician and health nurse through monthly consultations. Visits served to collect data on physical growth, breast feeding, food intake, and morbidity (Table II). Mother-infant

TABLE II. Subcohorts of the Puriscal Study, 1979–1983

Subcohort	Subcohort districts	Type of population	Field interventions
1.1 (115)[a]	Grifo Alto Barbacoas Candelarita	Rural dispersed	a. Visit by INISA's field worker within 10 days postpartum b. Contact with INISA's physician c. Monthly visits by INISA's field workers
1.2 (270)[a]	Mercedes Sur Desamparaditos San Antonio San Rafael	Rural dispersed	a. Monthly visits by health workers from Ministry of Health b. Occasional contact with INISA's physician
1.3 (220)[a]	Santiago	Rural concentrated and dispersed	a. Occasional contact with health personnel from Social Security Bureau, Ministry of Health, and INISA

[a]Number of infants born into subcohort.
Infants in all subcohorts were equally stimulated in the hospital (see text).

pairs of four other districts (Merccdes Sur, Desamparaditos, San Antonio, and San Rafael, constituting subcohort 1.2), equally rural and dispersed, were visited monthly by the staff of the Ministry of Health in coordination with INISA, to collect information on breast feeding and physical growth. Contact with INISA's physician and field staff was less than for subcohort 1.1. Mother-infant pairs of Santiago, which is the central district of Puriscal (subcohort 1.3) with rural dispersed and concentrated population, had more access to health resources of the region and the capital city. They could consult with INISA's personnel, but monthly visits were primarily coordinated through the staffs of the Social Security Bureau and the Ministry of Health.

Breast feeding was evaluated until complete weaning was effected, requiring prospective observation for 3 years. *Duration of breast-feeding*, whether the child was or was not receiving supplements, was expressed in months. *Age of weaning* was the month in which the child was definitely separated from the breast. Standard forms and procedures were used to collect data in all districts within the epidemiologic framework of a long-term prospective study [Mata, 1982].

RESULTS

Breast Feeding in the Hospital

The incidence of breast feeding in *well* (healthy) neonates was 95%; exceptions were imposed by complications requiring cesarean section or by illness in the mother. Some preterm and high-risk (*ill*) neonates who were separated from the mother were also breast-fed. All ill neonates received colostrum and milk during internment from the mother or from donors (pooled).

Abandonment of Newborns

A significant decline in the rate of abandoned infants was noted shortly after effecting rooming-in and other interventions (Fig. 1). The reduction was more marked for *well* than for *ill* infants, but the decrease in rate of abandonment of the latter was clear.

Early Neonatal Morbidity Attributed to Infection

Early morbidity (measured in the first week of life) declined abruptly after the interventions (Fig. 2), particularly for diarrhea and bronchopneumonia. Acute necrotizing enterocolitis did not appear after rooming-in, and human colostrum and milk were routinely administered to preterm and high-risk neonates. Evidently, the use of antibiotics significantly decreased. Changcs in early neonatal morbidity attributable to infection were not matched by a comparable decrease in congenital defects. Immaturity and asphyxia declined, although not significantly.

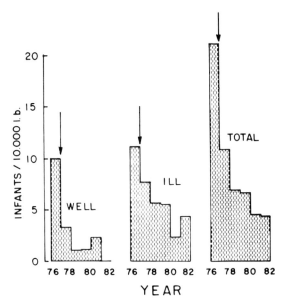

Fig. 1.   Abandonment of newborns in the hospital during the period 1976–1982. The arrows indicate the year in which rooming-in was started. Note the drastic reduction in abandonment of newborns, especially if they were healthy.

Early Neonatal Mortality Attributed to Infection

While the number of deaths attributed to infection was already low before the interventions were effected, a marked decline was nevertheless observed (Fig. 3). The most noticeable change was the disappearance of deaths due to diarrhea and meningitis.

Decline in Hyaline Membrane Disease (HMD)

A significant decrease in cases and deaths due to HMD was noted during the study period, especially during the years in which all interventions (rooming-in, colostrum, and early mother-infant stimulation) were operating simultaneously, that is, from 1979 onwards (Table III).

Duration of Breast Feeding After Hospital Discharge

This was evaluated in the cohort of Puriscal infants described. Data on the whole cohort (excluding infants whose families emigrated from the area) are compared in Table IV with data from the World Fertility Survey (WFS) for Costa Rica for 1976 [Ferry and Smith, 1983]. A significant increase in the mean (from 5 to 8.7 months) and median (from 1.8 to 6.9 months) duration of

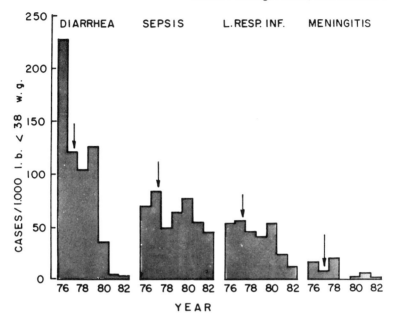

Fig. 2. Neonatal morbidity attributed to infection in the first week of life, as recorded in the hospital during the period 1976–1982. The arrows indicate the date (September 1976) at which rooming-in began. Note the marked decline in diarrheal disease, leading to its virtual disappearance.

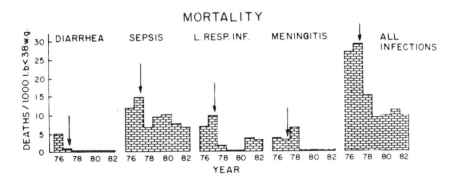

Fig. 3. Neonatal mortality attributed to infection in the first week of life, recorded in the hospital during the period 1976–1982. The arrows indicate the time in which rooming-in started. Note the disappearance of diarrhea as a cause of death.

TABLE III. Hyaline Membrane Disease (HMD) and Interventions, San Juan de Dios Hospital, Costa Rica

Year	Intervention[a]	Number of live births	Number of preterm infants ($<$ 38 wk gestation)	HMD, cases (rate per 1,000 preterm infants)			
				Observed cases	Observed minus expected[b] case rate, as %	Observed deaths	Observed minus expected[b] death rate, as %
1976	A	7,629	589(7.7)	154(261.5)		47(79.8)	
1977	B	8,582	618(7.2)	161(260.5)	− 0.4	37(59.9)	− 24.9
1978	B + C	8,931	597(6.7)	133(222.8)	− 14.8	33(55.3)	− 30.7
1979	B + C + D	8,638	437(5.1)	85(194.5)	− 34.5	41(93.8)	+ 17.5
1980	B + C + D	8,978	412(4.6)	67(162.6)	− 60.8	16(38.8)	− 51.4
1981	B + C + D	8,879	541(6.1)	36(66.5)	− 74.6	8(14.8)	− 81.4
1982	B + C + D	9,271	620(6.7)	62(100)	− 61.7	13(20.9)	− 73.8
% Change in rates 1976–1982			− 13	− 62		− 74	
Significance[c]				> 0.05	< 0.01		< 0.01

[a]Interventions as in Table I.
[b]The 1976 rates (261.5 and 79.8 per 1,000 live births) were assumed to be the expected values for 1977–1982.
[c]Test of equality, 1976 vs 1982.

breast feeding was evident in Puriscal infants in respect to the 1976 WFS data. Furthermore, differences were noted in the duration of breast feeding among the three subcohorts (Table IV): The more stimulated subcohort 1.1 showed the longest duration of breast feeding; duration was less in a similar rural dispersed population that had much less stimulation (subcohort 1.2). The rural concentrated or urban-rural subcohort 1.3 exhibited the shortest duration of breast feeding of the three groups, but still this was significantly greater than the preintervention figure. The bimodal frequency distribution of subcohort 1.1 probably resulted from exacerbation of breast-feeding efforts related to sustained emphasis and stimulus by the field staff.

Prevalence of Breast Feeding by Type of Delivery

Monthly prevalence rates of breast feeding by the type of delivery (four cases of *induced* delivery were excluded) revealed that the highest rates corresponded to *spontaneous* delivery, and the poorest to infants born by *cesarean* section (Table V). *Induced* deliveries were associated with some negative effect on the incidence of breast feeding.

TABLE IV. Duration of Breast Feeding (months) After Interventions, Puriscal, Costa Rica, 1976–1983

Population	Mean	Median
Costa Rica, WFS, 1972[a]	5.0	1.8
Puriscal, 1979–1983[b]		
Subcohort 1.1, RD more stimulated	12.6	11.4
Subcohort 1.2, RD less stimulated	7.8	7.9
Subcohort 1.3, RC, UR	7.6	5.9
Total cohort	8.7	6.9

[a]World Fertility Survey [Ferry and Smith, 1983].
[b]RD = rural dispersed; RC = rural concentrated; UR = urban-rural.

TABLE V. Percentage of Breast Feeding, by Type of Delivery and Age of Infant, Puriscal Cohort, 1979–1981

Age in months	Spontaneous (N = 189)	Induced (N = 245)	Cesarean (N = 80)
1	98.4	96.0	90.0
3	88.3	82.5	69.6
5	78.7	73.1	55.7
7	63.8	60.5	44.7
9	55.9	52.8	32.9
11	48.4	43.1	26.6

DISCUSSION

Premature weaning was already common in Costa Rica in the 1950s and undoubtedly contributed to the high rates of diarrheal disease, malnutrition, infant death, and demographic explosion recorded in that decade [Mata, 1981]. In spite of this situation, a sustained emphasis by governments on social development and improved nutrition and health had resulted in significant gains in the control of infectious diseases and infant deaths, particularly in the 1970s [Mohs, 1982].

Breast feeding continued its decline, and by the middle of the 1970s, measures to promote breast feeding through educational programs by the radio, television, and press emanated from the Social Security Bureau and the Ministry of Health, with collaboration of the Costa Rican Association of Demography. However, according to the World Fertility Survey (WFS), around 1976

26% of infants were never breast-fed [Ferry and Smith, 1983]. Furthermore, the 1978 nutrition survey [Ministerio de Salud, Costa Rica, 1978] revealed no significant changes since the preceding nutrition surveys of 1966 and 1975 [INCAP-OIR-MS, 1969; Díaz et al, 1975]. In fact, a decline in breast feeding was noted between 1975 and 1978, which raised questions about the effectiveness of such programs. According to the 1978 survey, 24% of infants from the rural areas were not breast fed or were weaned in the first days of life; by 3–6 months, about one-half had been weaned onto cow's and formula milks [Ministerio de Salud, Costa Rico, 1978].

Such a deterioration in infant feeding practices likely was the result of a) several years of drastic separation of mothers and infants immediately after delivery; b) formula-feeding in hospitals and clinics; c) many years of intense promotion of processed cow's milk for infants by the medical and commercial establishments; d) several years of governmental distribution of powdered milk to deliverying mothers; and e) cultural distortion of the role of the breasts and breast feeding.

Other Latin American nations evolving from traditional to modern lifestyles also experienced a decline in breast feeding, according to surveys conducted in the period 1975–1978 [Ferry and Smith, 1983]. The causes of the decline, as expected, are common to all nations; equivocal medical and hospital practices [Winikoff and Baer, 1980] have played a large role.

It is evident from the studies herein described that rapid transition that results in a significant increase in institutional delivery without the benefit of nontraumatic birth, rooming-in, and promotion of breast feeding undoubtedly has a deleterious effect on breast feeding and infant health. The Costa Rican case illustrates that the phenomenon is no longer urban, since the same is occurring in rural areas as instutitional delivery becomes universal.

Therefore, another approach to curtailing the decline in breast feeding must aim at drastic changes in the conditions under which women give birth [Winikoff and Baer, 1980]. The significant gains with interventions in a large general hospital of Costa Rica leave no doubt that they were justified not only in terms of improved benefit to the incidence of breast feeding and the health of suckling neonates, but also in terms of benefits to preterm and high-risk neonates that are derived from maternal stimuli and the provision of fresh human colostrum and milk.

A follow-up of neonates born in two Costa Rican hospitals with contrasting hospital practices showed that all infants separated at birth had been weaned by 9 months, whereas more than one-half of those exposed to rooming-in remained at the breast at 9 months of age [Mata et al, 1981]. The experience in this Costa Rican hospital linked rooming-in, breast feeding, and early mother-infant stimulation with a sharp decline in the rate of abandoned newborns, whether ill or healthy, but especially the latter, an observation of public health significance.

Field observations in a traditional village in the Guatemalan highlands demonstrated that almost all newborns received human milk from foster mothers shortly after birth. Weak neonates may be given drops of colostrum squeezed into their mouths. The survival rate of rural neonates that were able to suck within the first 24 hr was very high [Mata, 1978]. Furthermore, preterm and small-for-gestational-age rural infants grew adequately under extreme poverty in a microbially contaminated environment, provided they were breast-fed after birth and exclusively breast-fed for several months.

In the Costa Rican experience, the separation of preterm and high-risk neonates for medical reasons was partially compensated by maternal stimulation and the nutritional and anti-infection benefits of human colostrum and milk. The beneficial effect of early consumption of fresh human colostrum and milk rests on its unique anti-infection and nutritional components [Jelliffe and Jelliffe, 1978]. The theoretical and practical implications of feeding human milk to preterm infants have been discussed [Fomon et al, 1976] even though field experience has reiterated the desirability of giving human milk [Mata, 1978]. The administration of fresh human colostrum and milk had no side effects even if given as early as 1 hr after birth [Mata et al, 1982a, 1983].

Feeding of pooled human colostrum to neonates in an institutional setting has been done extensively by Larguía et al [1974, 1977] in Argentina, with striking reduction in diarrheal disease. Similarly, changes in medical practice leading to rooming-in in a Philippines hospital resulted in a reduction in morbidity and mortality of magnitude similar to that observed in Costa Rica [Relucio-Clavano, 1981].

The reduction in incidence and mortality due to hyaline membrane disease suggests a possible relationship with colostrum, particularly because the rate of cesareans did not increase and an improved detection of high-risk pregnancy was not established. It is possible that growth factors [Carpenter and Cohen, 1979; Klagsbrun, 1978] or substances like phospholipids in human colostrum and milk [Bracco et al, 1972] are required for synthesis of surfactant [Farrell and Hamosh, 1978], which plays a role in lung maturation.

The effect of hospital interventions in terms of prolongation of breast feeding and therefore in overall nutrition and health throughout infancy was outstanding [Mata et al, 1982c]. For instance, breast-fed Puriscal infants had a much lower rate of diarrheal disease and rotavirus infection than did artificially fed infants [Mata et al, 1981]. The protective role of breast feeding against diarrhea has been well proven, in industrial [Cunningham, 1979], transitional [Plank and Milanesi, 1973], and traditional societies [Lepage et al, 1981]. It was not surprising that Puriscal infants, who enjoyed a relatively clean environment, grew according to the WHO-recommended NCHS growth charts, whether they were normal at birth, preterm, or small for gestational age [Mata et al, 1982b]. Furthermore, virtually no stunting or wasting were diagnosed in the first two cohorts of infants, whereas infant mortality was very low in these cohorts [Mata et al, 1982c].

The hospital interventions apparently had a lasting effect in a cohort of rural mothers and infants that had close contact with the field team after hospital discharge (subcohort 1.1). The stimulus provided by field workers interested in breast feeding resulted in further gains in duration. Retrospective analysis showed that the prevalence of breast feeding of cohort infants was greater than that of the corresponding older siblings [Mata et al, 1982b, 1983].

While the rate and duration of breast feeding improved as a result of stimulation from field workers, it became quite evident that the most important health action consisted of early mother-infant stimulation and promotion of breast feeding immediately after birth. Indeed, the dramatic changes observed in a subcohort of mothers who received little stimulation, and in another subcohort living under rural-urban conditions, revealed how important it is to foster breast feeding in the hospital. Furthermore, the marked differentials in breast feeding with regard to the type of delivery attest to the need to reduce cesarean sections, anesthesia, and other interventions to a minimum compatible with good medical practice [Jelliffe and Jelliffe, 1978].

In the light of the present observations, change in hospital practice in Latin America is mandatory and has a higher priority than the orthodox approach of intervening after hospital discharge when the damage has already been done or may not be easily corrected. However, health interventions prior to delivery and after discharge by means of the communication media and the health infrastructure should not be neglected.

ACKNOWLEDGMENTS

The authors wish to thank the University of Costa Rica, the Social Security Bureau, the Ministry of Health, and the National Council of Scientific Research and Technology, Costa Rica. Support was also received from the Rockefeller Foundation, the US Agency for International Development, and the UK Overseas Development Agency.

REFERENCES

1. Bowlby J (1969): "Attachment and Loss." New York: Basic Books, Vol 1.
2. Bracco U, Hidalgo J, Bohren H (1972): Lipid composition of the fat globule membrane of human and bovine milk. J Dairy Sci 55:1375-1387.
3. Carpenter G, Cohen S (1979): Epidermal growth factor. Annu Rev Biochem 48:193-216.

4. Cunningham AS (1979): Morbidity in breast-fed and artificially fed infants. II. J Pediatr 95:685-689.

5. Díaz C, Brenes H, Córdoba M, García P, Quirós J (1975): "Encuesta Nacional Antropométrica y de Hábitos Alimentarios en Costa Rica." San José: Ministerio de Salud, Departamento de Nutrición.

6. Elliott K, Fitzsimmons DW (1976): "Breast-Feeding and the Mother." Ciba Found Symp, No. 46 (New Series). Amsterdam: Elsevier/Excerpta.

7. Farrell PM, Hamosh M (1978): The biochemistry of fetal lung development. Clin Perinatol 5:197-229.

8. Ferry B, Smith DP (1983): "Breast-feeding Differentials, WFS. Comparative Studies," No. 23. Voorburg: International Statistical Institute.

9. Fomon SJ, Avery GB, Beer AE, et al (1976): Human milk in premature infant feeding: summary of a workshop. Pediatrics 57:741-743.

10. Greiner T, Almroth S, Latham M (1979): "The Economic Value of Breast-Feeding." Monograph Series, No. 6. Ithaca: Cornell University.

11. INCAP-OIR-MS (1969): "Evaluación nutricional de la población de Centro América y Panamá. Costa Rica." Guatemala City: INCAP/PAHO/WHO.

12. Jelliffe DB, Jelliffe EFP (1978): "Human Milk in the Modern World: Psychosocial, Nutritional and Economic Significance." New York: Oxford University Press.

13. Klagsbrun M (1978): Human milk stimulates DNA synthesis and cellular proliferation in cultured fibroblasts. Proc Natl Acad Sci USA 75:5057-5061.

14. Klaus MH, Kennell JH (1976): "Maternal-Infant Bonding." St. Louis: C.V. Mosby.

15. Larguía M, Urman J, Ceriani JM, O'Donnell A, Stoliaro B, Martínez JC, Buscaglia JC, Weils S, Quiroga A, Irazu M (1974): Inmunidad local en el recién nacido. Primera experiencia con la administración de calostro humano a recién nacidos pre-término. Arch Argent Pediatr 72:109-125.

16. Larguía M, Urman J, Stoliar OA, Ceriani JM, O'Donnell A, Buscaglia JC, Martínez JC (1977): Fresh human colostrum for the prevention of E. coli diarrhea—a clinical experience. Environ Child Health 23:289-290.

17. Lepage P, Munyakazi C, Hennart P (1981): Breast-feeding and hospital mortality in children in Rwanda. Lancet 2:409-411.

18. Mata LJ (1978): "The Children of Santa María Cauqué. A Prospective Field Study of Health and Growth." Cambridge: MIT Press.

19. Mata L (1981): Epidemiologic perspective of diarrheal disease in Costa Rica, and current efforts in control, prevention, and research. Rev Latinoam Microbiol 23:109-119.

20. Mata L (1982): Estudio de Puriscal. I. Bases filosóficas, desarrollo y estado actual de la investigación aplicada en nutrición. Rev Méd Hosp Nac Niños (Costa Rica) 17:1-20.

21. Mata L (1983): Trends of diarrheal diseases, malnutrition and mortality in Costa Rica and role of interventions. Assignment Children 59/60:195-224.

22. Mata L, Jiménez P, Allen MA, Vargas W, García ME, Urrutia JJ, Wyatt RG (1981): Diarrhea and malnutrition: Breast-feeding intervention in a transitional population. In Holme T, Holmgren J, Merson MH (eds): "Acute Enteric Infections in Children: New Prospects for Treatment and Prevention." Amsterdam: Elsevier/North-Holland, pp 233-251.

23. Mata L, Allen MA, Araya JR, Carvajal JJ, Rodríguez ME, Vives M (1982a): Estudio de Puriscal. VIII. Efecto de intervenciones hospitalarias sobre la lactancia y la salud en el período neonatal. Rev Méd Hosp Nac Niños (Costa Rica) 17:99-116.

24. Mata L, García ME, Jiménez P, Sibaja A, Solís VJ, Vargas AC, Jiménez MM (1982b): Estudio de Puriscal. II. Crecimiento fetal y su influencia sobre el crecimiento físico posnatal. Rev Méd Hosp Nac Niños (Costa Rica) 17:21-36.

25. Mata L, Jiménez P, Castro B, García ME, Vives M, Jiménez S, Sánchez F (1982c): Estudio de Puriscal. IX. Estado nutricional y supervivencia del niño lactante. Rev Méd Hosp Nac Niños (Costa Rica) 17:117-139.

26. Mata L, Allen MA, Jiménez P, García ME, Vargas W, Rodríguez ME, Valerín C (1983): Promotion of breast-feeding, health, and growth among hospital-born neonates, and among infants of a rural area of Costa Rica. In Chen LC, Scrimshaw NS (eds): "Diarrhea and Malnutrition. Interactions, Mechanisms and Interventions." New York: Plenum, pp 177–202.

27. Mata L, Villegas H, Albertazzi C, Mohs E (1978): Crecimiento fetal humano en Costa Rica. Rev Biol Trop 26:431–450.

28. Ministerio de Salud, Costa Rica (1978): "Encuesta Nacional de Nutrición 1978." San José: Ministerio de Salud, Departamento de Nutrición.

29. Mohs E (1982): Infectious diseases and health in Costa Rica: The development of a new paradigm. Pediatr Infect Dis 1:212–216.

30. Plank SJ, Milanesi C (1973): Infant feeding and infant mortality in rural Chile. Bull WHO 48:203–210.

31. Relucio-Clavano N (1981): The results of a change in hospital practices. A paediatrician's campaign for breast-feeding in the Philippines. Assignment Children 55/56:139–165.

32. Winikoff B, Baer EC (1980): The obstetrician's opportunity: Translating "breast is best" from theory to practice. Am J Obstet Gynecol 138:405–412.

Malnutrition: Determinants and Consequences, pages 139–146
© *1984 Alan R. Liss, Inc., 150 Fifth Avenue, New York, NY 10011*

Breast Feeding Practices and Use of Supplemental Foods

Abraham Stekel, MD, Francisco Mardones-Santander, MD, and Eva Hertrampf, MD
Institute of Nutrition and Food Technology (INTA), University of Chile, Santiago 11, Chile

INTRODUCTION

The duration of breast feeding and the production of milk depend on a number of physiologic, nutritional, social, and cultural factors. Prolonged breast feeding is of critical importance in preventing infant mortality and morbidity in populations of low socioeconomic condition. However, women from these populations seem to produce less milk than women from a higher socioeconomic condition [Jelliffe and Jelliffe, 1978]. Breast feeding by Chilean mothers is of short duration. In the last few decades, Chile has been characterized by the existence of extensive programs of supplementary food distribution. In this chapter, we attempt to review the relationship between the availability of supplementary foods and the breast feeding practices among urban groups of middle-low socioeconomic condition in Chile.

DECLINE OF BREAST FEEDING IN CHILE

In Chile, as well as in many developing countries, the decline in breast feeding coincides with complex cultural, social, and economic changes. In these countries, the process of urbanization and industrialization has led to great urban concentration. In the large cities, immigrants from rural areas form the majority of the population. These are the people who have been most affected by cultural changes as well as by malnutrition, infection, and the psychosocial stress of the environment.

Chile began its urbanization early in this century, before industrialization was significant. In 1900, one-third of the population lived in cities, and in the

1930s, when industrialization began to acquire importance, half of the population lived in urban areas. Thus, urbanization in Chile was more advanced than in the majority of Latin American countries. It is estimated that in 1980, 80% of Chile's population lived in urban areas.

Mardones-Santander [1979] recently reviewed the history of breast feeding in Chile. As seen in Figure 1, the proportion of children from urban, low-class areas who were exclusively breast-fed at 3 months of age is similar in the various studies done between 1942 and 1977. The values range from 26.7% to 52%, the majority lying between 30% and 42%. There is no apparent historical trend over this period; in urban lower classes, there has not been a decrease since 1942 in the number of children breast-fed for a period of at least 3 months. It appears that the most significant decline to the present level occurred in the thirties, or perhaps even before that time [Mardones-Santander, 1979].

NATIONAL SUPPLEMENTARY FOOD PROGRAM (NSFP) IN CHILE

As previously stated, in the early 1940s the duration of breast feeding was already relatively short in women of a low socioeconomic condition living in urban areas. At that time, infant malnutrition was very prevalent and infant mortality was high (about 200 per 1,000 live births). When breast feeding was no longer possible, mothers used cereal flours as the main food for their infants [Araya, 1942].

The distribution of cow's milk was initiated at this time as a means of preventing the severe malnutrition and the high infant mortality resulting from the use of weaning foods of poor nutritional quality. A law passed in 1938 provided for this distribution program and during the forties the amount of cow's milk distributed through the government health system reached about 1 million liters per year, covering approximately 15% of children under 2 years of age [Mardones-Santander, 1979].

In 1954, the NSFP also began the distribution of powdered milk to pregnant women. The program, now reaching pregnant and lactating women and children under 6 years of age, gradually increased through the years (Fig. 2) and covered 81% of the population under 6 years of age in 1980 [Cruzat et al, 1982].

The delivery of food supplements is made through the National Health System (NHS), provided that the mother and child are up to date with their vaccinations and with their visits to the local health clinic. While there has been a continuous increase in food distribution by the NSFP, no further decline has occurred in the duration of breast feeding. The incidence of severe infantile malnutrition in Chile is now quite low. Infant mortality declined from 164.5 per 1,000 live births in 1945 to 23.4 in 1982.

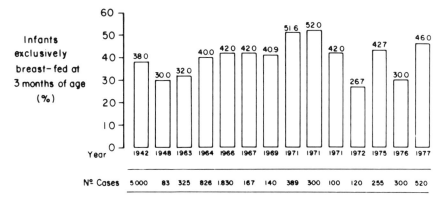

Fig. 1. Percentage of infants exclusively breast-fed for three or more months in urban areas of low socioeconomic condition in Chile, according to surveys performed between 1942 and 1977. Redrawn from Mardones-Santander [1979].

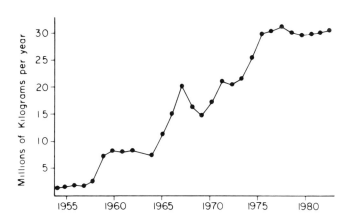

Fig. 2. Food distributed to infants, children under 6 years of age, and pregnant and lactating women by the Chilean National Supplementary Food Program.

PROMOTION OF BREAST FEEDING

Since the short duration of breast feeding continues to be a determinant of infant malnutrition in the Chilean setting [Mardones-Santander, 1980], a national program to promote breast feeding was set up in 1980 by the NHS [González et al, 1983]. The program, which includes the education of mothers by health personnel and the delivery of rice (3 kg per month) to underweight pregnant women, has apparently increased the duration of breast feeding as determined in a preliminary evaluation done in one health service area of the city of Santiago (Table I). Still, there is a need for a continuous effort to promote breast feeding, especially during the second trimester of life, when incidence is still low [González et al, 1983].

BREAST FEEDING DURATION AND AVAILABILITY OF SPECIAL SUPPLEMENTAL FOODS

In the last few years, the authors have been conducting pilot studies that involve the field evaluation of an iron-fortified milk formula and a fortified rice cereal, preceding the eventual incorporation of these products into the NSFP. The influence of the availability of these special products on duration of breast feeding is of interest.

Iron-Fortified Formula

Between 1978 and 1980 a study was conducted in the Central Area of Santiago to test the effect of substituting a special iron-fortified formula for the regular milk distributed to infants. Under the existing program, infants (or their lactating mothers) received 3 kg of full-fat powdered milk from 0 to 6 months of age and 2 kg from 6 to 24 months of age. This milk was packaged in polyethylene bags. Infants born in the seven health clinics in the area after August 1, 1978 received the fortified formula after weaning. This consisted of acidified full-fat powdered milk, fortified with iron and some vitamins. This product was packaged in attractive tin cans; oxygen-tight containers were needed for the adequate preservation of the iron-fortified product. The main objective of the study was to determine the effect of the new formula on iron nutrition status. A big concern, however, was that the appeal of the new formula might induce mothers to breast-feed for shorter periods of time; health personnel could consciously or unconsciously promote the new product.

Detailed follow-up studies were conducted in two cohorts of infants, those born in June–July 1978, who received the regular milk, and those born in August–September 1978, who received the fortified milk. The usual practice of encouraging breast feeding was followed in the two groups. Throughout the study a dietary survey was performed once a month by a registered nurse who visited each infant's house, so information on breast feeding was very reliable.

The duration of breast feeding in the two groups of infants was almost identical (Fig. 3). The percentage of infants exclusively breast-fed in the June–July group was 41.0% at 3 months, 23.5% at 6 months, and 16.0% at 9 months versus 41.2%, 26.7% and 16.5%, respectively, in the August–September group. Thus, in these urban communities characterized by low socioeconomic

TABLE I. Percentage of Breast-Fed Infants in Four Health Clinics of the Eastern Health Service in Santiago

Age (months)	Percentage of breast-fed infants		Percentage change
	1979 (N = 172)	1981 (N = 225)	
1	77.1	86.4	+ 12.0*
3	56.0	74.8	+ 33.6**
6	33.7	54.4	+ 61.4**

*P < 0.05.
**P < 0.001.

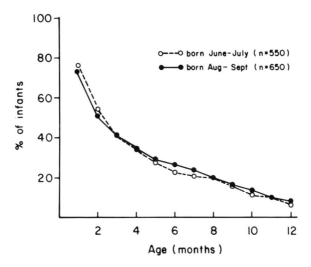

Fig. 3. Percentage of infants exclusively breast-fed at different ages in the Central Area of the city of Santiago. After weaning, infants born in June–July were given regular powdered milk; those born in August–September received a special iron-fortified formula.

conditions in which the population attends organized health clinics, the introduction of an attractive new food supplement had no influence on the duration of breast feeding.

Hemoglobin-Rice Cereal

When the mother's milk becomes insufficient to maintain normal infant growth, the usual practice in Chile is to introduce cow's milk given in a bottle, resulting in the rapid termination of breast feeding. The importance of supplementing breast feeding with solids, given in a way that will not interfere with breast feeding, is now well recognized. Ideally, these foods should have a high caloric density and an adequate protein quality. They should also provide the additional iron needed by breast-fed infants after 4–6 months of age.

An infant cereal developed in our laboratory has many of these characteristics. It consists of 95% extruded rice flour and 5% bovine hemoglobin concentrate. One hundred grams of this cereal provides 360 kcal, 11.6 gm protein, and 12.5 mg of heme iron. It is prepared as a gruel in a 20% dilution and it is fed with a spoon.

We have studied the influence of providing this cereal on the duration of breast feeding in infants attending a NHS clinic in Santiago. Healthy term infants who are being breast-fed at 3 months of age are admitted to the study. At this age, they are randomly assigned to two groups: One group receives 1,500 gm of cereal per month; the other serves as a control. Mothers in both groups receive powdered milk through the NSFP. For all infants, recommendations are given on the use of solid foods according to the usual local practices: fruits at 4 months; vegetable and meat soup at 5 months; eggs, cereals, and legumes at 6–7 months; and regular table food at 9–12 months. Pediatric care is delivered by a team of INTA pediatricians and nurses who continuously emphasize the importance of prolonged breast feeding. A nurse visits the home of each infant once a week and performs a morbidity survey and a dietary survey. She also stresses the importance of breast feeding and helps the mother to solve practical problems associated with it.

The duration of exclusive breast feeding was similar in the two groups of infants (Fig. 4). At 6 months of age, 91.5% of the infants in the cereal group and 94.2% of those in the control group were on breast milk; figures at 9 months were 73.4% and 69.2%, respectively.

The high prevalence of prolonged breast feeding in this study can be explained in part by the fact that this was a selected group of healthy term infants, being breast-fed at 3 months. In order to determine the influence of these factors, we selected from the Central Area study infants fulfilling the same criteria and followed their feeding record. It must be remembered that these infants were not involved in any special program to promote breast feeding. Prevalence of exclusive breast feeding in this subgroup of infants was higher than in the group as a whole (see Fig. 3), but much lower than in the infants in the cereal study (Fig. 5).

The tentative conclusion of the cereal study is that any effect that might derive from the availability of this special supplemental food is being obscured by the excellent results obtained in both groups as a consequence of the intensive dedication of the health team to the promotion of breast feeding.

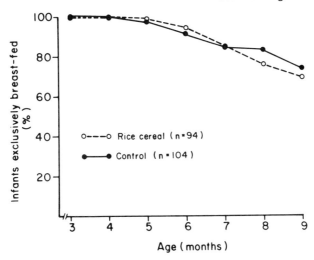

Fig. 4. Breast feeding in two groups of infants after enrollment in a special promotion program at 3 months of age. One group of infants received a rice cereal especially designed to supplement breast milk.

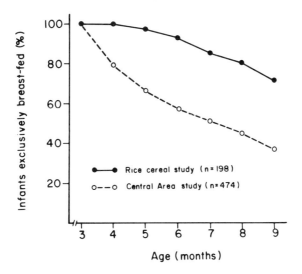

Fig. 5. Breast feeding after 3 months of age in two groups of healthy term infants in the city of Santiago. Infants in the rice cereal study were enrolled in a special breast feeding promotion program.

SUMMARY

In Chile, a decline in breast feeding has apparently occurred as a consequence of the process of urbanization; the decline preceded the beginning of massive programs of supplemental food distribution. The prevalence of breast feeding among urban groups of low socioeconomic condition in Chile has not changed significantly in the last 40 years. During the same period of time food distribution programs have markedly expanded. The duration of breast feeding in Chile can be significantly increased through specific programs of promotion and education. In the groups studied, the availability of supplemental foods does not seem to have had a marked influence on a mother's decision or potential to breast-feed.

ACKNOWLEDGMENTS

The following investigators from INTA participated in the field studies here reported: Marisol Cayazzo, Patricia Chadud, Gloria Heresi, Sandra Llaguno, Manuel Olivares, Fernando Pizarro and Tomás Walter.

This work was supported in part by grants from the Departamento de Desarrollo de la Investigación, University of Chile; the Chilean Ministry of Health; Nestlé Nutrition and the United Nations University.

REFERENCES

Araya P (1942): Alimentación artificial del lactante sano. Rev Chil Pediatr 13:716–767.

Cruzat A, González N, Mardones-Santander F (1982): Cobertura de los programas nutricionales y de salud en los sectores de menores ingresos. Rev Med Chile 110:585–592.

González N, Hertrampf E, Mardones-Santander F, Rosso P, Verdugo C (1983): Evaluación preliminar del impacto del Programa de Fomento de la Lactancia Materna. Rev Chil Pediatr 54:34–40.

Jelliffe DB, Jelliffe EFP (1978): The volume and composition of human milk in poorly nourished communities: A review. Am J Clin Nutr 31:492–515.

Mardones-Santander F (1979): History of breastfeeding in Chile. Food Nutr Bull 1:15–22.

Mardones-Santander F (1980): Algunos factores condicionantes del bajo peso de nacimiento. Rev Med Chile 108:839–853.

NUTRITION AND PERFORMANCE

Malnutrition: Determinants and Consequences, pages 149–150
© 1984 Alan R. Liss, Inc., 150 Fifth Avenue, New York, NY 10011

The Interrelationships of Diet and Exercise (Abstract)

Peter D. Wood, DSc
Stanford Heart Disease Prevention Program, Palo Alto, California 94304

Both the quantitative and the qualitative aspects of dietary intake will be considered in relation to physical activity level and health.

It is clear that caloric intake must *approximately* balance caloric expenditure for most people over prolonged time periods. There is ample evidence that very active individuals eat considerably more than sedentary individuals. Quite minor caloric imbalances lead to major weight gain (or loss) over years. It is becoming increasingly clear that weight control at a desirably modest body fat content is more easily attainable and better maintained at relatively high caloric flows (high activity level) than at low caloric flows (sedentary level). This is probably due in part to the favorable effect of both increased exercise level and increased food consumption on basal metabolic rate. Caloric balance maintained at higher (rather than lower) calorie intakes has many advantages related to health and adherence: A higher calorie intake predicts lower coronary disease rates, provides more micronutrients and fiber, and is more socially convenient. The accompanying higher (rather than lower) physical activity level also predicts lower coronary disease rates, promotes cardiovascular fitness, leads to a protective plasma lipoprotein pattern, and often results in an improved sense of well-being.

There is compelling (though not complete) evidence that the quality of the diet habitually consumed is related to long-term health. A diet that provides a low to moderate proportion of calories from fat, and is relatively high in complex carbohydrate and fiber, relatively low in salt and cholesterol, and at least adequate in vitamins and minerals seems to offer the best prospects of protection from the major chronic diseases (atherosclerosis and certain cancers), so far as we can tell at present. It is clear, in North America, that high levels of physical activity are often associated with consumption of increased amounts of less than optimally healthful foods. Although very active people typically have a "protective" plasma lipoprotein pattern, coronary disease is certainly not unknown in this group, so that improvement in dietary status is desirable even for the very active. The sedentary person about to become more active is poised, about to eat more. This provides an opportunity for nutritional improvement that should not be neglected. Preliminary evidence will be presented suggesting, for one population at least, that increased physical activity is accompanied, without prompting, by selection of a healthier diet.

This presentation develops these arguments, using data from epidemiologic studies and conditioning trials. The subject of nutrition in relation to exercise level is in its infancy: Areas where further work is urgently needed will be indicated.

Malnutrition: Determinants and Consequences, pages 151–163
© 1984 Alan R. Liss, Inc., 150 Fifth Avenue, New York, NY 10011

Effects of Overnutrition and Underexertion on the Development of Diabetes and Hypertension: A Growing Epidemic?

Ethan A.H. Sims, MD

Metabolic Unit, Department of Medicine, College of Medicine, University of Vermont, Burlington, Vermont 05405

INTRODUCTION

There are two main types of malnutrition. First, there is deficiency of calories or essential dietary elements and, second, there is excess of nutrients, which may contribute to chronic and costly disorders. The latter is seen when susceptible individuals are exposed to the affluence of the more fortunate members of Western societies and to an abundance of food without the need to work for it. In the United States there has been an increase in obesity, diabetes, and related cardiovascular disorders since pioneer days, although recently there has been a decline in the incidence of cardiovascular disease [Trowbridge, this volume]. There have been striking examples of racial groups, such as the Pima Indians of the US Southwest [Bennett et al, 1976] and the natives of Micronesia [Zimmet et al, 1977], who have adapted in the past to cycles of feast and famine and who now have developed a high incidence of diabetes and its complications. Japanese migrants and their offspring in Hawaii have a higher incidence of diabetes and of its vascular complications than their counterparts in Hiroshima [Kawate et al, 1979]. There is recent evidence that during the last decade what has been termed the epidemic of obesity and diabetes and the accompanying vascular disease has gained momentum in certain parts of this hemisphere. West [1978] has emphasized in his recent book the social forces that have brought this about in various parts of the world. There is a considerable common denominator of endocrine and metabolic derangement among obesity, non-insulin-dependent diabetes mellitus (NIDDM), and mild

TABLE I. Percentage Change in Age-Adjusted Death Rates
From 1970 to 1979

	All causes	Diabetes
Argentina	− 17	− 11
Canada	− 14	− 24
Puerto Rico	− 21	− 48
United States	− 17	− 26
Trinidad and Tobago	− 6	+ 73
Mexico	− 18	+ 33
Venezuela	− 17	+ 31
Costa Rica	− 38	+ 30
Chile	− 32	+ 12
Colombia	− 8	+ 6
Cuba	− 5	+ 3

From PAHO [1980], with permission.

to moderate "essential" hypertension [Sims and Berchtold, 1982], and thus many of the considerations of obesity and NIDDM, their treatment, and prevention apply to all three of these major health problems.

Both for planning management of individual patients and for developing policy regarding intervention it is important to consider the genetic influences that may be associated with susceptibility to obesity and to NIDDM and also the environmental factors that may bring them to the fore.

AREAS MOST AFFECTED BY THE CURRENT EPIDEMIC

The Pan American Health Organization of the World Health Organization has recently summarized changes in age-adjusted death rates from a number of diseases from 1970 to 1979. Table I is taken from their 1982 report. While death from all causes declined in each of the 11 countries selected, in seven there was an increase in death from diabetes, which was very marked in Trinidad-Tobago, Mexico, Venezuela, and Costa Rica. The actual estimated death rates are shown in Figure 1. There are many potential sources of error in such estimates, since stated single causes of death may be misleading, subtypes of diabetes are not considered, and criteria for diagnosis and method of detection vary. The figures are, however, consistent with the general impression of those working in these areas. The English-speaking Caribbean islands have been particularly affected [McGlashan, 1982]. The Honorable Billie A. Miller, Minister of Education for the Government of Barbados and former Minister of Health has reported to this Congress the conditions in this area. Obesity in males has increased to 19% in 1980 from 7% in 1969. Twenty percent of 10- to 14-year-olds are obese, with an increasing incidence in women following successive pregnancies. There is an increase in obesity-associated diseases, with a

RATE PER 100,000

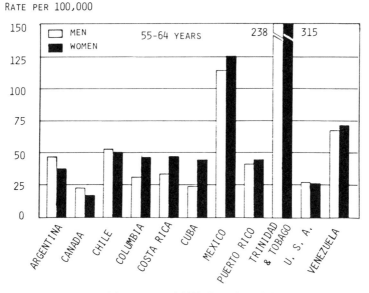

Fig. 1.   Death rates for diabetes, around 1978. From PAHO [1980], with permission.

29% incidence of hypertension in those over 35. Hypertension, increasing with age, is a major cause of death. At this Congress, Uauy [this volume] emphasized the negative contribution of urbanization to health and nutrition brought about by sedentary life styles, increased intake of animal foods, and availability of energy. There are increasing rates of mortality associated with obesity, atherosclerosis, and diabetes in Latin America [Valverde et al, this volume].

The increase in disorders associated with overnutrition is mainly an urban phenomenon. The study of Cruz-Vidal et al [1979] in Puerto Rico shows a high correlation with obesity in the moderately obese (up to 125% of ideal weight), but this does not hold for more severe grades of obesity, and they suggest that some elusive additional factor is operating. This factor could well be the lesser demands for physical exertion in the urban areas. In analyzing the increase in the Barbados area, Dr. Miller attributes the increase in obesity and diabetes to affluence secondary to influx of foreign dollars, to a shift from hard work in the sugar cane fields to light work in the towns, and to a reliance on imported food. The relative lack of fiber of the "junk" foods compared to native foods has also been emphasized.

TYPE OF DIABETES INVOLVED

A classification of diabetes into two main and quite different types has been developed by the US National Diabetes Data Group [1979], but to date available surveys of incidence have not made use of this differentiation. The increase is presumably in Type II diabetes, or NIDDM, which has a close association with obesity and increased insulin resistance as its major features and has only relative insufficiency of insulin. This is in contrast to Type I diabetes, which is now believed to be mainly secondary to autoimmune destruction of pancreatic β-cells, probably triggered by viral infection.

FACTORS CONTRIBUTING TO INCIDENCE OF NIDDM

There is increasing evidence of a strong genetic component in NIDDM. There is also evidence that persons with a certain body configuration are more susceptible to the disorders associated with insulin resistance. Finally there is evidence of a critical role of environmental factors.

Genetic Factors in NIDDM

The studies of the incidence of diabetes in identical twins has shown a strong concordance for NIDDM that greatly exceeds that for insulin-dependent diabetes [Tattersall and Pike, 1972; Zimmet, 1982]. Just what defect or defects are genetically determined has not been clarified. There have been no genetic markers for type II diabetes, but recently there has been promise that such may be identified. Variations in the DNA insertion sequences near the insulin gene, in the so-called 5' region, have been correlated with the incidence of NIDDM in whites, blacks, and Pima Indians [Rotwein et al, 1983]. Subsequent studies have both supported and refuted this correlation, although Owerbach et al [1983] have estimated from the pooled available data that the probability of an association is high ($p = 0.00036$ to be exact). However, when these markers were studied in Nauru, one of the islands in Micronesia where the incidence of NIDDM is extraordinarly high [83% in full-blooded natives], no correlation was found in those with or without diabetes [Serjeantson et al, 1983]. In those natives with foreign genetic admixture, the incidence dropped to 17%, suggesting a protective factor. Study by the same group of a kindred in Denmark with high incidence of maturity-onset diabetes of youth (MODY) also showed no linkage with the DNA insertion sequences. The Danish workers [Owerbach et al, 1982] have found a strong association between large DNA insertions, the U allele, and atherosclerosis. This rapidly developing field gives promise of considerable benefit in epidemiologic and other studies. Obtaining a family history of NIDDM is of value in estimating those at risk.

What Body Shape Makes a Person Most Vulnerable?

Twenty years ago Albrink and Meigs [1965] reported a relation of blood glucose and serum lipids with central distribution of body fat. At the same time Vague and co-workers [1969] noted a predisposition to diabetes of those with an upper trunk distribution of body fat, and this has recently been confirmed by others [Björntorp et al, 1971; Kissebah et al, 1982]. In recent studies of NIDDM [Bogardus et al, in press] we have found a high correlation between fasting plasma glucose and the fat distribution ratio of Ashwell et al [1978], an index of central obesity, but none with total body fat. Vague orginally suggested that the "cushingoid" distribution of body fat may be associated with increased adrenocorticoid secretion and the trunkal development with androgen secretion. It is of interest that Evans et al [1983] have now made a preliminary report of an increase in percentage free testosterone and a reduction in sex hormone-binding globulin in women with central obesity, increased abdominal adipocyte volume, and impaired glucose tolerance. Thus it seems quite possible that altered steroid secretion may be a factor both in the distribution of body fat and in the disturbance of carbohydrate metabolism. The type of obesity that most affects the upper and central portion of the body also corresponds to the hypertrophic obesity with onset later in life. In this there is predominantly adipoctye enlargement, in contrast to the hypertrophic-hyperplastic type, with more early onset, more generalized distribution of body fat, and predominantly an increase in cell number. This latter type is less associated with metabolic disorders and with hypertension, and in view of the hypercellularity it is often more difficult to treat. In fact, such efforts may be counterproductive.

Mechanisms of Insulin Resistance in Obesity and NIDDM

The most prominent feature of both obesity and NIDDM is resistance to the actions of insulin. However, before frank diabetes can develop, there must be a failure of compensatory increase in insulin secretion, giving a relative insulin deficiency. It is unclear whether the resistance or the impaired secretion is the primary factor. In NIDDM there is commonly a deficient first-phase insulin release, and the response to glucose may be impaired while that to arginine or secretin is preserved. This, however, may be a secondary effect, since Weir and Bonner-Weir [1982] have recently shown that in animals partial pancreatectomy can produce the same pattern of response in the remaining islet cells. In obesity and in NIDDM there may be a reduction in number of insulin receptors, but this does not always vary consistently with insulin resistance. Particularly in more severe NIDDM a postreceptor defect may be present. This may be at least in part secondary to insulin deficiency, since it is correctable, at least to the level found in uncomplicated obesity, by providing exogenous insulin. It seems likely, as suggested in a recent review by Weir [1982], that both peripheral resistance and defective insulin resistance may play a primary role and that the two defects augment each other.

When normal male volunteers without family history of diabetes or obesity deliberately gained weight by overeating, there was a decrease in glucose tolerance and an increase in serum insulin and in insulin resistance of muscle and of adipocytes [Sims et al, 1973]. Thus development of obesity by overeating and inactivity can contribute to development of latent diabetes or aggravate existing diabetes. But it cannot be said that the diabetes is simply a consequence of gluttony and overeating. Both the obesity and the carbohydrate intolerance may well be simply part of a larger syndrome. We will not know the answer until we understand the nature of the defects in this form of diabetes.

Sites of Insulin Resistance

Muscle constitutes a major site of insulin resistance in NIDDM. The liver is also a major and important site, since the output of glucose is characteristically high and is not suppressed by insulin to the same degree as in normals [Olefsky and Kolterman 1981; Rizza et al, 1981]. When carbohydrate disposal in response to insulin is improved by dietary therapy or the same plus exercise, a major effect is in restoration of responsiveness of the liver [Bogardus et al, in press]. One may well ask, if insulin resistance is so prominent in NIDDM, why are patients generally overweight? The answer is that adipose tissue is relatively more sensitive to the antilipolytic action of insulin [Howard et al, 1979].

Physical Fitness Vs Glucose Intolerance

Rosenthal et al [1983] have recently shown in normal subjects a high degree of correlation between the state of physical training, as indicated by $\dot{V}O_2$ max during bicycle ergometry, and the clearance of glucose during a euglycemic insulin clamp. In obese subjects Leon et al [1979] have found that those who were "unfit" by the same criteria had impaired glucose tolerance, and Berglund et al [1981] have reported the same in patients with NIDDM.

Effect of Physical Training on Diabetes

This topic has recently been reviewed by Kemmer and Berger [1983] and is the subject of recent symposia [Vranic et al, 1978a; Berger et al, 1982]. Over a decade ago Björntorp et al [1970] demonstrated that the plasma insulin concentrations of a group of middle-aged overweight men could be approximately halved by a course of physical training, indicating decreased insulin resistance. Serum lipids were reduced toward normal. Weight and body composition remained constant. More recently Leon et al [1979] found that a vigorous walking program only temporarily increased intake of food in a group of sedentary obese men, but that this gradually decreased so that they lost weight to below-pretreatment levels. High-density lipoprotein (HDL) cholesterol (the "good" cholesterol) levels were increased 16% after 16 weeks of exercise, and fasting blood glucose levels were significantly lower. Fasting insulin was reduced 43%. In a similar study of overweight women, Gwinup [1975] found that if a walking program exceeded 30 min a day, there was a net reduction of appetite and gradual loss of weight.

Effect of Physical Training Added to Dietary Therapy

Large-scale studies of the effect of added exercise alone on obesity, NIDDM, and other risk factors for cardiovascular disease are few and indecisive. The Chicago intervention study of the Stamlers [1980] in a program sustained over 5 years included increased physical activity, but it lacked a control group. A large-scale prospective study of the effect of a "prudent diet" as compared to that of insulin and oral hypoglycemic agents has been launched in England [Multi-Centre Study, 1983] but the words "physical activity" or "exercise" are not mentioned.

Bogardus et al [in press], in our laboratory, have compared the effect of a regimen of dietary therapy, including caloric intake of 450 kcal/m² and carbohydrate content of 60% with added fiber, in eight patients affected by NIDDM or glucose intolerance with a similar group of 10 who in addition took part in a program of physical training three times a week. This included stretching exercises, weight lifting, and anaerobic exercise sufficient to increase the VO_2 max 13%. There was no measureable change in body composition. Oral glucose tolerance was significantly improved in both groups. By means of the euglycemic hyperinsulinemic clamp procedure combined with indirect calorimetry and with measurement of splanchnic glucose production by dilution of 6,6-dideuteroglucose it was possible to show that the improvement in tolerance was accomplished in both groups by increasing the sensitivity of the liver to insulin so that the output of glucose was reduced. But, in addition, in the group with added exercise there was an improvement in the ability to dispose of glucose by nonoxidative routes, presumably by storage as glycogen. The exercised group also had a 30% increase in ability to dispose of glucose under the stimulus of insulin. This was considered a more physiologic response than that achieved through dietary restriction alone. The exercised participants appeared to achieve a sense of well-being that was definite but difficult to measure.

Impaired Adaptive Thermogenesis in Obesity and in NIDDM

It would be of advantage for animals and humans having difficulty obtaining adequate protein, minerals, or other constituents from food of poor quality to be able to retain the essential nutrients and to dispose of the excess calories in an inefficient manner, thus protecting against what might be a fatal obesity [Sims, 1976]. Such a concept was advanced many years ago, by the Germans Voit [1881] and Rubner [1902], but it has mainly been in disfavor since then. In our studies of experimental obesity marked variations in individual ability to gain weight were found [Sims, 1976], and most studies since then have shown an increase in resting metabolic rate of approximately 10% with overfeeding. In animals, overeating protein-deficient diets or "cafeteria" diets leads to an adaptive increase in thermogenesis. There has been defined a major role of brown fat in such caloric wasting. Other possible mechanisms of adaptive thermogenesis are futile cycling of substrate or change in cellular ion pumping [Danforth and Sims, 1983].

Rats given a cafeteria diet vary in their efficiency of weight gain. Some have an apparent adaptive thermogenesis or inefficiency of weight gain while over-feeding. Cunningham et al [1983] have found that rats that develop abnormal intravenous glucose tolerance during cafeteria feeding gain weight more efficiently than those with normal glucose tolerance. This finding is consistent with those in our laboratory by Ravussin et al [1983]. Indirect calorimetry was used to estimate the resting metabolic rate and route of disposal of substrate in normals, obese subjects without glucose intolerance, and in obese patients with glucose intolerance or Type II diabetes. A reduction in the thermogenic response to the insulin and glucose was found in the obese in contrast to the normals, and a considerably greater reduction was found in those with diabetes. The increased energy expenditure correlated with but was not entirely accounted for by glucose storage. The implication of the rat and human studies is that, as obesity and carbohydrate intolerance increase, weight gain becomes more efficient. This can form the basis of a vicious cycle in which increasing weight gain in turn leads to a greater efficiency of gain.

Enhanced Thermogenesis From Eating Plus Exercise and Effect of Obesity

Some very recent work indicates that the thermic response to exercise can be markedly affected by a preceding meal or meals. Obarzanek and Levitsky [1983] have submitted a preliminary report that subjects who overeat for a single day have a two-fold increase on the next day in the thermic response to treadmill exercise following a meal, whereas the resting metabolic rate and the thermic effect of the meal or the exercise separately was not affected. Segal and Gutin [1983] measured the thermic effect of food (910 kcal), of treadmill exercise, and of the two combined in lean and obese women. The workload was adjusted to the physical capacity of the subjects. While the thermic effect of the food was similar at rest for the lean and the obese, eating before the exercise increased the exercise metabolic rate by 11% in the lean but only by 4% in the obese. Exercise potentiated the thermic effect of food 2.5-fold in the lean, but only 1.01 times in the obese. The authors point out that exercise and eating stimulate metabolic cycles differently and that the net result of combining the two may be an amplification of the neural and hormonal responses to the separate stimuli of food and exercise. These two studies indicate that future attention must be given to the interrelation between eating and exercise, and they are also consistent with previous work suggesting that the obese are less sensitive to thermogenic hormones [Danforth and Sims, 1983].

The Burden of Guilt of the Susceptible

It is apparent from what has been discussed that there are subgroups of the population who are particularly susceptible to developing diabetes or hypertension and their cardiovascular complications when exposed to an abundance of food without the necessity to work for it physically. It is ironic that those people who have suffered the most from periodic famine and malnutrition now are those who suffer the most from exposure to relative affluence or to the Westernized structure of society. It is also apparent that these subgroups are subject to strong hormonal and metabolic forces and entrapping vicious cycles that make for perpetuation of their metabolic defects. These forces make maintenance of normal weight and activity more difficult than any lean person can comprehend. Such people are discriminated against because of their physical handicaps and have self-esteem damaged by repeated failures to maintain normal weight. It is easy to attach a label of laziness and gluttony, but to do so merely adds a burden of guilt to those already burdened.

Common Denominators of Obesity, NIDDM, and Hypertension

An association of hypertension and obesity has long been noted [Chiang and Perlman, 1969]. The interrelationships of these two conditions were first considered in detail at the first meeting on this subject, which was held in Florence only 3 years ago as a satellite meeting of the International Congress of Obesity. It is beyond the scope of this review to describe the suggested interrelationships in detail, but the reader is referred to the report of that meeting [Berchtold et al, 1981], and to other reviews and symposia [Sims and Berchtold, 1982]. A few general statements can be made. Patients with mild to moderate "essential" hypertension are in general significantly overweight and thus resistant to insulin and are thus hyperinsulinemic. At least in acute experiments, insulin causes renal sodium retention. Overeating per se both promotes hyperinsulinemia and increases the turnover of norepinephrine. Since catecholamines also can promote sodium retention this may be a contributor to hypertension. Dietary restriction and weight loss, even without restriction of sodium intake, can bring about a reduction in blood pressure. Physical training can also lower blood pressure, particularly in those who are hyperinsulinemic and hyperlipidemic.

WHAT CAN BE DONE TO COUNTER THE EPIDEMIC?

The problems of overnutrition must be recognized along with these of undernutrition. It must be recognized that a segment of any population cannot be expected to adapt to overnutrition and physical inactivity without incurring the penalties of obesity, NIDDM, and cardiovascular disease.

Perhaps these problems of overabundance may be relatively short-lived in the perspective of human history if the rate of population growth that has been predicted for the coming decades is realized and shortage of food becomes a more critical factor throughout the world. Then the tables may again be turned and those with the most developed mechanisms for conservation of energy will come into their own! In the interval, however, the problems associated with overabundance and inactivity must be dealt with. Clearly a variety of socioeconomic and environmental factors combine to bring about the increase in obesity, NIDDM, and their complications in certain areas of the hemisphere. Many of these are at least partially beyond the control both of individuals and of their policy makers. These factors include:

A shift of the population from rural, more physically demanding occupations and way of life to a less physically demanding urban way of life.

The gulf in many areas between the affluent and those with grinding poverty, with the affluent suffering from the overabundance.

An increase in money available to buy food in the form of petrodollars, tourist dollars, or the proceeds of a resurgence of local industry. This is combined with a shift from the use of native-grown, more complete foods to the use of convenience foods, often supplied by foreign international corporations.

Frequently, however, as in the United States, obesity may be prominent in the poorer economic groups. This is particularly true among black women [Sims, 1980]. Here boredom and discouragement may be playing a role.

With such a constellation of causes, to name only a few, it is obvious that no single measure can remedy a complex situation. As a matter of policy, perhaps some measures can be directed toward improving local agriculture and toward modifying economic forces. Probably the most effective agent will prove to be public education directed toward those most at risk and toward those who furnish their health care. The feasibility of undertaking efforts through the news media and by individual instruction of families has been shown in three relatively advanced communities in California by Farquahar et al [1977]. It is possible that such efforts could be cost-effective in other areas. It seems likely that measures to increase the level of physical activity in those at risk will be more effective than admonitions simply to reduce intake of food.

Admittedly, there is great difficulty in helping people to modify their life styles, and some hold that the effort is futile. Such, however, may be self-fulfilling prophesies, and a more positive approach is required. The Chicago study mentioned previously gives some encouragement. Psychologists and those concerned with more physiologic forms of intervention are developing new techniques [Martin and Dubbert, 1982; Dishman, 1982]. A coordinated approach is required by policy makers, educators, physicians, and other health professionals aided by those concerned with developing techniques for successful intervention.

SUMMARY

In some of the more developed areas of this hemisphere obesity and diabetes are endemic; in other regions there is an increase of epidemic proportions. The problems of overnutrition often occur in regions in which undernutrition is also a major problem. A segment of the population is genetically susceptible to the adverse effects of overnutrition and underexertion. Those who have become best adapted to the stress of caloric undernutrition may be the most susceptible.

ACKNOWLEDGMENTS

Supported in part by US Public Health Service grants GCRC RR-109 (Clinical Research Center) and AM 10254 (Dr. Sims).

REFERENCES

Albrink MJ, Meigs JW (1965): The relationship between serum triglycerides and skinfold thickness in obese subjects. Ann NY Acad Sci 131:673.

Ashwell M, Chinn S, Stalley S, Garrow JS (1978): Female fat distribution – A photographic and cellularity study. Int J Obes 2:289–302.

Bennett PH, Rushforth NB, Miller M, Lecompte PM (1976): Epidemiologic studies of diabetes in the Pima Indians. Recent Prog Hormone Res 32:333–376.

Berchtold P, Sims EAH, Brandau K (eds) (1981): Proceedings of a Symposium on Obesity and Hypertension. Int J Obes 5(Suppl 1):1–188.

Berglund B, Wajngot A, Efendic S (1980): The effect of physical training in young insulin dependent diabetics. Curr Prob Clin Biochem 11:176–178.

Berglund B, Wajngot A, Efendic S (1981): Decreased physical working capacity as an additional factor in the pathogenesis of maturity-onset diabetes. In Berger M, Christacopoulos P, Wahren J (eds): "Diabetes and Exercise." Bern: Hans Huber.

Björntorp P, Dejounge D, Söström L (1970): The effect of physical training on insulin production in obesity. Metabolism 19:631.

Bogardus C, Ravussin E, Robbins DC, Wolfe RR, Horton ES, Sims EAH (in press): Effects of physical training and diet therapy on carbohydrate metabolism in patients with glucose intolerance and non-insulin-dependent diabetes mellitus. Diabetes.

Chiang BN, Perlman LU, Epstein F (1969): Overweight and hypertension: A review. Circulation 39:403.

Cruz-Vidal M, Costas R, Garcia-Palmieri G, Sorlie PD, Hertzmark E (1979): Factors related to diabetes mellitus in Puerto Rican man. Diabetes 28:300–307.

Cunningham J, Calles J, Eisikowitz L, Zawlich W, Felig P (1983): Increased efficiency of weight gain and altered cellularity of brown adipose tissue in rats with impaired glucose tolerance during overfeeding. (Submitted for publication).

Danforth E Jr, Sims EAH (1983): Thermic effect of overfeeding: Role of thyroid hormones, catecholamines and insulin resistance. In Angel A, Hollander CH, Ronchari DAK (eds): "The Adipose Cell and Obesity: Cellular and Molecular Mechanisms." New York: Raven, pp 271–282.

Dishman RK (1982): Compliance/adherence in health-related exercise. Health Psychol 3:237–267.

Evans DJ, Hoffmann RG, Kalkhoff RK, Kissebah AH (1983): Relationship of androgneic activity to body fat topography, fat cell morphology, and metabolic aberrations in premenopausal women. J Clin Endocrinol Metab 57:304–310.

Farquhar JW, Wood PD, Breitrose H, Haskell WL, Meyer AJ, Maccoby N, Alexander JK, Brown BW, McClister AL, Nash JD, Stern MP (1977): Community education for cardiovascular health. Lancet 1:1192–1195.

Gwinup G (1975): Effect of exercise alone on the weight of obese women. Arch Intern Med 135: 676-680.

Howard BY, Savage PJ, Nagulesparan M, Bennion LJ, Unger RH, Bennett PH (1979): Evidence for marked sensitivity to the antilipolytic action of insulin in obese maturity-onset diabetics. Metabolism 28:744-750.

Kawate R, Yamakido M, Nishimoto Y, Bennett PH, Hamman RF, Knowler WC (1979): Diabetes mellitus and its vascular complications in Japanese migrants on the island of Hawaii. Diab Care 2:161-170.

Kemmer FW, Berger M (1983): Exercise and diabetes mellitus: Physical activity as a part of daily life and its role in the treatment of diabetic patients. Int J Sports Med 4:77-88.

Kissebah AH, Vydelingum N, Murray DJ, Evans DJ, Hartz AJ, Kalkoff RK, Adams PW (1982): Relation of body fat distribution to metabolic consequences of obesity. J Clin Endocrinol Metab 54:254-260.

Leon AS, Conrad J, Hunninghake DB, Serfass R (1979): Effects of a vigorous walking program on body composition, and carbohydrate and lipid metabolism of obese young men. Am J Clin Nutr 33:1776-1787.

Martin JE, Dubbert PM (1982): Exercise applications and promotion in behavioral medicine. Current status and future directions. J Consulting Clin Psychol 30(6):1004-1016.

McGlashan ND (1982): Causes of death in 10 English-speaking Caribbean countries and territories. Bull Pan-Am Health Org 16:212-223.

Multi-Centre Study (1983): UK prospective study of therapies of maturity-onset diabetes. I. Effect of diet, sulphonylurea, insulin or biguanide therapy on fasting plasma glucose and body weight over one year. Diabetologia 24:404-411.

National Diabetes Data Group (1979): Classification and diagnosis of diabetes mellitus and other categories of glucose intolerance. Diabetes 28:1039-1057.

Obarzanek E, Levitsky D (1983): One day of overeating enhances the thermogenic effect of exercise. Fed Proc 42:1189.

Olefsky JM, Kolterman OG (1981): Mechanisms of insulin resistance in obesity and non-insulin-dependent (type II) diabetes. Am J Med 70:151-168.

Owerbach D, Johansen K, Billesbolle P, Poulsen S, Schroll M, Nerup J (1982): Possible association between DNA sequences flanking the insulin gene and atherosclerosis. Lancet 2:1291-1294.

Owerbach D, Thomsen B, Johansen K, Lamm LU, Nerup J (1983): DNA insertion sequences near the insulin gene are not associated with maturity-onset diabetes of young people. Diabetes 25:18-20.

PAHO (1980): "Health Conditions in the Americas 1977-1980. Pan American Health Organization, World Health Organization. Scientific Publication Number 427.

Ravussin E, Bogardus C, Schwartz RS, Robbins DC, Wolfe RR, Horton ES, Danforth E, Sims EAH (1983): Thermic effect of infused glucose and insulin in man: Decreased response with increased insulin resistance in obesity and non-insulin-dependent diabetes mellitus. J Clin Invest (in press).

Rizza RA, Mandarino LJ, Gerisch JE (1981): Mechanisms of insulin resistance in man. Assessment using the insulin dose-response curve in conjunction with insulin-receptor binding. Am J Med 70:169-176.

Rosenthal M, Haskell WL, Solomon R, Widstrom A, Reaven GM (1983): Demonstration of a relationship between level of physical training and insulin-stimulated glucose utilization in normal humans. Diabetes 32:408-411.

Rotwein P, Chirgwain JL, Province M, Knowler W, Pettitt D, Cordell B, Goodman H, Permutt MA (1983): Polymorphism in the 5' flanking region of human insulin gene: A genetic marker for non-insulin-dependent diabetes. New Engl J Med 308:65-67.

Rubner M (1902): "Die Gesetze der Energie Verbrauchs bei die Ernährung." Translation by Joy RJT. Natick, MA: US Army Research Institute of Environmental Medicine, 1968.

Segal K, Gutin B (1983): Thermic effects of food and exercise in lean and obese women. Metabolism 32:581–589.

Serjeantson SW, Owerbach D, Zimmet P, Nerup J, Thoma K (1983): Genetics of diabetes in Nauru: Effects of foreign admixture. HLA antigens and the insulin-gene-linked polymorphism. Diabetes 25:13–17.

Sims EAH (1976): Experimental obesity, dietary induced thermogenesis and their clinical implications. J Clin Endocrinol Metab 5:377–396.

Sims EAH (1979): Definitions, criteria, and prevalence of obesity. In Bray G (ed): "Obesity in America." NIH Publication, No. 79-359.

Sims EAH, Berchtold P (1982): Hypertension and obesity: Mechanisms and management. J Am Med Assoc 247:49–52.

Sims EAH, Danforth E Jr, Horton ES, Bray GA, Glennon JA, Salans LB (1973): Endocrine and metabolic effects of experimental obesity in man. Recent Prog Hormone Res 29:457–496.

Stamler J, Forino E, Mojennier LM, Hall Y, Moss D, Stamler R (1980): Prevention and control of hypertension by nutritional-hygienic means: Long-term experience of the Chicago coronary prevention evaluation program. JAMA 243:1819.

Tattersall RB, Pike DA (1972): Diabetes in identical twins. Lancet 2:1120–1124.

Vague J, Boyer J, Jubelin J, Nicolino C, Pinto C (1969): Adipomuscular ratio in human subjects. In Vague J (ed): "Physiopathology of Adipose Tissue." Amsterdam: Excerpta Medica, pp 363–386.

Voit C (1881): Physiologie des Stoffwechsels. Hermanns Handb Physiol 6:209.

Vranic M, Horvath S, Wahren J (1978): Conference on diabetes and exercise. Proceedings of a conference on diabetes and exercise. California, March 13–17, 1978.

Vranic M, Horvath S, Wahren J (eds) (1978b): Proceedings of a conference on diabetes and exercise. Diabetes 28(Suppl 1):1–113.

Weir GC (1982): Non-insulin-dependent diabetes mellitus: Interplay between β-cell inadequacy and insulin resistance. Am J Med 73:461–464.

Weir GC, Bonner-Weir S (1982): Insulin secretion after partial pancreatecomy: Evidence for β-cell "Exhaustion." Diabetes 31:35A.

West KM (1978): "Epidemiology of diabetes and its vascular lesions." New York: Elsevier North-Holland, pp 1–579.

Zimmet P (1982): Type 2 (non-insulin-dependent) diabetes — An epidemiological overview. Diabetologia 22:399–411.

Zimmet P, Seluka A, Collins J, Currie P, Wicking J, Deboer W (1977): Diabetes mellitus in an urbanized isolated Polynesian population. The Funafuti survey. Diabetes 26:1101–1108.

Malnutrition: Determinants and Consequences, pages 165–178
© 1984 Alan R. Liss, Inc., 150 Fifth Avenue, New York, NY 10011

Body Composition and Physical Work Capacity in Undernutrition

M. Barac-Nieto

Department of Physiology, University of Rochester, Rochester, New York 14642 and Universidad del Valle, Cali, Colombia

This presentation deals with studies carried out a few years ago on the changes in body composition [Barac-Nieto et al, 1978b, 1979] and physical work capacity [Barac-Nieto et al, 1978a, 1980] that occur in chronically undernourished adult males.* The studies were carried out in 51 adult males, indigenous or *mestizos*, rural dwellers in the northern part of the state of Cauca, Colombia. All were unemployed general farmworkers from a depressed socioeconomic region. Social workers from the university established contacts, informed the subjects thoroughly of the purpose, methods, and procedures to be employed, and obtained written informed consent in each case [Barac-Nieto et al, 1978b].

The subjects were classified into three groups according to the severity of the nutritional compromise: mild (M), intermediate (I), and severe (S) [Barac-Nieto et al, 1978b]. The groups of severely undernourished subjects underwent nutritional repletion [Barac-Nieto et al, 1979], first for 45 days with an adequate caloric (2,240 kcal/day), low-protein (28 gm/day) diet, then for 74 days with an isocaloric, high-protein (100 gm/day) diet. The repletion diets contained 30% of the calories as fat and supplied the Recommended Dietary Allowances (National Academy of Sciences/National Research Council) of minerals and vitamins. The protein content was increased at the expense of the

---

*The studies were done at the Exercise Laboratory and the Metabolic Unit at the University Hospital at the Universidad del Valle, Cali, Colombia in collaboration with Dr. G.B. Spurr and M. Maksud from the Medical College of Wisconsin, Drs. H. Lotero, H. Dahners, and O. Bolanos from the Universidad del Valle, and with the cooperation of the nursing and technical staff at the Universidad del Valle.

carbohydrate content of the diet. Most (90%) of the protein was of vegetable origin but of high biological value (Colombia harina).

Figure 1 illustrates the means of several anthropometric variables in the three groups. Data obtained during nutritional repletion of the severely malnourished group are also shown. The group with mild nutritional compromise was somewhat younger than the others. All groups had similar heights. However, the body weight and skinfolds decreased with increasing severity of the nutritioinal compromise: A 10 kg body weight difference occurred between groups M and S. Upon repletion, the body weights in group S increased by an average of 10 kg. The skinfolds also increased upon repletion with the high-protein diet.

Figure 2 illustrates the means of some biochemical and metabolic variables in the various groups and upon repletion of group S. Serum albumin levels decreased with the severity of the nutritional compromise, reaching a mean value of 1.9 gm% in group S. Upon repletion with the high-protein diet the serum albumin levels increased to 3.8 gm%. Daily urinary creatinine excretion was

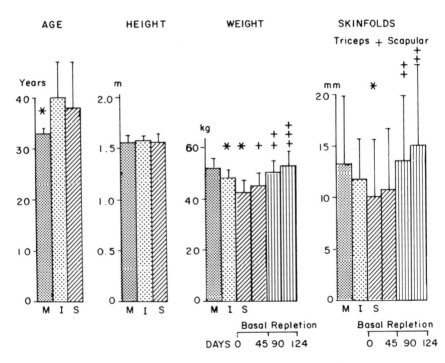

Fig. 1.   Anthropometry in adult males with mild (M), intermediate (I), or severe (S) nutritional compromise and during nutritional repletion with adequate calories (basal) and adequate protein (repletion).

also decreased in proportion to the severity of the nutritional compromise and only increased upon dietary repletion with the high-protein diet.

The body composition of the several groups was assessed 1) by measurements of the volume of distribution of tritiated water and thiocyanate, as indexes of the total and extracellular fluid volumes respectively, 2) by measurements of the daily creatinine excretion, an index of muscle mass, and 3) by the changes in N_2 balance with repletion, as an index of the changes in cellular proteins. Figure 3 summarizes the data.

While the extracellular water was unchanged with nutritional compromise or repletion, it increased when expressed as percentage of body weight, as the

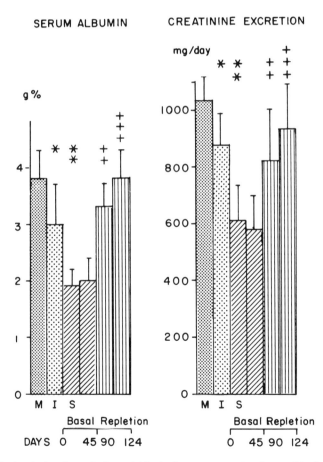

Fig. 2.   Biochemical and metabolic variables in threee groups of undernourished adult males and during nutritional repletion.

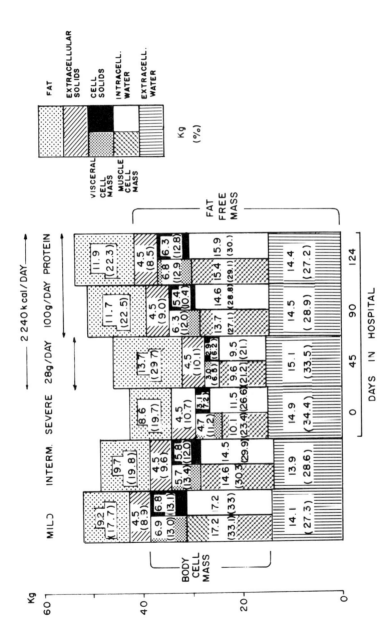

Fig. 3. Body composition in undernutrition and during nutritional repletion.

latter decreased with increasing nutritional compromise. Percentage extracellular water decreased as body weight increased with nutritional repletion.

By contrast, total body water decreased with increasing nutritional compromise and increased upon repletion, indicating that changes in intracellular water were occurring. The deficit in cell water in the severely undernourished group (about 6 kg) accounted for a large fraction of their deficit in body weight ($\cong 10$ kg). Upon repletion, increases in intracellular water ($+6$ kg) accounted also for most of the increase in body weight.

Cell solids and body cell mass (the sum of cell solids and intracellular water) were estimated in groups M, I, and at the end of the nutritional repletion period by assuming a constant cell hydration. In group S, and at the intermediate stages of repletion, cell solids were estimated from the measured N_2 balance (and hence from the average amount of protein retained per day during each stage of repletion). A deficit of 3.5 kg in cell solids occurred in group S. This deficit was corrected upon repletion with a high-protein diet. Thus, the deficit in body cell mass with nutritional compromise and its changes during repletion accounted for most of the changes in body weight observed in these subjects.

In group S, a significant increase in cell hydration (80% cell water) was estimated to occur. This increased cell hydration decreased to 76% with caloric repletion for 45 days and then to 71% upon repletion with a high-protein diet for 74 days.

Muscle mass, estimated from the daily creatinine excretion, represented 70% of the body cell mass at all stages of nutritional compromise and this proportion did not change upon nutritional repletion. The low creatinine excretion/intracellular water ratio observed in group S was accounted for by the increase in cell hydration observed in this group.

With increasing nutritional compromise muscle cells and nonmuscle cells in the body both were decreased and their relative proportions in the body cell mass were not markedly different at the different stages of undernutrition or during nutritional repletion. Thus, there was no evidence of specific wastage of muscle cells over that of other cells in the body with nutritional deprivation.

The extracellular solids, mostly skeletal components, were assumed to be a function of the height of the subjects and to be independent of nutritional status. Skeletal solids were also assumed to be invariant during the 4-month repletion period. Thus the percentage extracellular solids increased with decreasing body weight and decreased as body weight was restored by nutritional repletion.

Finally, body fat was lower by 0.6–1.1 kg in group S, representing, however, $\cong 20\%$ of their diminished body weights. Body fat increased markedly ($+5$ kg) with provision of an adequate caloric intake, while a low-protein diet was maintained, for 45 days. With subsequent protein repletion, the body fat stores did not vary significantly or they slightly decreased. Thus, when limited by the protein intake, an increase in the caloric intake resulted mostly in an increase in the body fat stores with little change in the body cell mass. Subsequent provision of a high-protein diet for 74 days resulted in a large increment in the body cell mass with little further change in the body fat stores. Thus the disposition of calories, that is, their storage or their use in growth and activity, was dependent on the simultaneous protein intake. A relative state of obesity ($\cong 30\%$ fat) can occur in undernourished subjects provided with adequate calories and a limited protein intake.

Oxygen consumption during maximal exercise was measured with a continuous treadmill test protocol of progressive intensity and the open-circuit technique for determinations of expired volumes and expired gas compositions [Barac-Nieto et al, 1978a, 1980]. Figure 4 illustrates the means of the data obtained. $\dot{V}O_{2\,max}$ was about 2.4 liters/min in group M and decreased with the severity of the nutritional compromise, reaching a mean value of about 1 liter/min in group S. Upon administration of adequate calories with maintenance of a low-protein diet for 45 days, $\dot{V}O_{2\,max}$ was unchanged. Repletion with 100 gm protein per day resulted in a progressive increase in the $\dot{V}O_{2\,max}$ to $\cong 1.8$ liters/min after 74 days on the high-protein diet. The difference in $\dot{V}O_{2\,max}$ between groups M and S was 52%. This difference partially decreased upon protein repletion. This effect of repletion occurred without changes in physical activity, which remained minimal throughout the stay of the subjects in the hospital ward.

The decrease in $\dot{V}O_{2\,max}$ with increasing severity of the nutritional compromise and its reversal upon protein repletion persisted when expressed per unit of body weight (Fig. 4, second panel), although the differences between groups were somewhat smaller in magnitude. This indicates that changes in body composition and not only in body mass profoundly influence the $\dot{V}O_{2\,max}$ in undernourished subjects. When normalized for the body cell mass, the differences in maximal O_2 consumption between groups were much reduced but still statistically significant. This decrease in the O_2-consuming capacity per unit of body cell mass could be accounted for, in part, by the increase in cell hydration found to occur in group S.

Finally, when normalized per unit of muscle cell mass (Fig. 4, third panel), the difference in $\dot{V}O_{2\,max}$ between groups M and S was only 18% but it was statistically significant. This indicates that most of the difference in absolute $\dot{V}O_{2\,max}$ between the groups was due to differences in the mass of muscle cells in the body. Only about 15% of the difference in $\dot{V}O_{2\,max}$ between groups M and S was accounted for by the decrease in the O_2 consumption capacity of the muscle cells themselves. This decrease in $\dot{V}O_{2\,max}$ per unit of muscle cell mass could be due to limiting O_2 delivery or to a decrease in the oxidative capacity of the muscle cells.

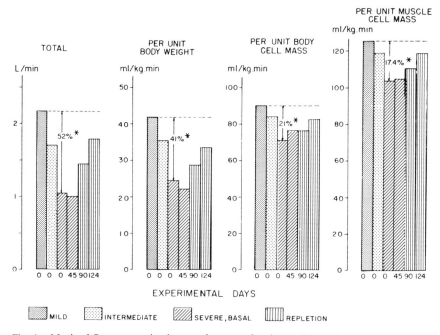

Fig. 4. Maximal O_2 consumption in several groups of undernourished adult males and during nutritional repletion.

The consequences of the reduction in $\dot{V}O_{2\ max}$ in undernutrition are illustrated in Figure 5. When working at submaximal loads representing an O_2 cost of 0.84 liter/min, the aerobic effort calculated as the ratio of the O_2 cost to the O_2 consuming capacity increased from 40% to 50% and to 80% of $\dot{V}O_{2\ max}$ with increasing severity of nutritional compromise. The percentage effort required to work at this level of O_2 consumption increased as the O_2 consumption capacity was reduced with nutritional compromise. Upon repletion with the high protein diet, the percentage effort at a $\dot{V}O_{2\ max}$ of 0.84 liter/min decreased progressively towards the value found in group M.

These increased efforts were also reflected in the heart rate responses to a submaximal load [Spurr et al, 1979] as shown in Figure 6. When working at submaximal loads representing an O_2 cost of 0.75 liter/min, the heart rate response to the workloads increased progressively with increasing severity of the nutritional compromise and decreased during protein repletion. The cardiovascular stress was progressively higher, the larger the reductions in O_2 consuming capacity and thus the larger the impingement of the submaximal workloads on the aerobic reserves of the subjects.

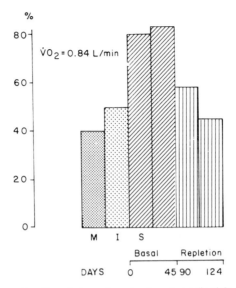

Fig. 5. Percentage aerobic effort during submaximal work at a fixed O_2 cost in several groups of undernourished adult males and during nutritional repletion.

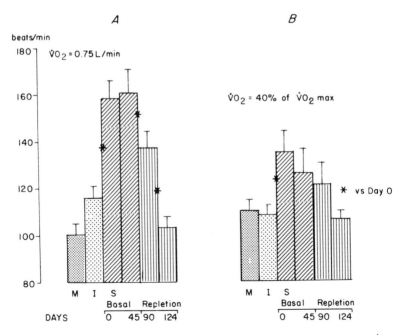

Fig. 6. Heart rates during exercise at a fixed O_2 cost (A) and at a fixed aerobic effort ($\dot{V}O_{2\,max}$) (B) in several groups of undernourished adult males and during nutritional repletion.

Also illustrated in Figure 6 (panel B) are the heart rate responses to a given effort level. At the same level of aerobic effort, in this case 40% of $\dot{V}O_{2\,max}$, the heart rate responses in groups M and I were similar. However, that in group S was significantly higher and returned towards normal upon dietary repletion. This higher cardiovascular stress in group S might reflect an adaptive response to the lower O_2-carrying capacity of blood in group S, which had a mean blood hemoglobin concentration of 10 gm%. Indeed, a significant negative correlation (Fig. 7) was found between the heart rate at 40% $\dot{V}O_{2\,max}$ and the blood hemoglobin concentration in the various groups and at the various stages of nutritional repletion. The responses of 88 gainfully employed, nutritionally normal, Colombian agricultural workers is also included here [Barac-Nieto et al, 1978a; Spurr et al, 1979]. Another important consequence of the reduced O_2-consuming capacity of the undernourished subjects is illustrated in Figure 8. In group M at workloads requiring an O_2 consumption of 0.84 liter/min, the maximal endurance (right panel) was 6.5 hr (estimated by exponential extrapolation of endurances measured at $\cong$ 80% and $\cong$ 90% loads) and was found to represent a 40% aerobic effort (left panel). In group I the same rate

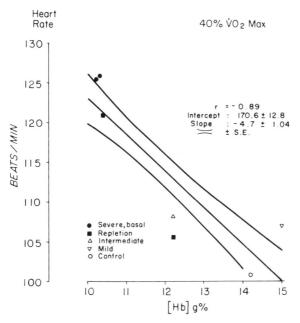

Fig. 7. Correlation between blood hemoglobin concentration and heart rate response during submaximal exercise at a fixed aerobic effort (40% of $\dot{V}O_{2\,max}$) in the various groups of undernourished adult males and during nutritional repletion.

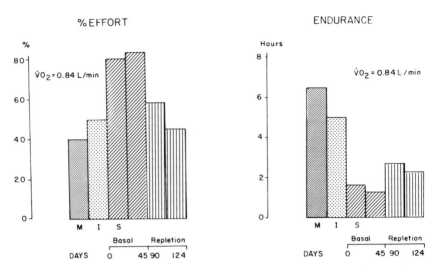

Fig. 8. Maximal endurance times and aerobic efforts during exercise at a fixed O_2 cost in several groups of undernourished adult males and during nutritional repletion.

of O_2 consumption represented a 50% effort (left) and could be endured for 5 hr (right). In group S, the same rate of O_2 consumption during submaximal work represented an 80% effort (left) and could be endured for only 1.5 hr (right). Thus, as the aerobic reserve decreased with nutritional compromise, a given rate of O_2 consumption could be endured for shorter and shorter times as the effort required increased progressively. Upon repletion, a partial and incomplete reversal of these changes occurred. After 45 days of repletion with a high-protein diet, work at 0.84 liter/min of O_2 consumption represented a 60% effort (left) and could be endured for 2.5 hr (right). After 74 days of protein repletion, the same rate of O_2 consumption during work represented a 45% effort (left) but could be endured only for a little over 2 hr (right). Thus a pronounced decrease in endurance occurred upon repletion. This effect of protein repletion on the endurance time can be better appreciated by comparing the endurance times at given level of aerobic effort (Fig. 9). Endurance at 80% aerobic effort decreased from about 97 min in groups M, I, and S, to about 42 min by the end of protein repletion of subjects in group S. This decrease in endurance was related to the nature of the repletion regimen rather than to differences in nutritional status: No differences in endurance at 80% effort were found between groups M, I, and S. A decrease in endurance occurred upon repletion of group S, which could be related to the prolonged inactivity of the subjects in this group during repletion [Saltin et al, 1968] or to diminished glycogen stores [Bergstrom et al, 1967] in the newly rebuilt muscles

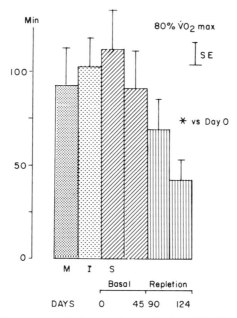

Fig. 9.   Maximal endurance times during exercise at a fixed aerobic effort (80% of $\dot{V}O_{2\ max}$) in several groups of undernourished adult males and during nutritional repletion.

of the repleted subjects. Thus, endurance at a given percentage effort can be drastically reduced by a repletion regimen such as that employed in our study. Similar decreases in endurance have been observed in experimental animals undergoing protein repletion [Hansen-Smith et al, 1977].

Another important variable that could be altered by undernutrition is the O_2 cost of a given task or its inverse, the gross work efficiency [Spurr et al, 1979]. We measured the O_2 cost of treadmill walking at various grades in each subject. The external work at each grade was calculated in kilograms-meters (kgm) per minute and related to the O_2 consumption measured at submaximal workloads. The O_2 cost of treadmill walking at 250 kgm/min was then estimated for each subject. The means for the several groups are illustrated in Figure 10.

The O_2 cost of treadmill walking at 250 kgm/min decreased from about 1 liter/min in group M to about 0.8 liter/min in group S and increased toward the value in group M upon protein repletion of the severely undernourished subject. A 1.16-fold increase in the efficiency of body translation upon walking on the treadmill on a grade was evident in group S. This increase in efficiency during body lifting and translation probably relates to the lower body mass present in the severely undernourished subjects.

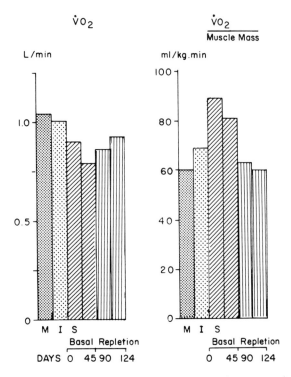

Fig. 10. O_2 cost at a fixed work load (250 kgm/min) during exercise on a treadmill in various groups of undernourished adult males and during nutritional repletion: Absolute values and normalization per unit of muscle cell mass.

When the O_2 cost to treadmill walking at 250 kgm/min is expressed per kilogram of muscle cell mass (Fig. 10, right), a different picture is observed. The O_2 cost per kilogram of muscle increases with increasing severity of nutritional compromise and decreases progressively with protein repletion. Thus, in spite of the lowered O_2 cost of the work performed, the decrease in muscle mass that occurs in the undernourished subjects is much greater than the decrease in the O_2 cost of work. At a given workload the O_2 consumption per unit of muscle mass increases significantly during protein calorie deficiencies. Indeed, the same amount of work has to be done with a smaller mass of muscle tissue. Thus, each unit of muscle has to generate more energy in spite of the increase in work efficiency that occurs in the undernourished subjects.

Thus, at a given workload, impingement on the reduced O_2-consuming capacity of muscle occurs at a higher level in the undernourished subjects, leading to an increase in aerobic effort and to a decrease in endurance that more

CAPACITY x EFFORT x EFFICIENCY x ENDURANCE = PRODUCTIVITY

	$\left(\dfrac{kcal}{min}\right)$	x	(%)	x	$\left(\dfrac{kcal}{kcal}\right)$	x	(min)	=	kcal	%
C	13.13	x	0.32	x	0.25	x	480	=	504	100
S	13.13 (0.4)	x	0.80	x	0.25 (1.16)	x	90	=	110	22
I	13.13 (0.64)	x	0.50	x	0.25 (1.04)	x	300	=	328	65
M	13.13 (0.83)	x	0.40	x	0.25 (1.00)	x	390	=	425	84

Fig. 11. Estimates of work output in control (C), and in mildly (M), intermediately (I), and severely (S) undernourished adult males. See text.

than offsets the small gain in gross work efficiency that occurs with undernutrition as a result of the lower body weight.

Some estimates of the magnitudes of these effects, based on the data derived from the present groups of subjects, are presented in Figure 11.

Physical work productivity is considered a function of 1) capacity, as measured by the maximal O_2 consumption expressed in kcal/min, 2) effort, measured as the percentage of $\dot{V}O_{2\,max}$ employed in a given task, 3) efficiency, measured as the inverse of the O_2 cost of the given task and expressed in kcal of external work per kcal of O_2 consumption, and 4) endurance, measured by the maximal time during which each effort level can be sustained.

Reasonable numbers for each of these variables are presented for a "control" group, derived from data obtained separately in healthy, employed Colombian agricultural workers [Barac-Nieto et al, 1978a; Maksud et al, 1976] and for the three groups with mild, intermediate, and severe nutritional compromise discussed here.

$\dot{V}O_{2\,max}$ and efficiency values in the control group have been modified by factors describing the changes observed to occur with undernutrition of various degrees. Percentage effort and endurance in the various groups are as derived from the data presented previously [Spurr et al, 1977] for normal Colombian agricultural workers (32% effort, 8 hr endurance) and the values presented here for undernourished subjects (group M: 40% effort, 6.5 hr endurance; group I: 50% effort, 5 hr endurance; and group S: 80% effort, 1.5 hr endurance) working at a $\dot{V}O_{2\,max} = 0.84$ liter/min. The work output per day is shown in kcal and in percentage of "control" values. A 15% reduction in work output is indicated for group M, a 35% reduction for group I, and a 78% reduction for group S.

Thus marked decreases in physical work output can occur as a consequence of the changes in body mass and body composition, and of the possible changes in muscle oxidative capacity that occur in undernutrition.

REFERENCES

Barac-Nieto M, Spurr GB, Maksud MG, Lotero H (1978a): Aerobic work capacity in chronically undernourished adult males. J Appl Physiol 44:209–215.

Barac-Nieto M, Spurr GB, Lotero H, Maksud MG (1978b): Body composition in chronic undernutrition. Am J Clin Nutr 31:23–40.

Barac-Nieto M, Spurr GB, Lotero H, Maksud MG, Dahners HW (1979): Body composition during nutritional repletion of severely undernourished men. Am J Clin Nutr 32:981–991.

Barac-Nieto M, Spurr GB, Dahners HW, Maksud MG (1980): Aerobic work capacity and endurance during nutritional repletion of severely undernourished men. Am J Clin Nutr 33: 2268–2275.

Bergstrom J, Hermansen L, Hultman E, Saltin BA (1967): Diet, muscle glycogen and physical performance. Acta Physiol Scand 71:140–150.

Hansen-Smith FM, Maksud MG, Van Horn DL (1977): Influence of chronic undernutrition on oxygen consumption of rats during exercise. Growth 41:115–121.

Maksud MG, Spurr GB, Barac-Nieto M (1976): The aerobic power of several groups of laborers in Colombia and the United States. Eur J Apl Physiol 35:173–182.

Saltin B, Blomqvist G, Mitchell JH, Johnson RL, Wildenthal K, Chapman CB (1968): Responses to exercise after bed rest and after training. Am Heart Assoc Monogr No. 23. Circulation 38, Suppl 7.

Spurr GB, Barac-Nieto M, Maksud MG (1977): Efficiency and daily work effort in sugar cane cutters. Br J Ind Med 34:137–141.

Spurr GB, Barac-Nieto M, Maksud MG (1979): Functional assessment of nutritional status: Heart rate response to submaximal work. Am J Clin Nutr 32:767–778.

Malnutrition: Determinants and Consequences, pages 179–185
© 1984 Alan R. Liss, Inc., 150 Fifth Avenue, New York, NY 10011

Nutrition and Behavior: A Review

Luis A. Ordóñez, PhD
Section of Neurochemistry and Behavior, Instituto de Medicina Experimental,
Universidad Central de Venezuela, Caracas, Venezuela

INTRODUCTION

Evaluation of the effects of nutrition on physiological status and maintenance of desirable body composition and function requires that attention also
be paid to whether nutrients affect behavior and/or mental function.

The Socioeconomic Setting

Whether nutrient intake affects behavior at any given time is a question that
has been explored for many years with ever increasing intensity, and is one to
which we have no clear-cut answer. Nevertheless, the fact that undernutrition
is a common occurrence in several areas of the world makes necessary the
generation of knowledge capable of allowing nutrition specialists to advise
governments on the best policies available to better the health status of their
populations.

As an example, Venezuela, which because of its oil revenues is a middle-of-
the-range country in its per capita income and is not known in particular for its
precarious nutritional or other health parameters, is probably facing several
major policy reorientations owing to its recent financial crisis — reorientations
that may profoundly affect the nutritional status of its population. Furthermore, the health status of the country may be very easily affected, because of
the now precarious socioeconomic situation of the Venezuelans. Between 35%
and 50% of the country's inhabitants live in the lowest socioeconomic group,
level 5 as defined by the Graffar [1956] scale, as compared to Belgium, where
only 8.6% of the population live at this level. Less than 5% of the people in
this Latin/American country are in the two highest socioeconomic levels, as
compared to Belgium, where 25% of the population enjoy such status.

If we remember at this point that Venezuela is an OPEC country and is therefore much better off economically than many underdeveloped countries of the world, we may envision the difficulties presented to the majority of nations in properly feeding their populations. If, furthermore, poor nutritional status affects behavior and/or mental functioning, care must be exercised in the allocation of resources to improve the health status of the population.

The Scientific Setting

On the basis of extrapolations from animal studies, authors have assumed for many years that nutritional insult during maturation causes irreparable brain damage to the human child [Dobbing, 1975], damage that is expressed mainly as mental retardation. However, nutrition is only one among many factors involved in the development of intelligence. Nevertheless, the behavioral adaptations found in the child subjected to malnourishment are extensive enough to impair its social development and, therefore, its mental performance [Chávez and Martínez, 1982]. Better information on these factors as well as on the effects of psychological stimulation is required in order to advise government agencies concerned with the quality of biological development of the population (eg, Intelligence Ministry of Venezuela).

Another very important area of study is in regard to whether, on a minute-to-minute basis, nutrients affect behavior. The finding by Wurtman and Fernstrom [1974] that the composition of the diet may affect brain levels of neurotransmitters suggests that mood and behavior may be affected by what we eat. Despite the many value judgments and cognitive maps already established regarding the issue of nutrition and behavior, researchers must continue to develop studies needed to orient public action on the nutritional status of the general population and on the specific needs of particular groups of individuals. It is the purpose of the present review to help define the problems that ought to be analyzed in this field, particularly from the point of view of developing countries.

EARLY UNDERNUTRITION AND MENTAL DEVELOPMENT

We have already commented that, on the basis of extrapolations from animal studies, authors have assumed for many years that undernutrition during brain development and maturation causes irreparable brain damage to the human child; however, nutrition is only one among many factors involved in the development of a child's intelligence, as seems to be shown by different studies.

Prenatal Nutrition and Psychological Development

Stein et al [1972] found no relation between prenatal exposure to famine and mental performance at age 19. In this study, based on the epidemiological data available on the Dutch famine of 1944–1945, the experience of famine was naturally isolated from other elements of the social environment. The study population, which comprised 120,000 males born during famine, and the males from control cities were evaluated at the time of military induction, leading the authors to conclude that "starvation during pregnancy had no detectable effects on the adult mental performance of surviving male offspring." Furthermore, it was found that "mental performance in surviving adult males from a total population had no clear association with changing levels of mean birth weight in a selected hospital sample of that population." Perhaps the most important finding was that "the association of social class with mental performance was strong."

In general, as shown in the review by Susser [1981] on prenatal nutrition and psychological development, it may be concluded that in the presence of good nutritional and social conditions in the postnatal environment, severe prenatal nutritional deprivation is unlikely to affect cognitive functions in the adult. Furthermore, in the case of overt chronic malnutrition extending into the prenatal period, "the data from existing studies do not exclude the possibility that a harsh social environment is a common cause both of malnutrition and of retarded performance on the usual cognitive measures." However, as Susser [1981] states, "This work on postnatal nutrition taken collectively suggests that under conditions of chronic malnutrition, postnatal nutritional state influences current affective state and somatic growth. Its influence on psychological test performance will be in interaction with the social environment. The data also suggest that diet supplementation improves the affective state and activity of a malnourished mother as well as of the offspring."

Postnatal Nutrition and Psychological Development

Another important study that sheds further light on the problem of nutrition and mental retardation [Koluchová, 1976] reports a follow-up of twin boys who from age 18 months until 7 years had been isolated and cruelly treated, such that on discovery they could barely walk, suffered from rickets, displayed abnormal behavior, and had IQ's in the 40's. When they were between ages 11 and 12 years, their speech was entirely adequate for their age; furthermore, between 12 and 14 years they reached and sustained IQ's of 100 and above. This case of severe deprivation, which began at an early age, shows that damage previously considered to be irreversible can be remedied.

Now I would like to bring your attention to the studies by Chávez and his group (reviewed by Chávez and Martínez [1982]) that illustrate the multiple variables involved in the relationship between nutrition and behavior.

Among many other interesting conclusions that could lead to public policy decisions, these authors advanced the opinion that "to have the child reach a weight of 8 kg in the first eight months of life should be the first objective in any preventive intervention in the field of malnutrition. This is what may be called the 'true birth' of the child; it means passing the barrier between what may be called an extra-uterine fetus before reaching that weight, and a true human being with capacities of its own."

In a study of children in an open-field test, it was observed that the only thing that the undernourished children did was to go toward the mother, cry, and demand to be picked up and taken away. They were afraid of the strange environment, they did not become interested in toys placed in the box, and their movements within the quadrilateral did not carry them beyond the area of the mother. The better-nourished children felt more confident; frequently went toward the toys, picked them up, and carried them to the mother and to the observers; and moved all around the quadrilateral.

Owing to the absence of adequate nutrients for growth, the amount of body mass in children living in environments of critical poverty is extremely limited, and as a consequence of the scarcity of energy intake, these children reduce their activity and their interaction with their environment. This adaptation is, in reality, a strong limiting factor in their potential for human expression.

In their neurological maturation studies, Chávez and Martínez [1982] conclude that moderate malnutrition affects the maturation of the central nervous system very little and in such a way that the children are not clearly abnormal. In another study [Waber et al, 1981], children who received food supplements performed better than those who did not, especially on subtests that primarily evaluated motor skills. The gains achieved in intellectual performance, however, although statistically significant, were still below those found in upper-class children. Thus, the authors stated "although intervention programs clearly benefit the recipients, they may be insufficient to counteract the effects of socioeconomic disparity" between lower- and upper-class children in developing countries.

SHORT-TERM EFFECTS OF FOOD CONSTITUENTS

Beyond the long-term effects of nutrition on human behavior previously referred to, there has recently developed a whole field of study that explores the short-term effects of food constituents on the mood and performance of the individual.

The first evidence that food constituents were capable of altering brain neurotransmitter composition originated in studies demonstrating that ingestion of the amino acid tryptophan elevated brain levels of serotonin [Fernstrom and Wurtman, 1971]. Since then, questions as to whether and, if so, how food and nutrients affect sleep, alertness, memory, pain, appetite, swings in mood, and motor activity are the subject of studies in several laboratories.

The rationale for these studies lies in the fact that several precursors of known brain neurotransmitters are essential nutrients [eg, tryptophan and tyrosine) or are present in low quantities in blood (ie, choline), their entrance into the brain being dependent upon their blood levels or those of other blood components (ie, other amino acids, hormones, etc.). Once in the brain, these nutrients enter the tissue cells and are converted into the specific neurotransmitters at the appropriate neurons and may in turn modulate the activity of these neurons, thus altering the functions in which they intervene. The neurotransmitters characterized by precursor dependence are acetylcholine, the catecholamines (dopamine and norepinephrine), serotonin, histamine, and glycine. Just to mention one example, the behaviors that have been linked to serotoninergic neurotransmission include sleeping, eating, locomotor activity, aggression, and pain sensitivity [Wurtman et al, 1981].

In a recent conference held at the Massachusetts Institute of Technology [Lieberman and Wurtman, 1982] on research strategies for assessing the behavioral effects of foods and nutrients in humans, reports were presented demonstrating "overwhelming evidence that L-tryptophan has a positive effect on sleep [Hartmann, 1982]" and on newborn behavior [Yogman et al, 1982]. Also, tryptophan was shown to increase subjective drowsiness and fatigue, and to decrease pain sensitivity, but unlike many hypnotics, it did not impair sensorimotor performance [Lieberman et al, 1982]. However, the effects of protein and carbohydrate meals on mood and performance were found to be related to age, sex, and time of day when food consumption occurred [Spring et al, 1982].

Although not definitive, the available evidence allows speculation as to whether in the future artificial intervention with food constituents will allow for treatment of certain disorders or for modulation of mood and behavior in large populations.

FINAL CONSIDERATIONS

I would like to conclude by citing two paragraphs from Chávez and Martínez [1982].

"There are two working hypotheses regarding the possibility that moderate malnutrition may be the cause of several problems in the school child and, especially, in the adult. There are those who feel that, after the initial effect of malnutrition, when the organism has achieved homeorrhesis, there is time for correction of the alterations in development, for achieving balance and normality.

On the other hand the majority of researchers believe that at least part of what is lost will not be recovered, depending on the timing, severity, and duration of malnutrition. The discussion is ironic at the present time, because, in poor environments, there is no possibility for improvement. Diet continues to be deficient throughout the rest of the life of those involved. The problem will only be solved when there is an investment of sufficient resources that are really directed toward a solution of the problem."

It has been thought that nutrition plays a fundamental role in brain development and therefore in intelligence. However, intelligence as a biological phenomenon is just a kind of adaptation, a system of behavioral characteristics appropriate to particular ecological niches. Therefore, in interpreting behavioral data obtained from nutritional studies, attention must be paid to value judgments that could favor some interpretations above others. Also, cognitive maps that tend to distort data interpretation by fitting new facts within previous experiences are to be avoided.

To expect similar results from children similarly aged, for example in relation to the most appropriate ages to enter given levels of the school system, without taking into consideration their general development based upon their socioeconomic and nutritional background is, in a sense, to act against an equality-oriented political system. Governments should consider these factors when deciding upon general policies.

REFERENCES

Chávez A, Martínez C (1982): "Growing Up in a Developing Community." México City: Instituto Nacional de Nutrición.

Dobbing J (1975): Malnutrition et developpement du cerveaux. Recherche 7:139.

Fernstrom JD, Wurtman RJ (1971): Brain serotonin content: Increase following ingestion of carbohydrate diet. Science 174:1023-1025.

Graffar M (1956): Une méthode de classification sociale d'echantillons de population. Courrier 6:445-459.

Hartmann E (1982): Effect of l-tryptophan on sleepiness and on sleep. In Lieberman HR, Wurtman RJ (eds): "Research Strategies for Assessing the Behavioral Effects of Foods and Nutrients." Center for Brain Sciences and Metabolism Charitable Trust, pp 12-29.

Koluchová J (1976): The further development of twins after severe and prolonged deprivation: A second report. J Child Psychol Psychiat 17:181-188.

Lieberman HR, Wurtman RJ (1982): "Research Strategies for Assessing the Behavioral Effects of Foods and Nutrients." Center for Brain Sciences and Metabolism Charitable Trust.

Lieberman HR, Corkin S, Spring BJ, Growdon JH, Wurtman RJ (1982): Mood, performance, and pain sensitivity: Changes induced by food constituents. In Lieberman HR, Wurtman RJ (eds): "Research Strategies for Assessing the Behavioral Effects of Foods and Nutrients." Center for Brain Sciences and Metabolism Charitable Trust, pp 69-93.

Spring B, Maller O, Wurtman J, Digman L (1982): Effects of protein and carbohydrate meals on mood and performance. In Lieberman HR, Wurtman RJ (eds): "Research Strategies for Assessing the Behavioral Effects of Foods and Nutrients." Center for Brain Sciences and Metabolism Charitable Trust, pp 106-131.

Stein Z, Susser M, Saenger G, Marolla F (1972): Nutrition and mental performance. Science 178:708-713.

Susser M (1981): Prenatal nutrition, birthweight, and psychological development: An overview of experiments, quasi-experiments, and natural experiments in the past decade. Am J Clin Nutr 34:784-803.

Yogman MW, Zeisel SH, Roberts CC (1982): Dietary precursors of serotonin and newborn behavior. In Lieberman HR, Wurtman RJ (eds): "Research Strategies for Assessing the Behavioral Effects of Foods and Nutrients." Center for Brain Sciences and Metabolism Charitable Trust, pp 44–68.

Waber DP, Vuori-Christiansen L, Ortiz N, Clements JR, Christiansen NE, Mora JO, Reed RB, Herrera MG (1981): "Nutritional supplementation, maternal education, and cognitive development of infants at risk of malnutrition. Am J Clin Nutr 34:807–813.

Wurtman RJ, Fernstrom JD (1974): Effects of the diet on brain neurotransmitters. Nutr Rev 32:7.

Wurtman RJ, Hefti F, Melamed E (1981): Precursor control of neurotransmitter synthesis. Pharmacol Rev 32:315–335.

EFFECTS OF URBANIZATION
AND DEMOGRAPHIC CHANGES

Malnutrition: Determinants and Consequences, pages 189–196
© 1984 Alan R. Liss, Inc., 150 Fifth Avenue, New York, NY 10011

Effects of Urbanization and Acculturation on Food Habits: Studies in Mexico

Maria Teresa Cerqueira, RD, MS

Direccion General de Educacion Para la Salud, Secretaria de Salubridad y Asistencia, Mexico City, Mexico

Food practices are intimately related to cultural habits. Both the culture and the socioeconomic situation of each individual and social group are elements that define the dietary patterns at any given moment. Thus, food habits as one of the many manifestations of cultural and social values are in a constant process of change. Some are discarded, others are renewed, still others are substituted. Food habits are a social process subject to the needs and specific economic and political interests of each society.

The profound changes in economic structure that are rapidly transforming Mexico from a basic agricultural society into a more industrialized one have required a large labor force "free" to be mobilized from the rural areas to the cities, where the industrial activity is concentrated. The changes not only affect the urban workers, but also have profound effects on the rural population. There is an interpersonal communication system between the urban and rural population groups, and also an increased exposure of both groups to the mass media, which constantly introduce new products, fashions and lifestyles.

In much of today's world, especially in Latin American countries, a great part of the rural population has migrated to the cities. Presently more than 50% of the Mexican population lives in urban areas.

The rural migrants come to the city in search of better economic and social opportunities, much as all migrants throughout history have done. However, once in the cities, these migrants usually have the lowest-paying jobs. This is in part due to their lack of training. Many are illiterate and have no experience other than their agricultural chores. They usually live in the outskirts of the city and build their homes of cardboard and leftover materials; a dirt floor is the general rule. They lack sewage disposal systems and a safe water supply. The neighborhoods do not have schools, transportation, or other public services; the price of food is usually much higher in the marginal areas than in other urban areas. The migrants no longer have their crops, the corn and beans that assured their survival. In the city they usually have only temporary, part-time, or seasonal jobs, and the work they get generally pays less than the minimum wage.

Many of the nutrition surveys and studies done in Mexico have focused on the characteristics of rural population groups. By the seventies, however, the demographic changes, especially those due to rural-urban migration, made it clear that the "new" marginal city areas required more attention. In 1976 a comparative study of changes in food habits in this "new" population group was initiated. The objective of this research project was to identify the dietary patterns of rural-to-urban migrants living in Mexico City and compare them with food habits of rural inhabitants.

RESULTS OF A STUDY OF A RURAL-TO-URBAN MIGRANT POPULATION (INSTITUTO NACIONAL DE NUTRICION, MEXICO, 1978–1980)

A group of 70 families originally from Guanajuato who had migrated to Mexico City within the last 10 years was chosen for this project. Another group of 75 families still living in the same villages that the migrant families came from was selected for the comparative analysis.

The results were alarming. Important changes were documented not only as related to food habits. The socioeconomic characteristics of the families were also changing rapidly. The rural families lived mainly on subsistance farming, and some of the men also worked at caring for livestock, helping on other people's farms, and other temporary odd jobs. The urban families no longer produced their basic foods. They became *consumers*. The income was obtained from unskilled labor, ie, cleaning, maintenance, etc. Generally these were temporary jobs. Forty-two percent reported earning the minimum wage and 58% less than the minimum.

The family composition was also different. While rural families had an average of seven children, their urban couterparts had only four. The type of housing was also undergoing important changes. While the majority (78%) of the rural families had one-room houses, 47% of the urban families had more than two rooms. Adults in the urban families were younger (20–40 years); families were of the nuclear type. Adults in the rural group were older (30–50 years); rural groups were composed more of extended families. In the rural areas most of the houses (93%) had electricity and radio, but none had drainage, running water, or gas for cooking. On the other hand many of the urban homes (20%) had drainage and running water, as well as television, and 65% had gas stoves for cooking.

TABLE I. Nutrient Intakes of Rural Families and Rural-to-Urban Migrant Families

Nutrient	Rural-to-urban migrant		Rural		
	M ± SD	% Adequacy	M ± SD		% Adequacy
Energy (calories)	2,134 ± 428	93	1,869 ± 431		71
Protein (gm)	72 ± 26 (13%)	100	58 ± 13	(11%)	82
Carbohydrates (gm)	236 ± 49 (43%)	—	351 ± 57	(70%)	—
Fat (gm)	131 ± 48 (47%)	—	42 ± 23	(20%)	
Calcium (gm)	440 ± 239	70	605 ± 279		91
Iron (mg)	10 ± 6	73	8.6 ± 3.9		60
Vitamin C (mg)	86 ± 21	170	82 ± 26		168
Retinol (μg)	581 ± 230	83	935 ± 208		94

Data are means and standard deviations of group values (men, women, children).
From Cerqueira et al [1980], with permission.

Another interesting change was that 20% of the urban mothers worked full-time outside the home; another 60% did odd jobs to help the family income. In rural areas the women worked in the fields at some intervals but did not have full-time, paying jobs away from home.

Most of the migrant families said they came to the city so that their children could go to school and have a better life. Our studies showed that 30% of the urban children had finished elementary school and 21% were in high school, whereas in the rural group 28% had finished elementary school and only 7% had gone on to high school.

Of course, food habits were radically different. To begin with, in the rural communities women spend most of the day preparing the tortillas (the main dietary staple). In fact, all of the rural families reported that they ate tortillas twice or three times daily. In contrast, only 21% of the urban families reported eating this staple more than once a day. The rural families consumed a mean 580gm of tortillas per capita daily and their urban cousins only 254gm. Urban dwellers ate more refined cereals, "junk foods," meat products, and much more fat, especially fried foods, and they used more salt and sugar. Results indicated that urban families satisfied their basic energy and protein needs. While the rural family's diet was deficient in energy and protein, the urban diet was deficient in calcium. Both were low in iron content (Table I).

The urban family's cholesterol intake (612 ± 235 mg/day) was high and the plasma levels (364 ± 180 mg/dliter) reflected this. They had greater access to animal food products; these were usually the "fatty meats," cold cuts (ham, sausage, bacon, lard) and also many fried foods. In contrast, rural people consumed animal food products sporadically and in much smaller quantities. Their cholesterol intake was 354 ± 109 mg/day, and plasma levels were 190 ± 47 mg/dliter.

The sodium intake had also changed. The urban families not only used salt for cooking and at the table in greater quantities than the rural folks (5.5 ± 2 gm/day vs 2.5 ± 1.5 gm/day), but also ate more canned and other processed foods and salty snacks. Particularly popular are the powdered consomme or cubes, which are 40% sodium. Consequently the urban families had a greater frequency of high blood pressure. Diastolic blood pressure was 100 ± 10 mm Hg, compared with 70 ± 10 mm Hg in the rural families.

RESULTS OF THE NATIONAL FOOD HABITS SURVEY (SECRETARIA DE SALUBRIDAD Y ASISTENCIA, 1980–1983)

A surveillance system to monitor food habits in the vulnerable population groups and to monitor growth and nutritional status, especially in children under 5 years of age, is a national priority. In 1980, a national survey of 47,000 families (43% in rural communities and 57% in marginal urban areas) was carried out to establish the baseline data. The survey focused on the dietary patterns of four basic population groups: infants, pregnant and lactating women, adolescents, and workers in the marginal urban areas. Findings in two of the groups are discussed below.

Infants

Of the 3,000 women with children under 6 months of age that were interviewed, only 49% in the rural areas and 30% in the urban areas were breast-feeding. Of the total group surveyed (7,600 women with children under 3 years of age), only 43% of the rural mothers and 36% of their urban counterparts had exclusively breast-fed their last child for at least 3 months.

Urban mothers tend to wean in the first 3 months of their child's life, whereas rural mothers still tend to wean after 6 months and many still breast-feed the traditional 12 months (Fig. 1).

Parallel to the tendency to abandon the practice of breast-feeding, the practice of introducing other milk (formula or whole milk) is growing. Both the urban mothers and the rural mothers tended to give other milk in addition to breast-feeding. Thus, one of the new patterns of infant feeding is that of mixed feeding.

The major reasons given for not breast-feeding were varied. Both the urban and rural mothers often said that it was due to a "lack of good milk." They claimed that their milk was of a poor quality or the child did not feel satisfied. These kinds of answers we grouped in a category labeled "Lack of knowledge and credibility," which also included advice and comments from friends, parents, and especially the godparents, basically because all discredited the value of breast-feeding. Responses of 61% of rural women and 46% of urban women were classified under "Lack of knowledge and credibility." Another

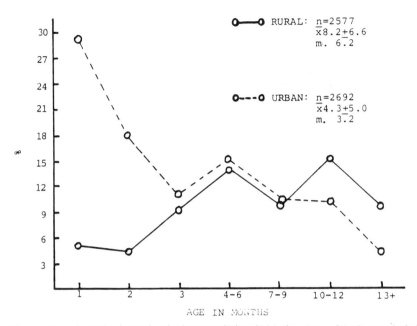

Fig. 1. Age of weaning in rural and urban populations in Mexico. Data of the Secretaria de Salubridad y Asistencia, 1980–1983.

important reason for the decline in breast-feeding by urban women was the lack of facilities for working mothers. In Mexico women workers with "social security" have a 45-day leave to have the baby and breast-feed. The time allowed for leave is inadequate and, in addition, most of the women do not have "social security." One of the most startling reasons given by the women interviewed was that they were following the doctor's advice; 19% of rural women and 15% of urban women indicated that they received medical advice against breast-feeding. Since radio and television advertisements to promote formulas are not permitted, the leading companies focus their publicity campaigns on printed materials directed to the physicians, especially those in private practice. On the other hand, it is also true that a great number of outdated and moralistic concepts about breast-feeding are still found throughout the country. Finally, illness of either the mother or infant was another reason given for not breast-feeding.

Survey results indicate that 52% of urban mothers gave infant formulas either as a substitute for or as a complement to human milk. In rural areas this was true of 38% of the mothers interviewed.

TABLE II. Adolescent Food Habits: Frequency of Eating Out

	Rural (%)	Urban (%)
Breakfast	13	52
Lunch	18	83
Dinner	7	19
Snacks	24	97

Sample of 7,500 boys and girls aged 12–18.
From Cerqueira et al [1983], with permission.

The urban group tended to give infants solid foods at an earlier age than did the rural mothers. The urban children also tasted "junk food" much earlier and with greater frequency than their rural counterparts. A majority of the urban group (52%) indicated that they regularly gave commercially prepared baby food to their infants; 24% of rural mothers indicated this practice as occasional. There were many children who were not given solid foods in their first year of life. Rural mothers are particularly reluctant to give beans, fruits, and vegetables. Urban mothers are apparently starting to introduce more of these foods, although they give fewer tortillas.

Adolescents

As a definite measure of the changing times we have the results of a survey of 7,500 adolescents. In rural areas the period of adolescence is very different from that in urban areas. Adolescents in rural areas are included in the agricultural activities, whereas in urban areas they continue in school for a longer period of time. In urban areas more adolescents eat outside the home (Table II). Since many schools have a breakfast program, this is probably the main reason that many of the youngsters ate this meal away from home.

The food preferences of this age group indicate that the urban group consumed much more processed or prepared food products and "junk foods" than did their rural counterparts. They ate more tacos, sandwiches, tamales, and other traditional items, which are now sold as "fast foods" at street stands (Table III).

CONCLUSIONS

The urban lifestyle affects the social and cultural values of all the city dwellers. However, the new immigrants have a particular need to feel part of the city, to integrate or at least not to be discriminated against or pointed out as inferior. Thus they readily adopt habits and patterns of conduct even though these do not always conform to their values.

TABLE III. Adolescent Food Preferences: Processed or Prepared Food Products Consumed at Least Three Times per Week

Food	Rural (%)	Urban (%)
Breakfast cereals	4	56
Breads/cakes	65	97
Cookies/crackers	83	99
Salty snacks	39	59
Cold meats	13	53
Cheese/yoghurt	17	45
Marmalade	24	78
Mayonnaise	9	94
Soft drinks	100	100
"Fast foods"	19	100

Sample of 7,500 adolescents.
From Cerqueira et al [1983], with permission.

On the one hand, women are now becoming part of the labor force. This means a change in roles, less time for cooking and preparing foods, especially traditional dishes. Children go to school for a longer period of time. This means traveling certain distances away from home, having to make new friends, sharing the group "likes" and "dislikes" in order to be accepted. It means eating out more often, smoking cigarettes (only 24% of all teenagers interviewed did not smoke), and trying alcoholic beverages (52% indicated they drank "socially").

For babies, it means having less of mother's milk, eating from a bottle and probably in a crib instead of mother's arms, being with other people at an earlier age, spending less time with the mother and older siblings, and eating commercially prepared baby food more often.

For the adults, it means more fat in their diets, much more salt and cholesterol, and higher incidences of obesity and high blood pressure.

For all of the family it means a greater risk of accidents, at home, in the street, at work. Although medical services are closer and of better quality, the cities have one of the highest infant death rates. In adolescents the death rates are higher owing to the violence, accidents, alcoholism, and drug addiction that are also more common than in rural communities. Urban adults have greater chances of a heart attack or cancer than their rural counterparts.

Finally, a brief look at some of the factors that play a leading role in these drastic changes. The process of adoption of a habit begins with identifying a need. Housing, jobs, food, education, transportation, water, drainage, medical care, social acceptance, etc, are real needs (identified and felt). However, in the complicated urban life, needs can be created (by manipulation through advertising) to generate consumption and to maintain certain economic interests.

Thus we have a lifestyle that obligates people to eat out and to buy prepared and refined food products, because there is no time to cook or eat at home. We have a need for social acceptance. Breast-feeding may be old-fashioned, and so are the tortillas. Many doctors recommend infant formulas and an early introduction of solid foods. Smoking and drinking not only are sophisticated, they promise social, economic, and sexual success.

Urban workers have money to buy food, and a wide variety of products compete for their salary via radio, television, magazines, store announcements, and other media. This new population group is not only the labor force for the struggling process of industrialization, but also the consumers needed to keep it alive.

After analyzing the data and reaching these conclusions, a few questions arise: Are science and technology really at the service of mankind? Are these changes permanent or temporary? Are food habits really so stubborn, so difficult to change? Whether the new patterns are superficial conduct or whether they will be incorporated as social and cultural values is difficult to say. One thing we know for sure, we cannot turn back time. Our responsibility, then, is the future. Where are we going? What kind of a society do we want?

REFERENCES

Cerqueira MT, Torre MP, Moncada C, Valverde M (1980): "Estudio de Hábitos Alimentarios en Población Migratoria Rural–Urbana." Monografía. Mexico City: Instituto Nacional de la Nutrición.

Cerqueira MT, Torre MP, Valverde M (1983): "Encuesta Nacional de Hábitos Alimentarios. Sistema de Vigilancia." Mexico City: Secretaría de Salubridad y Asistencia (preliminary data).

Malnutrition: Determinants and Consequences, pages 197–205
© 1984 Alan R. Liss, Inc., 150 Fifth Avenue, New York, NY 10011

Changes Over Time in Food Intakes of a Migrated Population

Hilary Creed Kanashiro, BSc, SRD, MPhil, and George G. Graham, MD
Instituto de Investigacion Nutricional, Apartado 55, Miraflores, Lima, 18, Peru

A survey carried out in 1972 identified differences among the nutrient intakes and growth rates of children in the capital city of Lima, the Andean highlands, and the thinly populated jungle areas of Peru [Amat y Leon Chavez, 1977]. Other surveys [Adrianzen et al, 1973; Graham et al, 1980] found urban children to be taller and heavier than rural children at all ages after infancy.

The population studied here for dietary intake and growth was part of a group of families living in Lima who had had at least one severely malnourished child. The majority had migrated from the highlands (some from other coastal areas) and had been in Lima for at least 7 years prior to the first dietary survey.

The growth of these children seemed less a function of the severity of the early malnutrition than of the quality of the home environments during the ensuing years [Graham, 1968; Graham and Andrianzen, 1972]: Within a few years after discharge from the hospital there was little difference in the growth status between the ex-patients and their siblings who had not been clinically malnourished [Graham and Andrianzen, 1971]. Some of the children had been adopted into homes of higher socioeconomic status and achieved greater "catch-up" growth [Graham and Andrianzen, 1972].

Preliminary analysis of longitudinal socioeconomic and anthropometric data indicated that the per capita disposable income was one of the most important determinants of achieved growth [Graham, 1972]. To assess the importance of this relationship a detailed dietary survey was carried out with a subsample of families from the longitudinal study.

THE 1972–1974 SURVEY

Study Population

The children followed in the longitudinal study were those hospitalized for acute malnutrition between the years 1961 and 1971 and their siblings, from 167 families. Twenty-six families were selected for the dietary survey, six of whom were families into which ex-patients had been adopted. Four families lived in the inner city, the rest in the shanty towns surrounding Lima.

Methodology of the Dietary Survey

The first study was carried out in 1972–1974. A 7-day individually weighed food survey method was chosen to obtain reliable estimates of the food and nutrient intake of the individual members of the family. All surveys were carried out by the same person, who was present in the house for an average of 7 hours a day, during the preparation and consumption of each of the main meals. Each food item that was included in the preparation of the meals was weighed, as were the dishes and foods served and left over by each member of the family present. Items consumed between meals were also weighed if the surveyor was present; otherwise they were estimated by recall, as was food consumed out of the house [Creed and Graham, 1980].

The nutrient contents of the diets consumed were calculated with the use of food tables derived principally from the 1974 revision of "The Composition of Peruvian Foods" [1969].

Results of the 1972–1974 Survey

The intakes of animal protein, β-carotene, and fat were associated with superior linear growth, particularly among males and despite seemingly adequate protein intakes. In females the energy intake, as a percentage of the recommendation for height-age, was a prominent factor associated with height quotient, and the percentage of energy from fat was associated with weight quotient [Graham et al, 1981a].

Progressively higher energy and total protein "adequacies" and higher intakes of animal protein, fat, calcium, carotene, riboflavin, and vitamin C were associated with increasing per capita expenditure for food. After adjustment for relative size and total energy requirement, all of the increase in total protein intake was found to be due to animal protein; vegetable protein consumption remained constant. In the poorer families of the group there was a modest increase in carbohydrate intake; otherwise all the remaining increase in total energy intake was due to fat [Graham et al, 1981b].

With more income available for food there was relatively little change in the consumption of cereals, roots or tubers, which together provided 50% of the energy needs. Families who were significantly better off consumed three times as much fruit and twice as much vegetables. Increases in energy intake were from milk, meat, and separated fats [Graham et al, 1981c].

TABLE I. Energy, Protein, and Fat Intakes of 162 Persons From 26 Families, Estimated in 1972–1974, Contrasted With Same Intakes of 99 Persons From 17 of the Same 26 Families in 1979–1980

	1972–1974	1979–1980
No. of families	26	17
No. of persons	162	99
Age (years): Mean ± SD	15.2 ± 14.2	17.8 ± 14.8
Range	0.1–67.0	0.9–73.6
Dietary intakes: Mean ± SD		
Energy (MJ/day)	7.0 ± 2.1	7.4 ± 2.5
Total protein (gm/day)	41.1 ± 12.1	42.2 ± 16.0
Animal (gm/day)	14.7 ± 8.1	11.6 ± 9.1
Vegetable (gm/day)	26.2 ± 7.9	30.5 ± 13.1
Total fat (gm/day)	42.1 ± 21.1	33.3 ± 15.9

THE 1979–1980 SURVEY

Since 1975 Peru has experienced severe inflation, devaluation of currency, the discontinuation of subsidies on foods and other commodities, and a significant loss of buying power. To study the effect of these drastic economic changes on food habits and nutrient intakes a resurvey was conducted over a period of 7 months between 1979 and 1980 with the same group of families as those studied 1972–1974.

Study Population

Seventeen of the original 26 families were available and willing to participate in the follow-up survey. Of these 17, two were families who had adopted the ex-patients. Ninety-nine subjects were included in the second survey.

Methodology

It was decided on the basis of the first survey that a 3-day individually weighed survey would be adequate as the intakes measured in the 7-day survey had not varied much from day to day. For the second survey two weekdays and one weekend day were chosen. Otherwise the methods were identical.

Results and Comparison With the Initial Survey

The uncorrected intakes from the two surveys are outlined in Table I. The mean age of the subjects in the second survey was 2.6 years greater, explaining the moderate increase in mean energy intakes. Despite this factor, important decreases in animal protein and total fat intakes are apparent.

For the 1972–1974 survey, the data from the 17 families who were resurveyed and the nine families who were not are compared in Table II. Included in these nine families are four of the adoptive families; it is apparent that as a

TABLE II. Data (1972–1974) From 17 Families Who Were Resurveyed in 1979–1980, Compared With Data (1972–1974) From 9 Families Who Were Not

	17 Families	9 Families	P Value
Per capita expense for food (soles): Mean ± SD	11.0 ± 6.3	18.0 ± 9.9	<0.001
Protein intake (% energy requirement): Mean ± SD	8.5 ± 1.8	9.3 ± 2.1	<0.05
Iron (mg/4.19 MJ): Mean ± SD	5.2 ± 0.8	5.9 ± 1.2	<0.001
β-Carotene (μg/4.19 MJ): Mean ± SD	852 ± 547	1244 ± 545	<0.001
Other carotenes (μg/4.19 MJ): Mean ± SD	174 ± 104	311 ± 296	<0.001
Energy sources (% indiv. req.): Mean ± SD			
Corn	1.8 ± 1.6	0.8 ± 0.6	<0.01
Roots	6.2 ± 3.4	8.0 ± 3.3	<0.02
Carrots	0.2 ± 0.2	0.5 ± 0.8	<0.01
Vegetables	1.1 ± 0.4	1.8 ± 0.6	<0.001
Meat	3.8 ± 3.3	5.8 ± 4.2	<0.01
Fowl	0.9 ± 1.1	1.4 ± 1.2	<0.05
Fish	1.1 ± 1.2	0.6 ± 0.6	<0.05

Data (from children over 2 and under 19 years of age) are included only when significantly different by two-tailed t test.

group they were better off, spending more money on food and consuming more protein, iron, and carotenes through more meat, poultry, carrots, and other vegetables. Because of these differences the subsequent analyses are limited to the 17 families who participated in both surveys.

Changes in the mean family intakes between the two surveys are shown in Table III. Mean energy intakes as percentages of estimated individual requirements had increased minimally but not significantly. The most notable changes are the significant decreases in total fat intake, particularly separated fats, and an increase in the proportion of energy provided by cereals.

Mean total protein intakes had increased marginally owing to the higher average age of the subjects present: There was a dramatic and significant decrease in the percentage of animal protein due to a reduction of meat and milk consumption. This was compensated by an increase in fish and vegetable proteins.

In the following analyses only the 48 children between 2 and 19 years of age present in both surveys are included. Table IV shows that there were slight but not significant increases in the height and weight quotients of these children. The ratio of weight to height quotients remained essentially unchanged.

In Table V it is apparent that the families spent approximately 28% more per person on food. The 1979–1980 per capita expenditure for food was converted to the 1972–1974 currency values by dividing by the official deflator in-

TABLE III. Sources of Diet Energy and Protein for 17 Families in 1979–1980 Compared With Same in 1972–1974

	1979–1980		Change from 1972–1974		P value[a] of paired t
	Mean	SD	Mean	SD	
Mean total energy intake as percentage of individual requirements[b]	91.3	21.3	0.7	19.4	
Percentage of energy intake from:					
Protein	9.7	1.2	−0.1	1.2	
Fat (all)	16.6	4.9	−6.2	6.3	<0.001
Separated fats	8.9	4.5	−4.7	3.6	<0.001
Cereals (all)	51.1	8.2	4.3	8.4	<0.05
Rice	18.1	7.5	2.0	6.6	
Wheat	29.4	9.4	3.0	11.7	
Potato	5.3	2.9	0.6	3.2	
Cane sugar	13.2	4.5	1.7	4.1	
Fruits	1.9	1.9	−0.2	1.7	
Vegetables	1.5	1.0	0.2	0.9	
Percentage of protein intake from:					
Animal sources	26.6	13.5	−7.1	10.3	<0.02
Meat	8.7	7.3	−6.1	9.7	<0.02
Milk	7.4	7.1	−2.0	9.2	
Fish	10.7	9.5	2.7	9.1	
Legumes	8.5	7.4	−1.1	7.6	
Cereals (all)	50.9	12.8	5.4	11.9	

Each family value is the mean for all children who were 2–19 years of age on each occasion.
[a]Statistically significant (<0.05) P values only are listed.
[b]FAO/WHO recommendations, modified for Peruvian heights and weights.

TABLE IV. Changes in Age and Anthropometric Indices of 48 Children (28 boys, 20 girls) From 17 Families Who Were Present and Between 2 and 19 Years of Age in Both Surveys (1972–1974 and 1979–1980)

	1972–1974		1979–1980		Change	
	Mean	SD	Mean	SD	Mean	SD
Age (years)	7.4	2.6	13.7	2.7	6.3	0.4
Height quotient[a]	102.4	14.6	105.5	15.3	3.6	14.6
Weight quotient[a]	102.8	18.9	104.5	16.0	1.8	17.0
WQ/HQ	1.01	0.10	1.00	0.15	−0.01	0.14

[a]Height (or weight) age, on median of Peruvian data, as a percentage of chronologic age.

TABLE V. Multiplier Factor for Increase in Food Prices 1972–1974 to 1979–1980 (deflator index was 7.42)

Rice	9.1	Evaporated milk	9.7
Pasta	11.7	Cheese	9.5
Bread	10.9	Beef	7.4
Potato	8.1	Chicken	7.4
Legumes	8.4–16.2	Fish	7.4
Sugar	12.1	Eggs	6.4
		Cooking oil	9.0
		Margarine	5.4

Daily per capita expenditure for food increased from 10.4 ± 6.2 to 13.3 ± 5.6 soles (corrected).

TABLE VI. Nutrient Intakes in 1972–1974 and 1979–1980 of 48 Children (17 families) Who Were Present and Between 2 and 19 Years of Age During Both Surveys

	1972–1974		1979–1980		Change		P value[a] of
	Mean	SD	Mean	SD	Mean	SD	paired t
Expenditure (soles/day)[b]	10.4	6.2	13.3	5.6	2.9	7.1	< 0.01
Energy intake (MJ/day)	6.7	1.6	8.4	2.8	1.6	2.4	< 0.001
Percentage of indiv. requirement	90.8	15.4	90.7	28.8	− 0.1	28.1	
Percentage protein	9.6	1.0	9.4	1.4	− 0.2	1.5	
Percentage fat	20.8	6.7	15.4	4.9	− 5.4	6.1	< 0.001
Fat intake (gm/day)	38.2	18.7	35.5	18.7	− 2.6	19.3	
Protein intake (gm/day)	38.4	9.2	47.1	17.5	8.8	15.3	< 0.001
Animal protein (gm/day)	11.8	5.7	10.3	7.9	− 1.5	7.5	
Percentage of total protein	30.1	9.1	21.2	13.4	− 8.9	13.7	< 0.001
Vegetable protein (gm/day)	26.4	5.9	36.8	14.5	10.5	13.1	< 0.001
Calcium (mg/4.19 MJ)	160	51	139	48	−21	66	< 0.05
Iron (mg/4.19 MJ)	5.2	0.9	5.2	2.6	0.0	2.6	
Thiamin (mg/4.19 MJ)	0.38	0.05	0.38	0.07	0.00	0.07	
Riboflavin (mg/4.19 MJ)	0.53	0.11	0.46	0.08	− 0.07	0.12	< 0.001
Niacin (mg/4.19 MJ)	6.0	1.1	6.2	1.1	0.2	1.4	
Ascorbic acid (mg/day)	50	31	63	44	13	39	< 0.02
Retinol equivalents (μg/day)	347	193	387	379	39	400	

[a]Statistically significant (< 0.05) P values only are listed.
[b]Daily per capita expenditure for food in 1979–1980 was converted to 1972–1974 soles by dividing actual amounts by a deflator index of 7.42.

TABLE VII. Changes Between 1972–1974 and 1979–1980, in Important Sources of Energy in the Diets of 48 Children Who Were Between 2 and 19 Years of Age in Both Surveys

| | 1972–1974 | | 1979–1980 | | Change | | P value[a] of |
	Mean	SD	Mean	SD	Mean	SD	paired t
Cereals	45.8	8.5	49.4	17.0	3.5	16.6	
Rice	15.4	6.2	16.9	9.4	1.5	7.9	
Wheat	25.8	5.2	28.5	14.9	2.7	15.7	
Bread	15.1	5.1	17.9	11.1	2.8	12.8	
Pasta	8.3	4.8	8.9	7.3	0.5	7.7	
Potato	3.8	2.8	4.5	2.4	0.7	2.4	< 0.05
Sweet potato	1.2	1.7	0.3	0.9	− 0.9	2.0	< 0.001
Sugar	10.3	3.9	10.7	7.0	0.4	6.8	
Legumes	3.3	1.5	3.3	3.3	0.0	3.6	
Fruit	1.8	1.7	1.5	1.9	− 0.3	1.8	
Vegetables	1.2	0.4	1.3	1.1	0.2	1.2	
Meat	3.3	3.2	1.5	2.3	− 1.8	2.7	< 0.001
Eggs	0.7	0.7	0.3	0.5	− 0.5	0.9	< 0.001
Fish	1.2	1.3	1.6	1.8	0.4	2.1	
Milk	2.8	3.1	1.4	2.1	− 1.4	3.4	< 0.01
Separated fats	12.2	6.9	8.5	5.8	− 3.7	7.3	< 0.001
Butter	1.3	1.8	1.7	2.5	0.4	2.2	

Data are percentages of estimated individual energy requirements, as derived from FAO/WHO recommendations modified to size of Peruvian children.
[a]Statistically significant (< 0.05) P values only are listed.

dex of 7.42. It can be seen that during the same interval the majority of food prices increased considerably more. In 1979–1980 the family expenditure on food represented 65.5 ± 10.4% of disposable income; in 1972–1974 it was less than 60% on the average.

The children present in both surveys were 6.3 ± 0.4 years older at the time of the second survey and this accounts for the significant increases in total energy and protein intakes as shown in Table VI. When the intakes are expressed as a percentage of individual requirement the changes are not significant. Despite the greater ages, there were actual decreases in the total intakes of fat and animal protein and these changes were highly significant when expressed as percentages of energy intake and total protein intake. In the nutrient densities there were significant differences in calcium and riboflavin because of decreased milk and meat intakes.

Table VII analyzes the sources of nutrients for the same children. The major increase is in the consumption of cereals. In spite of a significant increase, potato consumption remains relatively low. Sweet potatoes are consumed as an "extra" accompaniment to other dishes and the sharp drop was undoubtedly due to a large increase in cost. Meat, egg, and milk consumption all decreased by 50% or more, whereas fish consumption increased by 33%. Fish was the one major item that was consumed preferentially by the poorer families of this population. It can be seen here that in the second survey fish had become the most important source of animal protein, whereas previously it was third after meat and milk. Fish remained much cheaper than meat (one-quarter to one-fifth of the price) and the shifts in consumption were almost certainly dictated by the real decreases in buying power, particularly for food. The great decrease in separated fat consumption was probably determined by cost, and a decrease in the consumption of fried foods was observed.

DISCUSSION

Inflation and devaluation of currency, with a disproportionate increase in the cost of food, produced important changes in the diets of children from poor families in Lima, Peru between 1972–1974 and 1979–1980. The fact that relative heights and weights did not deteriorate for the children present in both surveys suggests that the adaptations in eating habits were nutritionally appropriate. It is interesting that the first survey, a cross-sectional survey, suggested that both quantity and quality of food intake were affected by buying power and were associated with achieved growth, particularly the intakes of animal protein, total fat, and β-carotene, yet the decreases in animal protein and total fat were not sufficient to affect anthropometric indices. It may be that food budgets had been stretched tighter in 1979–1980 but were still not at a breaking point, and that the nutrient intakes found on both surveys were equally adequate to support the rates and nature of the growth found in this population: moderate stunting with normal to excessive weight-for-height.

Some important policy implications of this study are that food prices and availability significantly influence consumption patterns and the sources of nutrients in the diet, that Peruvian homemakers display considerable and appropriate flexibility in their food-buying practices, and that it is important to monitor the growth of children as an indicator of nutritional status.

REFERENCES

— (1969): "Composición de Los Alimentos Peruanos." Lima: Instituto de Nutrición.

Adrianzen TB, Baertl JM, Graham GG (1973): Growth of children from extremely poor families. Am J Clin Nutr 33:926–930.

Amat y Leon Chavez C (1977): "Niveles de Vida. Analisis de la situacion Alimentaria en el Peru." Lima: Ministerio de Economia y Finanzas.

Creed HM, Graham GG (1980): Determinants of growth among poor children. I. Food and nutrient intakes. Am J Clin Nutr 33:715–722.

Graham GG (1968): The later growth of malnourished infants: Effects of age, severity and subsequent diet. In McCance RA, Widdowson EM (eds): "Calorie Deficiencies and Protein Deficiencies." London: J & A Churchill, pp 301–316.

Graham GG (1972): Environmental factors affecting the growth of children. Am J Clin Nutr 25:1184–1188.

Graham GG, Adrianzen TB (1971): Growth, inheritance, and environment. Pediatr Res 5:691–697.

Graham GG, Adrianzen TB (1972): Late "catch-up" growth after severe infantile malnutrition. Johns Hopkins Med J 131:204–211.

Graham GG, MacLean Jr WC, Kallman CH, Rabold J, Mellits ED (1980): Urban-rural differences in the growth of Peruvian children. Am J Clin Nutr 33:338–344.

Graham GG, Creed HM, MacLean Jr WC, Kallman CH, Rabold J, Mellits ED (1981a): Determinants of growth among poor children: nutrient intake-achieved growth relationships. Am J Clin Nutr 34:539–554.

Graham GG, Creed HM, MacLean Jr WC, Kallman CH, Rabold J, Mellits ED (1981b): Determinants of growth among poor children: Relation of nutrient intakes to expenditure for food. Am J Clin Nutr 34:555–561.

Graham GG, Creed HM, MacLean Jr WC, Rabold J, Mellits ED (1981c): Determinants of growth among poor children: Effect of expenditure for food on nutrient sources. Am J Clin Nutr 34:562–567.

Malnutrition: Determinants and Consequences, pages 207–219
© 1984 Alan R. Liss, Inc., 150 Fifth Avenue, New York, NY 10011

Effects of Dependence on Seasonally Available Food

Marina Flores, MS, and Rafael Flores, MAP

Pan American Sanitary Bureau (M.F.) and Institute of Nutrition of Central America and Panama (INCAP) (R.F.), Guatemala City, Guatemala

INTRODUCTION

The solar system provides our planet with a natural seasonal cycle that produces changes in the climatic conditions. The geographical location of a country determines the degree of intensity of those changes. Furthermore, the topography of the soil protects against or modifies the severity of the effects of winds and rainfalls on the valleys and plains. This diversity of conditions, due to natural changes, allows the flora and fauna to grow profusely during certain periods of the year. Man has learned the right place and best time to obtain the best yield for different products. Therefore, to secure a good harvest the farming pattern in each region follows seasonal climatic changes. The availability of food products affects the food consumption pattern of communities and the nutriture of individuals. If "Nature" is so prodigal, it is difficult to accept that hunger and malnutrition exist in some areas as a result of insufficient food or lack of resources to produce it. Bonderstam [1981] has indicated that in Ethiopia hunger is basically caused by nonnatural factors resulting from economic or political events. However, natural disasters, such as floods, droughts, or earthquakes, in developed as well as in underdeveloped countries, can aggravate hunger. Natural disasters can be predicted sometimes and negative nutritional consequences may be diminished if appropriate measures are taken.

Countries with major nutritional problems in the Western Hemisphere are those located in the tropics, where the economy relies mainly on agriculture. Malnutrition is the result of the system of land tenure and modes of production. Countries are compelled to cultivate food crops for local consumption and produce cash crops for the international trading market to obtain currency for manufactured products and other commodities. Most domestic food products are in the hands of small farmers, whereas the cash crops are produced on large plantations run by modern capitalist farmers. These plantations generate great demand for a seasonal labor force. For small farmers and agricultural laborers the seasonal availability of foods may vary accordingly, owing to the availability of work and the agricultural cycle of their products. Thus, families without land to cultivate or income to buy foods run a high risk during certain time periods of suffering from malnutrition.

In addition, poor environmental conditions, poor social infrastructure, high illiteracy rates, and lack of health and medical facilities contribute to a high rate of malnutrition and mortality. Moreover, these countries are suffering from external penetrating forces creating political unrest, which precipitates hunger problems into starvation and death.

SEASONAL NUTRITIONAL STUDIES IN DIFFERENT LATITUDES

Food is abundantly available the year round in well-developed countries. The high degree of urbanization and industrialization allows individuals to obtain and consume sufficient amounts of fresh or processed foods. In countries such as the United States the excellent food distribution and communication systems, as well as the number of modern supermarkets, make all kinds of foods available to different states. Moreover, the agricultural system, price and economic policies, and social welfare programs allow families to maintain diets adequate in both quality and quantity.

Orr and Clark [1930], in their review of 12 nutritional studies carried out in Europe and the United States, reported a seasonal effect on the growth of children. The findings suggested a higher increase in height during March and June and a minimum gain in winter months. In their review of more recent studies in developed countries, Valverde et al [1982] concluded that a pattern of seasonal growth similar to that described by Orr and Clark has been observed.

Fjeld and Summer [1982] illustrated the seasonal changes in food patterns in the United States. They indicated that the new trend in food demand is the purchase of more fresh fruits and vegetables. This is confirmed by a survey conducted among 1,350 households in which 60% of families purchased food, at least once, directly from farmers' markets. Price savings and the desire for good-quality food support this trend. Therefore, seasonal fluctuations are likely to appear in the food consumption patterns of families. A study conducted in California, of ten fruits and vegetables available in supermarkets during the year indicated that eight of them are cultivated locally and show seasonal fluctuation in consumption. All eight items were avoided when not in season, but were consumed in great amounts during the growing season because of their freshness and flavor.

Relatively few studies on the seasonal effect on nutritional status in developed countries are to be found in the literature. The reasons may be that basic foods are available all year round and nutritional problems are confined to a few special population groups. In Canada [CDNHW, 1973], a national nutrition survey was conducted during two seasons in 1971–1972. Clinical evidence of serious nutritional deficiencies was not found; on the contrary, overconsumption of energy was a general finding. Beaton [1981] reported on nutritional status in Canada, where obesity, as in the United States, was a major problem in the adult population. Only in a few Canadian Indian groups were some nutritional deficiencies found. The Eskimos exhibit low levels of serum ascorbic acid, which may be associated with the lack of fruits and vegetables. The findings in regard to the incidence of clinical signs of vitamin C deficiency are a subject of much discussion.

Seasonal studies in developing countries, particularly in Asia and Africa, are abundant. Most of these studies present information on the seasonal effects on growth and mortality of young children. In an anthropometric study conducted in the Congo [Pagezy, 1982], the existence of seasonal hunger already described by other investigators was confirmed. During the rainy season, from the end of September to the middle of December, people complain of hunger, despite the fact that the basic food (mandioca) is available throughout the year. The reason is that, during these rainy months, animal food disappears because of the suspension of fishing and hunting. The anthropometric results among the male adults showed weight losses during the season, but the degree of the weight change followed an occupational pattern.

Longhurst and Payne [1981] have summarized the information available in 1979 regarding the incidence of malnutrition as related to seasonal food shortages and deficits in energy intake among adults and children. These authors indicate that childhood growth is affected both by changes in food supply and by infectious diseases. Malnutrition is the consequence of both problems. Some studies in Gambia [Marsden and Marsden, 1965] show an increase of mean weights during the dry months but no marked changes during wet months, when the incidence of malnutrition is higher. However, the authors have reported other findings of no changes in weight in either of the seasons.

The observations of Schofield [1974] from 25 African villages showed that energy requirements were met during the dry season but that intake dropped to 85% during the wet season. The review by Annegers [1973] of studies in West Africa concluded that there was a higher energy intake in November and December, which corresponds to the harvest period.

Children in Uganda [Rutishauser, 1974] showed a higher energy and protein intake during the rainy season, when food was abundant. Valverde et al [1982] cited Slooff [1978], who indicated that in his studies among small children in Kenya he did not find differences in food consumption between wet and dry seasons. The lack of such an effect on these communities was attributed to the fact that there are two harvest periods per year and, in addition, people were able to generate income from other, nonagricultural activities.

SEASONAL FINDINGS IN MESOAMERICA

While countries located in some parts of the Western Hemisphere enjoy the benefits of four seasons, those in the tropics are limited to two seasons. In Central America, the rainy season begins in May and ends around October. The dry period includes the months from November to April. Cultivation of basic food products follows the cycle of dry or wet seasons, defining them as preharvest and postharvest for these crops. Consequently, a positive effect on food consumption is expected as a result of the corn harvest, which is the staple food for most of these countries. The analysis of factors affecting nutritional status of rural populations in El Salvador and Costa Rica, presented by Valverde et al [1982] clearly shows the dependence of food availability on the labor cycle. Corn and beans are scarce from June to August in these countries, and farmers do not have income because it is not the labor season. By the middle of August, the corn harvest arrives, followed by beans, and both are abundant if the weather and other agricultural factors are normal. Unfortunately, there is a seasonal pattern of disease when the incidence of diarrhea increases with the early rains, usually in May. To compensate for some of the detrimental effects of the seasonal shortage of food, families have to use a different system of marketing or trading to obtain at least the minimum amounts of basic foods. In some communities, men or entire families have to migrate to larger plantations or sell some products in order to obtain the benefit of some income to pay for food supplies obtained by credit.

Rawson and Valverde [1976] reported information about seasonal effects in Costa Rica, where farm families depend on labor demand during the harvest period of the large coffee plantations to pay their debts. The coffee harvest in Costa Rica presents a more serious problem in regard to the nutritional status of small children, owing to the practice of leaving the children at home with an older sibling in the absence of both parents during the labor season. The same observation was made in the coffee plantations of El Salvador.

Trowbridge and Newton [1979] presented information, gathered from 1974–1976, on anthropometric measurements and morbidity of children in a coastal area of El Salvador. They found the highest prevalence of malnutrition, as measured by weight-for-height, during June, and the lowest during March. No specific seasonal trends were observed when weight-for-age or height-for-age were used as measures. The highest incidence of diarrhea was observed during the first part of the rainy season, from May to July. This period coincides with the scarcity of food near the cotton- and coffee-growing areas. Field studies conducted on coffee farms in Guatemala in 1977–1978

TABLE I. Nutritive Value and Adequacy of the Family Diets: Rural Village of Quezaltepeque, El Salvador, 1954

Energy and nutrients		Daily intake levels per person		% Adequacy[a]	
		February	September	February	September
Energy	kcal	1,967	2,380	99	121
Protein	gm	52	58	92	102
Calcium	mg	1,000	1,000	108	95
Iron	mg	29	39	281	378
Vitamin A	UI	638	438	17	11
Thiamine	mg	1.0	1.0	123	138
Riboflavin	mg	0.6	1.0	46	60
Niacin	mg	10.0	11.0	104	106
Vitamin C	mg	55	35	89	57

Total number of families, 60.
[a]Recommended dietary allowances, INCAP 1953.

[Valverde, 1979] showed that 21.5% of children were below 90% of the standard for weight in families where the household head was employed all year, whereas 25.5% were below 90% of the standard in those families where the father was not working all year. When the author compared the results obtained during preharvest with postharvest periods, no significant differences were found in the distribution of children with second- and third-degree malnutrition. In general, Valverde's analyses of increments of weight and height, for each seasonal period, did not show any specific growth pattern.

The food consumption data in Central American countries show seasonal dietary differences. Family dietary surveys have been conducted, and results are presented in the following tables for El Salvador, Panama, and Honduras.

Table I presents results of a dietary survey carried out during the dry season and repeated during the rainy season in small rural villages of El Salvador in 1954 [Castillo and Flores, 1955]. People increased their consumption of foods and nutrients during the rainy or postharvest season.

Table II shows information on food consumption by 38 families studied during the dry and rainy seasons in a rural community of Panama. Again, an increment in the consumption of the staple food was found in the rainy season [Sogandares and Barrios, 1955]. The staple food in this case is not corn but rice complemented with bananas.

In the case of Honduras [CSPE, 1981], figures given in Table III correspond to averages for the three main rural areas representing the entire country. The results are similar in regard to the increases of the staple food (corn) in the rainy, or postharvest, period. In addition, a high increment is also observed in the postharvest period in the consumption of dairy products.

TABLE II. Food Consumption Per Person Per Day in Rural Area of
Veraguas, Panama, 1952–1953

Foods	First survey (gm)	Second survey (gm)
Dairy products[a]	47	116
Eggs	8	9
Meats	83	82
Beans	54	54
Green vegetables	6	54
Fruits	36	38
Roots and tubers	42	50
Bananas	36	83
Corn	72	67
Wheat bread	9	13
Rice	171	268
Sugar	53	44
Fats	35	26

[a]In terms of liquid milk.

CASE STUDY: SEASONAL INTAKES AMONG RURAL GUATEMALAN CHILDREN

Food consumption surveys were conducted in families in rural areas of Guatemala during two periods of 1977, as part of a study conducted from 1975 to 1977 evaluating the vitamin A sugar fortification program [Arroyave et al, 1979]. To secure a representative sample of the rural population, 12 localities were selected according to a geographical distribution of the main agricultural regions in the country. The 12 sites were drawn from a list of communities with populations ranging from 1,000 to 2,000 inhabitants. Thirty families with children were selected at random in each community for each period. Children's food consumption for 24 hr was obtained by recording the available food for the family and weighing or estimating the portions given to the selected child.

Before presenting the results it is pertinent to describe the social structure of the rural family economy. Guatemala is one of the countries where agriculture has been oriented toward the production of coffee, sugar, and cotton because of the high income from these crops. In order to secure their food supplies the large majority of the rural population need to combine two sources of income. The first is the cultivation of their own small plots of land and the second is the salaries derived as wages on large plantations. The labor demand of those plantations fluctuates according to the type of crop; this implies that the cash crop agriculture system works with high rates of temporary unemployment. The combination of the intensive seasonal demand of the modern farming sec-

TABLE III. Food Consumption in Rural Area of Honduras (1978–1979)
(grams per person per day)

Foods	Preharvest, May–June	Postharvest, October–November
Dairy products[a]	193	226
Eggs	27	16
Meats	25	37
Beans	64	64
Green vegetables	15	34
Fruits	30	16
Bananas	74	46
Roots and tubers	9	10
Corn	217	260
Sorghum	51	7
Wheat bread	7	8
Rice	30	35
Sugar	34	30
Fats	17	16

[a]In terms of liquid milk.

tor with the very low productivity of the microfarm of the traditional farming sector presents a complicated problem for the economy of the rural family [Hintermeister and Blas, 1980]. The introduction of new technology for the cultivation of the cash crops — for instance, a new variety of coffee to increase the number of plants per unit of land — represents a greater demand for labor for shorter periods, thereby accentuating the seasonal fluctuation of labor demand. Thus, the low utilization of the labor force during long periods of the year results in poor living conditions in the rural area.

The results of the surveys of food consumption were analyzed to find the seasonal effect on food intake. Data are presented in Table IV on the average amounts of foods consumed in the two periods investigated. The foods consumed in small amounts do not differ from period to period. Changes are observed in the figures for dairy products, fresh vegetables, and corn tortillas at the family level and in children. Both groups consumed less fruit in the second period. Very poor families, during the first season, had to use sorghum to complement their corn consumption. The differences are of greater magnitude when consumption figures are presented by communities. To illustrate this point, the consumption of the basic food "corn tortilla" is presented in Table V. In the smallest, more rural communities, families consume more corn because they subsist mainly from this food. All figures are lower during the preharvest season (April and May), with an increased consumption in postharvest periods (November and December). The only community not showing an increment is Jícaro, the town with the higher degree of urbanization. The data

TABLE IV. Food Consumption in Rural Area of Guatemala, 1977 (grams per person per day)

	At family level		At child level	
Foods	April–May	October–November	April–May	October–November
Dairy products	82	104	96	123
Eggs	14	14	14	14
Meats	28	26	12	14
Beans	51	42	22	23
Green vegetables	48	81	22	52
Fruits	53	43	69	40
Roots and tubers	6	10	4	8
Corn – tortillas	468	536	217	249
Sorghum – tortillas	15	0	6	0
Wheat bread	16	16	17	18
Rice	16	11	8	8
Other cereals[a]	8	6	6	5
Sugar	47	51	37	41
Fats	6	4	3	3

[a]Including Incaparina.

on children do not show the same seasonal trend as that observed in families; there are some increases in the second period whereas in other the consumption decreases.

The information on the nutritive value of family and children's diets, as presented in Table VI, shows an increase in intake levels during the second period. Only the figures for retinol show a decrease, at family and child levels, where there is great variability in the intakes.

To explore whether the increase in food consumption, which occurred in postharvest periods, was reflected in calorie and nutrient intakes, analyses of variance (Anova) were performed with periods and communities and the interaction between periods and communities as independent variables. For the analyses, intakes by families and children of energy, total protein, animal protein, and retinol were taken as dependent variables.

At the family level there was no interaction between period and communities ($P > 0.05$). There was a difference between periods in neither energy nor nutrients; however, differences among communities were significant ($P < 0.05$). This indicates that the variability among communities in the country is very important and merits consideration. In the case of retinol, analyzing all families together, differences between periods were statistically significant, showing a decrease during the second period.

In regard to children, there were no interactions between communities and periods for the intakes of energy, total protein, and animal protein; however, there were differences among communities and between periods ($P < 0.05$).

TABLE V. Consumption of Corn Tortillas Per Person Per Day in Rural Area of Guatemala, 1977

	At family level		At child level	
Communities	April–May (gm)	October–November (gm)	April–May (gm)	October–November (gm)
Villages				
6. San Rafael Sacatepéquez	828	867	422	504
5. Buena Vista	748	801	285	278
7. Saquitacaj	539	614	213	283
12. Santa Fe	518	632	276	236
11. Cahaboncito	463	566	176	276
1. El Barrial	282	433	130	174
3. San Juan, Zacapa	327	333	140	146
Towns				
10. San Carlos Alzatate	472	583	210	247
2. Sta. María Ixhuatán	404	475	179	181
8. La Libertad	355	429	174	222
9. Cubulco	343	409	163	128
4. El Jícaro	347	330	124	153

TABLE VI. Dietary Intakes in Rural Area of Guatemala, 1977 (per person per day)

		At family level[a]		At child level[b]	
Energy and nutrients		April–May	October–November	April–May	October–November
Calories		1,730	1,811	984	1,096
Total protein	gm	52.7	54.2	29.3	31.7
Animal protein	gm	9.5	9.8	7.1	8.3
Calcium	mg	895	978	523	613
Iron	mg	13.8	12.9	6.8	7.6
Retinol (equivalent)	μg	279	156	170	141
Thiamine	mg	0.9	1.0	0.5	0.6
Riboflavin	mg	0.5	0.6	0.4	0.5
Niacin (equivalent)	mg	9.3	10.9	4.7	5.2
Vitamin C	mg	47	37	39	24

[a]Total number of families, 720; total number of children, 716.
[b]Total number of children, 716.

By means of the Bonferroni method [Neter and Wasserman, 1974] with the results of the Anova, it was found that differences greater or equal to 57 kcal, 1.9 gm total protein, and 1.6 g of animal protein could be considered as statistically significant, owing to the size of the present study sample and the lack of interaction. As for retinol, the interaction was significant ($P < 0.05$), meaning

TABLE VII. Energy Intake of Preschool Children in Rural Area of Guatemala, 1977 (kcal per child per day)

Communities	April–May	October–November	X̄
1. El Barrial	1,228	1,209	1,218
2. Santa María Ixhuatán	984	1,132	1,059
3. San Juan Zacapa	930	1,042	985
4. El Jícaro	1,092	1,230	1,160
5. Buena Vista	914	1,002	957
6. San Rafael Sacatepéquez	1,162	1,351	1,258
7. Saquitacaj	798	1,151	978
8. La Libertad	975	1,037	1,006
9. Cubulco	1,071	1,125	1,098
10. San Carlos Alzatate	996	1,068	1,032
11. Cahaboncito	699	1,017	867
12. Santa Fe	1,199	1,178	1,188
Mean	1,009[a]	1,130	

[a]Periods are statistically significant ($P < 0.05$).

that children in some communities changed their intake and in others did not. Utilizing the Bonferroni method again, it was found that children in three communities diminished their intake significantly ($P < 0.05$). No statistical change was observed in the rest of the communities.

Anthropometric observations of the same children showed no significant differences between periods, on the basis of weight-for-height and weight-for-age indicators ($P > 0.05$); nevertheless, there was a significant decrease when height-for-age was used ($P < 0.05$). This decrease may reveal a deterioration in the second period, even when energy intakes increased in the second period. This is probably due to the fact that the increment of 121 calories was not sufficient to maintain nutritional status of the children.

Results regarding the statistical analyses of the intake of children, for energy, total protein, animal protein, and retinol are presented in Tables VII–X.

CONCLUSIONS

1. There is a seasonal variation in food availability in different countries, but the effects on food consumption and nutritional status of the people are not very clear, even in poor rural areas. Changes appear in type, quality, and quantities of food components of diets in each season. Some foods replace others of the same nature, resulting in similar energy and protein intakes.

2. Dramatic seasonal effects during critical periods, as expected in poor areas, are not observed owing to the ability of families to generate some income, by means of different social or economic mechanisms. There is also an extra-

TABLE VIII. Total Protein Intake of Preschool Children in Rural Area of Guatemala, 1977 (grams per child per day)

Communities	April–May	October–November	X̄
1. El Barrial	36.8	37.0	36.9
2. Santa María Ixhuatán	28.4	34.4	31.5
3. San Juan Zacapa	24.0	27.5	25.7
4. El Jícaro	30.8	34.8	32.8
5. Buena Vista	26.6	29.9	28.2
6. San Rafael Sacatepéquez	34.9	38.0	36.5
7. Saquitacaj	24.6	35.6	30.2
8. La Libertad	27.5	30.4	29.0
9. Cubulco	31.6	35.5	33.5
10. San Carlos Alzatate	29.6	33.5	31.5
11. Cahaboncito	21.1	31.0	26.3
12. Santa Fe	32.8	36.4	34.6
Mean	29.2[a]	33.7	

[a]Periods are statistically significant (P < 0.05).

TABLE IX. Animal Protein Intake of Preschool Children in Rural Area of Guatemala, 1977 (grams per child per day)

Communities	April–May	October–November	X̄
1. El Barrial	10.4	12.7	11.6
2. Santa María Ixhuatán	5.4	9.2	7.3
3. San Juan Zacapa	7.0	8.7	7.8
4. El Jícaro	10.8	13.5	12.1
5. Buena Vista	1.4	1.9	1.6
6. San Rafael Sacatepéquez	4.7	4.5	4.6
7. Saquitacaj	5.4	6.2	5.8
8. La Libertad	8.2	8.4	8.3
9. Cubulco	12.0	16.8	14.4
10. San Carlos Alzatate	6.6	5.4	6.0
11. Cahaboncito	5.2	7.0	6.2
12. Santa Fe	8.0	10.1	9.0
Mean	7.2[a]	8.8	

[a]Periods are statistically significant (P < 0.05).

ordinary metabolic process of adaptability that allows individuals to survive on a reduction of energy intake, maintaining their nutritional well-being.

3. In rural areas of developing agricultural countries, the social and economic structures, as well as agricultural and marketing systems and policies, may have worse consequences than seasonal cycles. Low purchasing power of families in these areas, and the poor or nonexisting health and medical ser-

TABLE X. Retinol Intake of Preschool Children in Rural Area of Guatemala, 1977
(μg per child per day)

Communities	April–May	October–November	$\overline{X}$
1. El Barrial	349[a]	211	278
2. Santa María Ixhuatán	298[a]	89	192
3. San Juan Zacapa	137	142	140
4. El Jícaro	159	178	168
5. Buena Vista	101	121	110
6. San Rafael Sacatepéquez	116	153	135
7. Saquitacaj	102	130	117
8. La Libertad	167	127	147
9. Cubulco	220	215	217
10. San Carlos Alzatate	135	90	113
11. Cahaboncito	71	64	67
12. Santa Fe	519[a]	279	397

[a]Periods are statistically significant ($P < 0.05$). Interaction between communities and periods are also significant.

vices, will have a more detrimental effect, especially during abnormal seasonal changes.

4. It is important to invest more time in continuing this type of study, to elucidate the main natural and nonnatural factors that affect the nutritional status of the people, especially young children, in each month of the year. In each country, the knowledge of the most critical period and the most affected area will help to orient policy makers to plan and select effective measures for solving and, even better, preventing any detrimental effects on the health and nutrition of the population.

REFERENCES

Annegers JF (1973): Seasonal food shortages in West Africa. Ecol Food Nutr 2:251–257.

Arroyave G et al (1979): "Evaluation of Sugar Fortification With Vitamin A at the National Level." PAHO, Scientific Publication 384. Washington, D.C. Pan American Health Organization.

Beaton GH (1981): Nutritional Conditions in Canada. In "Nutrition in the 1980s; Constraints on our Knowledge." Proceedings of the Western Hemisphere Nutrition Congress VI, held in Los Angeles, California, August 10–14, 1980. New York: Alan R. Liss, pp 221–235.

Bondestam L (1981): Understanding hunger and predicting starvation. Food Nutr Bull 3(4):1–4.

Castillo AS, Flores M (1955): Estudios dietéticos en El Salvador. II. Cantón Platanillos, Municipio de Quezaltepeque, Departamento de la Libertad. In Bol Of Sanit Pan, Suplemento No. 2. Publicaciones Científicas del Instituto de Nutrición de Centro América y Panamá. Washington, D.C., Oficina Sanitaria Panamericana, pp 54–65.

CDNHW (Canadian Department of National Health and Welfare) (1973): "Nutrition, a National Priority." A report by Nutrition Canada, of the National Survey to the Department of National Health and Welfare. Ottawa, Canada: DNHW.

CSPE (Consejo Superior de Planificación Económica) (1981): "Encuesta Sobre Consumo de Alimentos Realizada en la Ciudad de Tegucigalpa y las Regiones de: Occidente, Sur y Litoral Atlántico de la República de Honduras. Primer Informe." Tegucigalpa, Honduras: Secretaría Técnica del Consejo Superior de Planificación Económica, Diciembre, 1981.

Fjeld CR, Summer R (1982): Regional seasonal patterns in produce consumption at farmers markets and supermarkets. Ecol Food Nutr 12:109–115.

Hintermeister A, Blas J (1980): Guatemala, estacionalidad y subempleo en el sector agropecuario. Guatemala (PREALC-OIT): Impresos Industriales, pp 1–42.

Longhurst R, Payne P (1981): Review of evidence and policy implications. Seasonal aspects of nutrition. In Chambers R, Longhurst R, Pacey A (eds): "Seasonal Dimensions to Rural Poverty." London: Frances Pinter.

Marsden PD, Marsden SA (1965): A pattern of weight gain in Gambia babies during the first 18 months of life. J Trop Pediatr 10:89–99.

Neter J, Wasserman W (1974): "Applied Linear Statistical Models." Homewood, Ill: Richard D. Irwin, pp. 594–595.

Orr JB, Clark ML (1930): Seasonal variation in growth of school children. Lancet 2:365–367.

Pagezy H (1982): Seasonal hunger, as experienced by the Oto and Twa of a Ntomba village in the Equatorial Forest (Lake Tumba, Zaire). Ecol Food Nutr 12:139–153.

Rawson I, Valverde V (1976): The etiology of malnutrition among preschool children in Rural Costa Rica. J Trop Pediatr Environ Child Health 22:12–17.

Rutishauser IHE (1974): Factors affecting the intake of energy and protein by Ugandan preschool children. Ecol Food Nutr 3:213–222.

Schofield S (1974): Seasonal factors affecting nutrition in different age groups and especially preschool children. J Dev Study 11:22–40.

Sloof R (1978): Health and disease of under fives in Machakos District, Kenya. In "Seasonal Dimensions to Rural Poverty." A Conference Organized by the Institute of Development Studies and the Ross Institute of Tropical Hygiene, held in Sussex, Great Britain, July 3–6, 1978.

Sogandares L, Barrios G de (1955): Estudios dietéticos en Panamá. I. La Mesa, Provincia de Veraguas. In Bol Of San Pan, Suplemento No. 2. Publicaciones Científicas del Instituto de Nutrición de Centro América y Panamá. Washington, D.C., Oficina Sanitaria Panamericana, pp 38–46.

Trowbridge FL, Newton LH (1979). Seasonal changes in malnutrition and diarrheal disease among preschool children in El Salvador. Am J Trop Med Hyg 28(1):135–141.

Valverde V (1979): Functional Classification of Undernourished in Guatemala. Family socioeconomic characteristics and seasonal effects on the nutritional status of children living in coffee farms in Western Guatemala. PhD Thesis. London: University of London.

Valverde V, et al (1982): Seasonality and nutrition status. A review of findings from developed and developing countries. Arch Latinoam Nutr 32:521–540.

Malnutrition: Determinants and Consequences, pages 221–229
© *1984 Alan R. Liss, Inc., 150 Fifth Avenue, New York, NY 10011*

Adapting to Cultural Changes in Food Habits

Magdalena Krondl, PhD, **Nina Hrboticky,** MSc, **and Patricia Coleman,** MS
Department of Nutritional Sciences, Faculty of Medicine, University of Toronto, Toronto, Ontario, Canada M5S 1A8

Immigrants settling in Canada and the United States present a challenge to health professionals concerned with the prevention of nutritional disorders. The exposure of these groups to the Western food environment with comparatively easy access to items high in energy, fat, and sodium has been shown to increase the risk of major diseases, such as heart disease, obesity, periodontal disease, and cancer, which are prevalent in the host country [Marmot et al, 1975; Yano et al, 1979; Hankin et al, 1970; Schaefer et al, 1980; Calloway and Gibbs, 1976; Haenszel and Kuritara, 1968; Muto, 1977; Toshio, 1978; Wenkham and Wolff, 1970; Draper, 1974]. Adolescent newcomers in particular may be tempted to increase consumption of pleasant-tasting sweet and salty foods at the expense of nutritionally superior items. The "pleasure" connotation of these foods may have been introduced to groups such as West Indians and some Oriental countries through the strong influence of the North American media and tourism.

At this stage of development, with increasing independence, exposure to school environment and peer influence, the adolescents are likely to change their lifestyle and diet [McElroy and Taylor, 1966]. This is of special interest, since adaptation of food habits of adolescents may affect their health as well as that of the next generation.

With increased immigration such as is occurring in Ontario, where 17% of the population in 1981 [Statistics Canada, 1981] was other than British or French, the founding cultural groups, as compared with 11% in 1941 [Dominion Bureau of Statistics, 1946], the nutritional implications are considerable.

The main objective of this chapter is to describe changes in food habits of adolescents following immigration, focusing on the items found most likely to be affected—the popular "pleasure" foods and the less popular vegetables [Randall and Sanjur, 1981]. Factors influencing these changes will be reported. In addition, the concept of food perceptions and their relative influence on food use as a measure of nutritional behavioral change will be discussed. Since Western food guides [Hertzler and Anderson, 1974] may not be relevant to populations of other cultures, this concept may serve as an alternative means of assessing dietary intake of immigrant groups. Generally food intake data are evaluated in terms of nutrient requirements, which tends to mask the problem of excesses of nutrients and may not warn nutrition educators of potential dietary imbalance.

BACKGROUND

The numerous variables involved in food selection are recognized now as an important area of study [Freedman, 1977]. Nutritional anthropologists are endeavoring to link the complex areas of nutrition behavior to food resources and cultural values. Krondl and Boxen [1976] suggested a conceptual framework in which the basic variables were divided into utility and nonutility stimuli. This model was refined to incorporate research related to food meanings and classification of foods according to attitudinal values [Krondl and Lau, 1982]. The overall process of food selection was visualized as a barrier between food availability and food use with a set of food perceptions delineated as the barrier components. Food perceptions were considered as a blend of three factors: 1) the external and internal realities, 2) the messages of the stimuli that are conveyed by the nervous system to the integrative centers where thinking and evaluation take place, and 3) the resultant interpretations of the messages with feedback from past experiences [Lau et al, in press]. Since 1978, systematic study has been undertaken to test this cultural anthropology model with well-defined target groups and to determine the strength and direction of relationships between food perceptions and food use [Reaburn et al, 1979; Krondl et al, 1982a,b].

Heterogeneity Among Immigrants

Adaptation to the North American diet will differ from culture to culture depending on the immigrants' desire and opportunity to assimilate, degree of traditional family influence, and similarity of established values to those in the Western host country. In addition, socioeconomic status within the country of origin and noted assimilation trends within the immigration group will affect dietary acculturation [Reitz, 1981]. The value system especially is important. It is rooted in ecological, religious and philosophical beliefs well documented in Occidental and Oriental cultures. The West and East differ in the concept of a balanced diet. The West is concerned with the nutrient content. The East em-

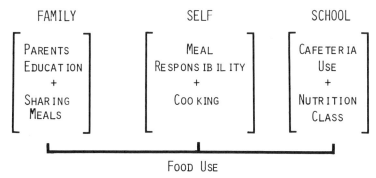

Fig. 1.   Intergroup comparison of food behavior.

braces the idea of Yin and Yang [Libasse, 1974]. According to Myrdall [1968] more spiritualism and ascetic detachment are represented in the Asian value system than in that of the Western "New Man" showing preparedness for change and alertness to opportunities.

Comparison of Four Cultural Groups

In the intergroup comparison of food-related behavior, subjects were adolescents between 14 and 16 years of age. They were selected through purposive sampling from three schools in Metropolitan Toronto. The immigrant populations consisted of 35 Northern and Central Europeans, 34 West Indians, and 38 Chinese (mainly from Hong Kong). The West Indian population was pooled from Jamaica, Barbados, Guyana, Dominican Republic, Trinidad, and Grenada, the majority being from Jamaica. The current population of the West Indies descended originally from immigrant Europeans, Africans, Indians, and Chinese who came to their islands from the 17th century to the present. Thus they are not culturally homogeneous but in this study represent the values prevailing in the island countries. The host country sample was made up of 213 adolescents representing third-generation British-Canadians. The number of girls and boys was approximately the same in all groups with the exception of the Chinese sample, which had boys only. The mean length of time in Canada was similar for all the immigrant populations.

In the intergroup comparison of food behavior the roles of family, self, and school were examined (Fig. 1). Two variables involved the family. First was the *parents' education*, the only information allowed to be obtained that would indicate socioeconomic status of the family. The mother's education was important because of the implied potential occupation and the implied ability to assimilate.

The Chinese students had the lowest percentage of parents with postsecondary education. The educational level of the parents of the West Indian students was higher than that of the Chinese parents but lower than that of the British-Canadian and European parents. The percentage of mothers having postsecondary education was highest among the Europeans; the educational level of the fathers was highest among the British-Canadians.

The second factor studied was the *sharing of meals*. This gave an idea of the space for interaction of the adolescent with the family. Data related to social environment at meal time indicated that over 40% in each ethnic group ate breakfast alone; this was most common among the West Indians (54%). Chinese students ate lunch with their parents most frequently. Dinner was generally family-oriented among all groups; the West Indian students had a slightly higher incidence of eating alone.

The amount of responsibility for their own meals and for cooking at home gave us some idea of the degree of food involvement by the adolescents themselves. Adolescents in all groups had little *responsibility for their meals*. They were mostly responsible for their breakfast and lunch. But when we looked at the responses for all meals the West Indians scored highest. Frequency of cooking at home, the other index of food involvement, was found to be highest among the Chinese, followed by West Indians. Greater responsibility for their own meals and for cooking at home may lead to greater opportunity for nutritionally undesirable food choices among the Chinese and West Indian adolescents.

Finally, the *use of the school cafeteria* indicated the degree of influence of the Canadian food environment on the adolescent. In regard to frequency of cafeteria use and type of lunch purchased, intergroup differences were evident. The Chinese were the highest consumers of hot lunches or à la carte items; next were the West Indians. British-Canadian students frequently supplemented their lunches from home with items purchased in the cafeteria; Europeans followed this practice as well but on a less regular basis.

A *nutrition quiz* was employed to determine how much the adolescent learned, presumably at school, of nutrition concepts. Awareness of nutrition concepts prevalent in the host country was assessed with an eight-item questionnaire. The items included energy, iron, calcium, vitamin C and D, fiber, salt, and heart disease. Lack of awareness of current nutrition concepts was apparent in the case of the West Indians, who scored lowest for six of eight items. Chinese students were not consistent in their nutrition awareness in comparison to the British-Canadians and the Europeans, but achieved similar scores. European adolescents scored highest.

The effects on food use of the many factors that must be considered in intercultural studies [Goode et al, 1981] were reflected among the "pleasant" foods: wieners, potato chips, and French fries (Table I). These are items considered nutritionally poor when used indiscriminately. Higher frequency of use of these foods was found among the West Indians and Chinese adolescents than

TABLE I. "Pleasant" Foods in the Diets of Four Adolescent Cultural Groups

Food	Culture[a]	n	Daily	Weekly	Less than weekly	Intergroup difference[b]
				Use frequency (%)		
Wieners	British-Canadian (BC)	210	1	33	66	
	European (E)	35	0	23	77	BC/WI, BC/C
	W. Indian (WI)	33	12	32	56	E/C, C/WI
	Chinese (C)	38	0	55	45	
Potato chips	British-Canadian	213	5	45	50	
	European	34	0	35	65	BC/C, E/C
	W. Indian	34	11	56	33	
	Chinese	38	3	55	42	
French fries	British-Canadian	211	8	52	40	
	European	35	9	46	45	BC/WI, C/WI
	W. Indian	34	27	44	29	
	Chinese	38	3	50	47	

[a]All groups are first generation immigrants, except for British-Canadians.
[b]Chi-square, $P < 0.05$.

among the British-Canadians and Europeans. The Europeans were seen to be less susceptible to nutritionally negative influences on dietary behavior.

The higher educational level of the mother among West Indians and the higher nutritional knowledge of the Chinese did not offset the effect of the factors of self-involvement with food, the use of the cafeteria, and the economic level of the country of origin, all of which appeared to encourage the more frequent use of "pleasant" foods.

In contrast, the higher educational level of the European mothers coupled with the higher nutrition knowledge of the student, the lower degree of food involvement and use of school cafeteria, as well as higher economic level of country of origin, seemed to impede the use of "pleasant" foods.

COMPARISON OF TWO GENERATIONS OF A SINGLE CULTURAL GROUP

Food-use frequency and food perceptions, specifically prestige, healthfulness, and taste, were combined to assess the effect of duration of exposure to the new environment on the use of specific foods, emphasis being placed on "pleasant" foods and vegetables (Fig. 2). The Chinese adolescents involved in the intergroup comparison were selected also for the intergenerational comparison with 38 first-generation and 16 second-generation Chinese boys.

In concordance with the findings of other studies [Grivetti and Paquette, 1978; Ho et al, 1966; Jerome, 1975], it was found that the core foods repre-

DURATION OF RESIDENCE IN CANADA

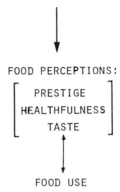

FOOD PERCEPTIONS:

PRESTIGE

HEALTHFULNESS

TASTE

FOOD USE

Fig. 2.   Intergenerational comparison of food behavior.

TABLE II. Perceptions of "Pleasant" Foods Used More Frequently by Second-Generation Chinese Boys (Kendall's tau b coefficients)

"Pleasant" foods	Frequency of use	Perceptions		
		Taste	Prestige	Healthfulness
Cakes/pastries	− 0.33*	− 0.28*	− 0.12	0.18
Salami	− 0.31*			
Cold cereals	− 0.27*			
Potato chips	− 0.22*	− 0.21	− 0.27*	0.11

Kendalls' tau b coefficients indicating intergenerational differences. Negative tau b indicate higher use and/or more positive food perception rating. Positive tau b indicate lower use and/or more negative food perception rating.
*P < 0.05.

senting dietary staples, or foods used more than three times a week, changed little regardless of duration of residence. When first- and second-generation adolescent Chinese were compared, the majority (65%) of changes found were among the peripheral and marginal foods used on a monthly or yearly basis. The degree of change may appear of little significance, but the type of change is important because it indicates the incorporation of "pleasant" foods, which are high in sugar, salt, and fat.

Table II indicates the increased use of cakes, salami, cold cereals, and potato chips by the second-generation Chinese. This change is significant specifically in view of the higher use of potato chips by first-generation Chinese than by other cultural groups. The trend to the use of "pleasant" foods coincided with the decreased use of certain vegetables (Table III). Many vegetables have

TABLE III. Extent of Decrease of Vegetable Use by Second-Generation Chinese Boys (Kendall's tau b coefficients)

Vegetable	Extent of decrease in frequency of use
Radishes	0.33*
Squash	0.31*
Peppers	0.30*
Brussels sprouts	0.29*
Celery	0.28*
Tomatoes	0.24*

For further details see Table II.
*P < 0.05

been reported as unpleasant in taste, possibly because of their bitter components. The element of pleasantness in an environment of high availability of foods is a factor that is of importance to nutritionists concerned with change in food habits.

The behavioral phenomenon is reinforced with increased rating of perception of taste and prestige, which are significant in the case of certain foods shown in Table II. Ratings of perception of taste and prestige give evidence that "pleasant" foods increase in desirability with increased length of exposure. This was not balanced by an appropriate change in perception of healthfulness that would discourage the extensive use of these foods.

CONCLUSIONS

The wide variety of foods available in large metropolitan centers in Canada presents a problem of nutritionally appropriate choices to immigrant populations. Specifically, adolescents may be vulnerable to excess consumption of foods pleasant in taste and high in salt, fat, and sugar content. This is of concern since adolescents are in the process of forming habits that affect their health and that of succeeding generations. An intergroup comparison of food-related behavior of Europeans, West Indians, Chinese, and British-Canadians has shown that the higher educational level of the mother among West Indians and the high nutrition knowledge of the Chinese did not offset the undesirable effect of other factors affecting food choices. They include the self-selection of foods at home or in the school cafeteria and the lower economic level of the country of origin. These factors appeared to increase the frequency of use of "pleasant" foods such as wieners, French fries, and potato chips. This trend increases with longer exposure to the new environment. An intergenerational comparison of Chinese students indicated that more frequent use of "pleasant" foods and decreased use of vegetables occurred in the second generation. The greater frequency of use was accompanied by the higher rating of perception of taste and prestige but not of the healthfulness of these foods. This suggests the need for providing appropriate nutrition information to immigrant populations, warning of the potential risks of excessive use of "pleasant" foods at the expense of vegetables.

REFERENCES

Calloway DH, Gibbs JC (1976): Food patterns and food assistance programs in Cocopah Indian community. Ecol Food Nutr 5:183–196.

Dominion Bureau of Statistics (1946): "Eighth Census of Canada 1941."

Draper HH (1977): The aboriginal diet in modern perspective. Anthropologist 79:309–316.

Drewnowski A, Greenwood RC (1983): Cream and sugar: Human preference for high-fat foods. Physiol Behav 30:629–633.

Freedman RL (1977): "Nutritional anthropology: An overview." In Fitzgerald JK (ed): "Nutrition and Anthropology in Action." Assen/Amsterdam: van Gorcum, pp 1–23.

Goode JG, Curtis K, Theophano J (1981): Group-shared food patterns as a unit of analysis. In Miller SA (ed): "Nutrition and Behavior." The Franklin Institute Press, pp 19–30.

Grivetti LE, Paquette MB (1978): Non-traditional ethnic food choices among first generation Chinese in California. J Nutr Ed 10:109.

Haenszel W, Kuritara M (1968): Studies of Japanese migrants. Mortality from cancer and other diseases among Japanese in the United States. J Natl Cancer Inst 40:43–68.

Hankin J, Reed, Labarthe D, Nichaman M, Stallones R (1970): Dietary and disease patterns among Micronesians. Am J Clin Nutr 23:346–357.

Hertzler AA, Anderson HL (1974): Food guides in the United States. J Am Dietet A 64:19–28.

Ho GP, Nolan FL, Doods ML (1966): Adaptation to American dietary patterns by students from Oriental countries. J Am Diet Assoc 58:277–280.

Jerome NW (1975): On determining food patterns of urban dwellers in contemporary United States society. In Arnott M (ed): "Gastronomy: The Anthropology of Food and Food Habbits." Paris: Mouton, pp 91–111.

Krondl MM, Boxen GG (1976): Nutrition behavior, food resources and energy. In Arnott M (ed): "Gastronomy: The Anthropology of Food and Food Habits." Paris: Mouton, pp 113–120.

Krondl M, Lau D (1982): Social determinants in human food selection. In Barker LM (ed): "The Psychobiology of Human Food Selection." Westport, Conn: Avi, pp 139–152.

Krondl M, George R, Coleman P (1982a): Factors influencing food selection of adolescents in different social environments. Nutr Q (Dairy Bureau of Canada) 6:38–43.

Krondl M, Lau D, Yurkiw MA, Coleman PH (1982b): Food use and perceived food meanings of the elderly. J Am Diet Assoc 80:523–528.

Lau D, Krondl M, Coleman P (in press): Psychological factors affecting food selection. In Galler JR (ed): "Nutrition and Behavior." New York: Plenum.

Libasse PT (1974): Two for the cellular seesaw. Sciences 14:15–20.

Marmot MG, Syme SL, Kagan H, Cohen JB, Belsky J (1975): "Epidemiologic studies of coronary heart disease and stroke in Japanese men living in Japan, Hawaii and California. Am J Epidemiol 106:514.

McElroy J, Taylor J (1966): Adolescents' values in selection of foods. J Home Ec 58:651.

Muto S (1977): Dietary sweet: Exposure and preference among Japanese children and in laboratory rats. In Weinffenbach JW (ed): "Taste and Development: The Genesis of Sweet Preference." Bethesda, Maryland: US Department of Health and Welfare.

Myrdall J (1968): "Asian Drama." New York: The Twentieth Century Fund.

Randall E, Sanjur D (1981): Food preferences — Their conceptualization and relationship to consumption. Ecol Food Nutr 11:151–161.

Reaburn J, Krondl M, Lau D (1979): Social determinants in food selection. Am Diet Assoc 74: 637–641.

Reitz JG (1981): "Survival of Ethnic Groups." New York: McGraw-Hill Ryerson.

Schaefer O, Timmermans JFW, Matthews AR (1980): General and nutritional health in two Eskimo populations at different stages of acculturation. Can J Publ Health 71:397–405.

Statistics Canada (1981): Census 1981 Population, Mother Tongue.

Toshio O (1978): Anthropometric and disease pattern changes in the Japanese population: Nutritional or other? In Margen S, Ogar RA (eds): "Progress in Human Nutrition." Westport, Connecticut: Avi, Vol 2.

Wenkham SN, Wolff RJ (1970): A half century of changing food habits among Japanese in Hawaii. J Am Diet Assoc 57:29–32.

Yano K, Blackwelder WC, Kagan A, Rhoads GG, Cohen JN, Marmot MG (1979): Childhood cultural experience and the incidence of coronary heart disease in Hawaiian, Japanese men. Am J Epidemiol 109:440.

NUTRITION AND
THE IMMUNE RESPONSES

Malnutrition: Determinants and Consequences, pages 233–244
© 1984 Alan R. Liss, Inc., 150 Fifth Avenue, New York, NY 10011

Nutritional Factors in Immune Response

Susanna Cunningham-Rundles, PhD
Laboratories of Clinical Immunology and Human Immunogenetics, Memorial
Sloan-Kettering Cancer Center, New York, New York 10021

Impaired nutrition is the single most common cause of acquired immune deficiency in the world today. In impoverished environments poor nutrition and chronic contact with infectious agents combine to undermine healthy development throughout life. In affluent environments suboptimal nutrition may affect critical metabolic functions, including the immune response, without discovery, since malnutrition has received comparatively little attention in economically developed cultures. Exceptions to this have been malnutrition secondary to disease (specifically cancer), and requirements in neonatal development and in aging, where efforts have been focused on essential nutritional support.

Specific knowledge of the critical interaction between nutritional factors and immune mechanisms, however, has been difficult to obtain because of the complexity of factors involved. Some effects of nutritional status on immune response may be primary, having specific and direct impact on immune response. Other effects may be secondary, arising from negative effects of malnutrition on other organ systems that have immune regulatory functions or from negative effects on all cellular metabolism including the immune system. In many states of malnutrition primary and secondary effects act in concert in producing the clinical presentation. The development and use of animal models, although inevitable and invaluable, has rather uncertain application to human nutrition, in which genetic and environmental factors are more complex and less defined. With the recent development of newer techniques and more sensitive methodology in the fields of immunology, genetics, and epidemiology, greater clarity may be expected and one can anticipate rapid changes in this field.

The immune system has been regarded, somewhat artificially, as being composed of two separate systems, humoral and cellular, and investigation into the nature of immune impairment in specific nutritionally defined states has depended upon use of parametric assessment of immune function. It should be borne in mind, however, that this approach is useful only to the degree that the tested response in vitro mirrors the actual challenge in vivo or the potential to respond to actual environmental challenge. Thus, specific, unrecognized deficits in immune response may underlie susceptibility to specific types of infections in undernourished persons or susceptibility to infections presenting in particular modes.

MALNUTRITION AND DISEASE RESISTANCE

Severe malnutrition leading to maramus or kwashiorkor has been invariably associated with both bacterial and viral infections, gastrointestinal malfunction, and skin rashes. The relationship of these clinical observations to impaired immunity has been well appreciated for many years and extensively reported [1–6]. The principal infections found in severe protein-calorie malnutrition (PCM) are listed in Table I. Many of these, specifically tuberculosis, herpes, *Pneumocystis carinii* pneumonia, measles, and malaria are intracellular pathogens, so that a critical role for the cellular immune arm of the immune system has been postulated, since the cellular immune system evolved in association with this need. These findings have been strengthened by studies of histopathology in children dying of protein-calorie malnutrition [7] in which marked thymic atrophy was found in nearly all cases. Similarly, other postmortem studies of kwashiorkor and marasmus have revealed marked loss of normal thymic architecture, and atrophy of peripheral lymphoid tissues with a tendency toward preservation of diffcreuliated B cells in the spleen [8,9].

Animal model studies of protein deficiency in early life have confirmed clinical observations that protein deficiency alone produces markedly reduced cellular proliferation in lymphoid organs and ultimately atrophy [10]. This condition occurs frequently in underdeveloped cultures during the weaning period, and some workers have considered weaning rather than birth to be the period of greatest dangei to survival.

In recent animal studies, malnutrition during suckling followed by intermittent feeding during weaning was found to produce both cell-mediated and humoral deficiency, whereas malnutrition during suckling alone did not have a significant effect [11]. Clearly, the relative protection of infants by breast milk would be highly dependent upon both quantity and quality as well as factors affecting its availability. The work of Hanson [12] has shown that IgA antibodies in breast milk persist during lactation, in contrast to IgA antibodies produced at other mucosal surfaces, which are known to be relatively short-

TABLE I. Principal Infections in Protein-Calorie Malnutrition

1. *Mycobacterium tuberculosis*
2. *Herpes simplex*
3. *Pneumocystis carinii* pneumonia
4. Measles
5. Malaria
6. Diarrheal disease caused by numerous enteropathogenic, enterotoxic strains of *E. coli, Shigella,* and rotoviruses
7. Schistosoma and other parasitic infections

lived. Milk antibodies supply passive humoral protection to the infant against endogenous bacteria, including coliform bacteria, viruses, and foodstuffs at a period when the immune system is immature and therefore vulnerable to attack. During the period of birth until puberty, thymus weight normally increases, and in the absence of nutritional support thymic atrophy becomes a major consequence, blocking essential maturation of the immune system.

Protein-calorie malnutrition acts indirectly on the immune system, as this state affects all cellular metabolism. However, since the maturation of a fully functioning immune system must occur during the postbirth period, nutritional status is critical for immune system differentiation and development so that failure directly compromises survival.

The role in PCM of environmental pathogens and infections spread by contact, food, or water is central for several reasons. Direct damage to infected tissues weakens the host. In the case of agents causing diarrheal disease, for example, direct loss of protein is a cause of PCM and nutritional repletion is difficult. In addition, the limited reserve capacity of the immune system may become rapidly exhausted by intense antigenic stimulation. Finally microbial and viral agents are in themselves powerful immune regulators that affect immune network interactions and modify biological response to subsequent antigenic signals. In addition to causing protein loss, diarrheal disease may be associated with selective malabsorption of nutrients and vitamins required for normal immune functioning and may result in specific depletion of cofactors critical for differentiated immune expression. The relationship between intestinal flora and local intestinal lymphoid tissue in healthy persons leads to a stimulation of lymphoid cells in Peyer's patches by organisms colonizing the intestinal tract that subsequently migrate to other lymphoid organs [13], leading therefore to the development of an active immune response. For example, the initial development of spontaneous cytotoxic cells, natural killer cells, has been found to reflect this process [14]. Decreased production of secretory IgA in saliva and nasopharyngeal secretions has been found to be markedly reduced in PCM [15,16]. McMurray and co-workers have reported specific loss of normal levels of secretory IgA in moderately malnourished children

[17] and an apparently compensatory increase in serum IgA which appeared to be related to reduced production or function of the secretory component. The loss of secretory IgA would be expected to leave mucosal surfaces unprotected against adherence of microorganisms and also to permit penetration by macromolecules. Although these children were uninfected at the time of study, parallel observations by Bell et al [10] suggest that following infection elevated immunoglobulin production including secretory IgA occurs. Thus, the critical interface between nutritional impairment and susceptibility to infection may be sequence-dependent, since after the initiation of infection primary differences between well-nourished and critically undernourished persons may become temporarily blurred. Related animal model studies by Lim et al [18] have shown that mice fed a low-protein diet had lower intestinal IgA than controls in early life but that the imposition of the same diet in older mice did not affect intestinal IgA. These data are also in agreement with clinical observations that malnutrition in early life is particularly deleterious.

Chandra [19] has observed that undernutrition increases frequency of infections, specifically of mucosal surfaces, and has reported impaired secretory IgA antibody response to poliovirus and measles vaccines. Thus a link between susceptibility to infections and reduced secretory IgA is suggested.

Despite the correlation between serum albumin and survival in severe infections in African children, definition of the exact cellular basis of deficient immune response has been elusive. Whittle et al [20] have reported a higher susceptibility of cells from undernourished uninfected children to measles virus in vitro than from healthy children, but found similar cellular cytotoxicity against measles-infected targets during infection. Since children who were malnourished and subsequently died of measles had lower killing ability than did survivors who were also undernourished, one may speculate that after the onset of infection absolute functional response may not reflect survival potential, possibly for the simple reason that greater killing or effector target binding of higher affinity would be required to eliminate a more widespread infection. Since in most cell-mediated testing, lower limits are established based on healthy controls, one is not necessarily able to ascertain what level of activity would be required effectively to eliminate infection in a significantly physiologically compromised host.

Although loss of interferon production to Newcastle disease virus in marasmus has been reported [21], it was not found in older children [20] challenged with measles virus. Thus, specificity of immune deficits may vary markedly according to age, associated infections, and the nature of the challenge. Since the characterization of cytotoxic mechanisms now known to mediate host defense has become more complex [22], assessment of these mechanisms in vitro in a more complete way can be applied in future studies of this type.

The host defense mechanisms that have been reported to be deficient in PCM are briefly outlined in Table II. Defects in polymorphonuclear leukocyte

**TABLE II. Deficient Host Defense Mechanisms in
Protein-Calorie Malnutrition**

1. Lymphocyte proliferation in autologous plasma
2. Delayed-type hypersensitivity
3. Total hemolytic complement
4. Inflammation and chemotaxis
5. Antibody production

and monocyte chemotaxis result in failure to localize pathogens and secondarily impede activation of amplification systems. Failure of monocyte chemotaxis has been particularly associated with kwashiorkor and marasmus [23]. Overall clearance by phagocytes may be reduced as a result of lymphoid atrophy; some workers [24] have reported a compensatory increase in single-cell functioning. Since monocyte functioning is critical for antigen processing and T-B lymphocyte cooperativity, quantitative reduction in this function would be expected to have an important impact on host defense and immune response. Many of the reported losses of lymphocyte proliferative activity in PCM have not been observed in cultures with serum or plasma from control subjects, suggesting that toxic materials or lack of nutritional elements may affect the observed lack of response. Anticomplementary activity possibly associated with endotoxin has also been reported [25]. Studies on prospective analysis of the possible effects of mild to moderate nutrition by McMurray et al [26] have shown loss of ability to undergo a primary immunization to dinitrochlorobenzene in children experiencing the progressive effects of undernutrition in early life. Other workers have reported that malnourished children failed to develop a positive Mantoux test reaction following BCC vaccination but that in vitro response was normal [27].

Taken as a whole, studies in protein-calorie malnutrition confirm that cellular and humoral immunity are compromised. The studies provide evidence that timing, duration, and environmental setting are determinative in the long-term consequences of undernutrition.

Malnutrition continues to be a relatively common occurrence in hospitalized patients. Disease states that have been associated with acquired malnutrition are listed in Table III. In many of these conditions positive correlations between skin test responses to recall antigens and impaired nutritional state have had predictive value for survival [28–30]. Improved survival and good nutritional status have been found to correlate in children with localized lymphoma or solid tumors (Donaldson et al [30]), but no correlation was seen in advanced disease.

Nutritional support of the surgical patient can be assessed for effect on immune response in a way that nutritional support of the cancer patient cannot be. The relationship of diet and cancer is quite complex, and little clarity has been obtained in this field to date. Neoplastic cellular growth must be main-

TABLE III. Disease States Associated With Acquired Malnutrition and Immunocompromise

1. Trauma
2. Lymphoreticular malignancies
3. Breast cancer
4. Bronchogenic cancer
5. Hepatic disease, including cirrhosis, chronic alcoholic disease, and viral hepatitis
6. Renal disease maintained on hemodialysis
7. Osteogenic sarcoma

tained by nutritional support derived from the host, and the differential nature of this support as distinct from that required by the host is not known. Clearly, the basis of malnutrition in the cancer patient must similarly be understood at least to some degree before meaningful observations can be made on the effect of nutrition on tumor immunity.

NUTRITIONAL FACTORS AND IMMUNE RESPONSE: MECHANISMS OF ACTION

Acquired immune deficiency may develop in association with either acute severe undernutrition, or chronic mild malnutrition occurring at times of weakened resistance. The resulting immunodeficiency state, if compounded by the establishment of an infecting process, may have long-term consequences even if repletion can be achieved. Efforts to clarify the mechanism of specific nutritional action on immune response have produced qualitative information at best. This appears to be the case not because nutritional factors act only in general ways to provide substrates for more structured biological events, but because of the inherent difficulties in identifying the critical processes.

One approach to this problem has been to study the interaction of single nutrients in defined settings. The following discussion will focus on examination of the role of zinc in immune response, both as an example of a specific, critical interaction and as a method of approach to more general issues applicable to the field of nutrition and immunity.

Several lines of investigation have suggested that zinc has a specific and critical effect on immune function. Both the development and the maintenance of normal cellular immune function have been found to require zinc. Some of the extensive literature in this field has been summarized in reviews [31–33]. Zinc deficiency in man was first reported by Prasad et al [34] as a major limiting factor in the nutrition of children and adolescents in Iran, which was found to be directly associated with growth retardation and gonadal dysfunction. Halsted et al [35] successfully treated a group of Iranian persons with zinc deficiency and clinical features nearly identical to those of Prasad's group, and then achieved resolution of impairment with zinc alone. In both these studies, immunodeficiency associated with zinc deficiency was inferred from observations of increased incidence of infection but no direct link was established. Brummerstedt et al [36] was the first to observe an association between zinc deficiency and grossly abnormal thymic development in the A-46 lethal mutation in cattle. Lethality was directly attributable to failure to absorb zinc from the gastrointestinal tract. Moynahan [34] similarly found that the congenital syndrome *Acrodermatitis enteropathica* was produced by failure of zinc absorption. Children with this genetic defect had markedly increased susceptibility to infection and marked immunodeficiency disease, all features of which could be resolved by zinc repletion [37].

Systematic investigations of zinc and immunity have been carried out by a number of workers. Fraker et al [38] have demonstrated that in mice, zinc is essential to the development of the T cell, specifically those T cells that interact with B lymphocytes to produce an antibody response to T-dependent antigens. These results have been confirmed and extended by Fernandes et al [39]. Basic studies have been summarized by Good et al [31]. Related studies in the rat by Gross et al [40] have also shown zinc deficiency to be associated with immune impairment.

In human studies zinc has been found to be a mitogen in vitro, stimulating peripheral blood lymphocytes to undergo cell division [41]. Cunningham-Rundles et al [42] have reported that zinc stimulation in vitro produces the differentiation of B cells, leading to antibody secretion.

The effect of zinc on the development and expression of cytotoxic cells has been less clear. Fernandes et al [39] have reported low natural killer (NK) activity in zinc-deficient mice, and Chandra and Au [43] have reported increased NK activity in a somewhat different system.

Since in previous studies [42] we found a synergistic effect of zinc acting in concert with other B-cell-activating agents, a study of the effect of zinc on the natural killer system has recently been undertaken. The results of these experiments are briefly described in the following discussion to illustrate the effect of a single nutritional factor on immune function.

Addition of zinc to freshly isolated peripheral blood lymphocytes taken from healthy volunteers and mixed with tumor target cells (K562) caused inhibition of the cytotoxicity normally seen. The effect was found to be caused by a protective effect of zinc acting to impede target lysis; it was rapidly diluted out by reducing the concentration of the added zinc.

In contrast, strong enhancement of interferon-mediated natural killer activity was seen when zinc was added at a concentration of approximately 5×10^{-4} M. These experiments are described elsewhere in more detail [44]; they suggest that zinc prevents the gradual loss of interferon-induced activity, which occurs as a normal consequence of signal metabolism, not by directly activating NK cells but perhaps by prolonging the life of newly matured NK cells or by enhancing the efficiency of target lysis. The presence of interferon in lymphocytes cultured for 6 days was found to be typically associated with a sixfold or greater NK activity compared to that of cultures where interferon was not present. When zinc was added as well, strong enhancement was observed and this effect was proportionately stronger at lower effector target ratios.

Figure 1 shows the enhancement of α-interferon-boosted NK activity in relation to the concentration of zinc used. The marked change in lysis at lower effector-target ratios appeared to occur in a narrow concentration range, the most striking of which is illustrated here. At other concentrations of zinc, the slope of the line was not changed from that seen with interferon alone. Different donors were found to have an essentially similar optimal concentration effect, but the amount of the augmentation varied. In about one-third of cases, enhancement was 5–6 times that of cells cultured with interferon alone.

In the recently identified acquired immunodeficiency syndrome (AIDS) [45, 46], many patients have been found to have reduced natural killer activity or none [47]. In addition, many patient lymphocytes cannot be induced in vitro by interferon. This condition of lack of precursor NK cells has been frequently observed among people at risk for AIDS [48]. In Table IV are shown results obtained with lymphocytes from four such persons. As shown, only Cases 1 and 4 showed normal NK augmentation. Zinc alone did not affect NK activity. In contrast, 3 of 4 cases showed enhancement of NK activity when zinc was used to coactivate the system.

The results presented here in light of the previous discussion may serve to clarify some of the issues involved in studying the interaction between nutrition and immunity. As shown, nutritional factors may act pharmacologically on the immune system to affect critical processes. This kind of effect is inherently different from modes of activity in which zinc-dependent enzyme reactions are negatively affected by zinc deficiency. Conversely, if zinc has an immunomodulating role, one might expect that zinc deprivation would lead to the development of altered immunoregulation that might be reversed by another immunomodulating agent. Gross et al [49] have observed that levamisole was able to improve the response of zinc-deficient rat spleen lymphocytes to phytohemagglutinin while having no effect on pair-fed controls.

Dardenne et al [50] have recently demonstrated that zinc is essential for the biological activity of thymic hormone, and Bach [51] has suggested that zinc affects the immune system in four different ways: 1) as part of essential metalloenzymes, eg, thymidine kinase; 2) as a component of biologically active mediators, eg, thymic hormones; 3) as a membrane stabilizer, eg, interaction with cytochalasin B [52]; and 4) as a mitogen.

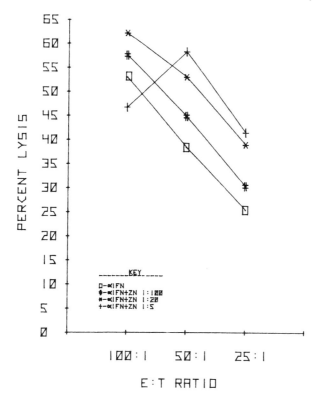

Fig. 1. Peripheral blood mononuclear cells were activated or not, as shown by key, for 6 days and then tested in a standard 4-hr chromium-release assay (see also note to Table IV). Results are shown for three effector-target ratios.

TABLE IV. Effect of Zn^{++} on Activated NK Activity in Persons at Risk for Acquired Immunodeficiency Disease Syndrome (AIDS)

Case	None	α-IFN	Zn^{++}	α-IFN + Zn^{++}
1	7.4	17.3	0.3	33.6
2	0.3	6.5	-1.7	9.7
3	7.3	0.0	0.5	30.8
4	9.7	28.3	1.3	38.5

Peripheral blood mononuclear cells activated with α-IFN following overnight preculture to deplete endogenous NK. α-IFN was added at a concentration of 800 units/10^6 lymphocytes and zinc at 2.5×10^{-4} M. The target was the erythroleukemia cell line K562. The effector-to-target ratio was 100:1 and the assay was a 4-hr chromium release assay. Data are shown as percentage specific release.

The specificity of the interaction of nutritional factors with the immune system depends upon nutritional state, since the metabolism of a factor during acute shortage of supply must be different from the metabolism of the same factor during moderate shortage of supply. Hence, the level of activity of nutritional factors must be considered in investigating mechanisms of action. Finally, pharmacological effects need to be differentiated from physiological requirements. The essential activity of the immune system is response to challenge. This activity requires intact lymphoid architecture and cellular machinery, much of which can be developed only after birth and therefore competes for nutritional support. The response process itself involves intense amplification and differentiation of cell populations interacting with each other and with signals, all of which again require vigorous cellular metabolism and nutritional support. Measurement of immune processes reflects current concepts of these interactions [53] and must be reworked to reflect actual environmental settings. The immunoregulatory effect of nutritional factors on immune response may occur in the presence of normal nutritional support as well as in its absence, and it therefore defines a critical area for future investigations.

ACKNOWLEDGMENTS

The excellent technical assistance of Mrs. K.M. Smith is gratefully acknowledged.

These studies were supported in part by NIH NCI CB 08748-17, The Richard Molin Memorial Foundation for Cancer Research, and NIH PO I CA 29502-04.

REFERENCES

1. Scrimshaw NS, Taylor LE, Gordon JE (1968): Interactions of nutrition and infection. WHO Monogr Ser, No. 57.
2. Chandra RK (1972): Immunocompetence in undernutrition. J Pediatr 81:1194–1200.
3. Suskind R, Sirisinha S, Vithayasai V, Edelman R, Damrongsak D, Charopatara C, Olson RE (1976): Immunoglobulin and antibody response in children with protein-calorie malnutrition. Am J Clin Nutr 29:835–841.
4. Edelman R (1975): "Cell-Mediated Immunity in Protein-Calorie Malnutrition." New York: Academic, pp 377–381.
5. Schlesinger L, Stekel A (1974): Impaired cellular immunity in marasmic infants. Am J Clin Nutr 27:615–620.
6. Mata LF (1975): Malnutrition-infection interactions in the tropics. Am J Trop Med Hyg 24:564–574.
7. Purtila DT, Connor DH (1975): Fatal infections in protein-calorie malnourished children with thymolymphatic atrophy. Arch Dis Child 50:149–152.
8. Mugerwa JW (1971): The lymphoreticular system in kwashiorkor. J Pathol 105:105–109.
9. Smythe PM, Brereton-Stiles GG, Grace HJ, Mafoyane A, Schorland M, Coovadja M, Loening WEK, Parent MA, Vos GH (1971): Thymolymphatic deficiency and depression of

cell-mediated immunity in protein-calorie malnutrition. Lancet 2:939–943.

10. Bell RG, Halzell LA, Price P (1976): Influence of dietary protein restriction on immune competence. II. Effect on lymphoid tissue. Clin Exp Immunol 26:314–326.

11. Wade S, Lemonnier FB, Delorme J (1983): Early nutritional experiments: Effects on the humoral and cellular immune responses in mice. J Nutr 113:1131–1139.

12. Good RA, Hanson L (1982): Infections and undernutrition. Nutr Rev 40:119–128.

13. Parrott DMV (1981): Lymphocyte circulation outside the lymphoid system. In deSousa M: "Lymphocyte Circulation." New York: Wiley, pp 99–122.

14. Huh NHY, Kim YB, Koren HA, Amos DB (1981): Natural killing and antibody-dependent cellular cytotoxicity in specific pathogen-free miniature swine and germ-free piglets. II. Ontogenic development of NK and ADCC. Int J Cancer 28:175–182.

15. Chandra RK, Newberne PM (1977): "Nutrition, Immunity and Infection: Mechanisms of Interactions." New York, London: Plenum.

16. Sirisinha S, Suskind R, Edelman R, Asvapaka C, Olson RE (1975): Secretory and serum IgA in children with protein-calorie malnutrition. Pediatrics 55:166–170.

17. McMurray DN, Rey H, Casazza CJ, Watson RR (1977): Effect of moderate malnutrition on concentrations of immunoglobulins and enzymes in tears and saliva of young Colombian children. Am J Clin Nutr 30:1944–1948.

18. Lim TS, Messiha N, Watson RR (1981): Immune components of the intestinal mucosa of aging and protein-deficient mice. Immunology 43:401–407.

19. Chandra RK (1975): Reduced secretory antibody response to live attenuated measles and poliovirus vaccines in malnourished children. Br Med J 2:583–585.

20. Whittle HC, Mee J, Webinska J, Yakubu A, Onuora C, Gomwalk N (1981): Immunity to measles in malnourished children. Clin Exp Immunol 42:144–151.

21. Schlesinger L, Ohlbaum A, Grez L, Stekel A (1976): Decreased interferon production by leukocytes in marasmus. Am J Clin Nutr 29:758–761.

22. Cunningham-Rundles S (1981): Cell-mediated immunity. Immunodermatology.

23. Coovadia HM, Soothill JF (1976): The effect of protein restricted diets on the clearance of ^{125}I-labeled polyvinyl pyrrolidone in mice. Clin Exp Immunol 23:373–377.

24. Freyre EA, Chabes A, Peornape O, Chabes A (1973): Abnormal Rebvek skin-window response in kwashiorkor. J Pediatr 82:523–526.

25. Suskind R, Edelman R, Kulapongs P, Pariyanonda A, Sirisinha S (1976): Complement activity in children with protein-calorie malnutrition. Am J Clin Nutr 29:1089–1092.

26. McMurray DN, Loomis SA, Casazza LJ, Rey H, Miranda R (1981): Development of impaired cell-mediated immunity in mild and moderate malnutrition. Am J Clin Nutr 34: 68–77.

27. Satyanarayana K, Bhaskaran P, Seshu VC, Reddy V (1980): Influence of nutrition on post-vaccinial tuberculin sensitivity. Am J Clin Nutr 33:2334–2337.

28. Bansal VK, Popli S, Pickering J, Ing TS, Vertuno LL, Hano JE (1980): Protein-calorie malnutrition and cutaneous anergy in hemodialysis maintained patients. Am J Clin Nutr 33:1608–1611.

29. O'Keefe SJ, El-Zayadi AR, Carraher TE, Davis M, Williams R (1980): Malnutrition and immunocompetence in patients with liver disease. Lancet 2:615–617.

30. Donaldson SS, Wesley MN, DeWeys WD, Suskind RM, Jaffe N, VanEys J (1981): A study of the nutritional status of pediatric cancer patients. Am J Dis Child 135:1107–1112.

31. Good RA, Fernandes G, Cunningham-Rundles C, Cunningham-Rundles S, Farofalo JA, Rao KMK, Incefy GS, Iwata T (1980): The relation of zinc deficiency to immunologic function in animals and man. In Seligman M, Hitzig WH (eds): "Primary Immunodeficiencies." INSERM Symposium 16. Amsterdam: Elsevier/North-Holland.

32. Chandra RK (1980): Single nutrient deficiency and cell-mediated immune responses. Am J Clin Nutr 33:736–738.

33. Prasad AS (1979): Clinical, biochemical and pharmacological role of zinc. Ann Rev Pharmacol Toxicol 20:393–426.
34. Prasad AS, Halsted JA, Nadimi M (1961): Syndrome of iron deficiency anemia, hepatosplenomegaly, hypogonadism, dwarfism and geophagia. Am J Med 31:532–540.
35. Halsted JA, Ronaghy HA, Abadi P, Haghshenass M, Amirhakimi GH, Baraket RM, Rheinhold JG (1972): Zinc deficiency in man, the Shiraz experiment. Am J Med 53:277–283.
36. Brummerstedt E, Flagstad T, Andresen E (1971): The effect of zinc on calves with hereditary thymus hypoplasia (lethal tract A46). Acta Pathol Microbiol Scand (Sec A) 79: 686–687.
37. Moynahan EJ (1974): Acrodermatis enteropathica: A lethal inherited zinc-deficiency disorder. Lancet 2:399–400.
38. Fraker PJ, Haas SM, Luecke RW (1977): The effect of zinc deficiency on the young adult A/J mouse. J Nutr 107:1889–1895.
39. Fernandes G, Nair M, Onoe K, Tanaka T, Floyd R, Good RA (1979): Impairment of cell-mediated immunity functions by dietary zinc deficiency in mice. Proc Natl Acad Sci USA 76(1):457–461.
40. Gross RL, Osdin N, Fong L, Newberne PM (1979): Depressed immunological function in zinc-deprived rats as measured by mitogen response of spleen, thymus and peripheral blood. Am J Clin Nutr 32:1260–1265.
41. Kirchner H, Ruhl H (1970): Stimulation of human peripheral blood lymphocytes by Zn^{++} in vitro. Exp Cell Res 61:229–230.
42. Cunningham-Rundles S, Cunningham-Rundles C, Dupont B, Good RA (1980): Zinc activation of human B lymphocytes. Clin Immunol Immunopathol 16:115–121.
43. Chandra RK, Au B (1980): Single nutrient deficiency and cell-mediated immune responses. 1. Zinc. Am J Clin Nutr 33:736–738.
44. Cunningham-Rundles S (1983): New findings on the role of zinc as a biological response modifier. In Laurent P, Bienvenu J (eds): "Markers of Inflammation." Walter de Gruyter (in press).
45. Siegal FP, Lopez C, Hammer GS, Brown AE, Kornfeld SH, Gold J, Hassett J, Hirschman SZ, Cunningham-Rundles C, Adelsbert BR, Parham DM, Siegal M, Cunningham-Rundles S, Armstrong D (1981): Severe acquired immunodeficiency in male homosexuals manifested by chronic perianal ulcerative herpes simplex lesions. N Engl J Med 305:1439–1444.
46. Masur H, Michelis MA, Greene JB, Onorato I, Vande Sfouve RA, Holzman RA, Wormer G, Brettman L, Lange M, Cunningham-Rundles S (1981): A community acquired outbreak of Pneumocystis carinii pneumonia: Initial manifestation of cellular immune dysfunction. N Engl J Med 305:1431–1438.
47. Cunningham-Rundles S (1983): Analysis of cellular immune deficiency in acquired immunodeficiency syndrome. In Ma P, Armstrong D (eds): "Yorke Proceedings of AIDS Symposium" (in press).
48. Cunningham-Rundles S, Safai B, Metroka C, Krown SE, Rubin BY, Stahl WE (1983): Lymphocyte effector function in vitro in the Acquired Immunodeficiency Disease Syndrome. In Friedman-Keen AE (ed): "Progress in AIDS." Paris: Masson (in press).
49. Gross RL, Osdin N, Long L, Newberne PM (1979): In vitro restoration by levamisole of mitogen responsiveness in zinc-deprived rats. Am J Clin Nutr 32:1267–1271.
50. Dardenne M, Wade S, Nabarra B, Bach JF (1983): Thymic hormones and zinc deficiency. In Laurent P, Bienvenu J (eds): "Markers of Inflammation." Walter de Gruyter (in press).
51. Bach JF (1981): The multifaceted zinc dependency of the immune system. Immunol Today 225–227.
52. Roo RMK, Schwartz SA (1980): Zinc modulates mitogenic responses of human lymphocytes by affecting structures influenced by cytochalasin B. Clin Immunol Immunopathol 16:463–473.
53. Cunningham-Rundles S (1982): Effect of nutritional status on immunological function. Am J Clin Nutr 35:1202–1210.

Malnutrition: Determinants and Consequences, pages 245–251
© 1984 Alan R. Liss, Inc., 150 Fifth Avenue, New York, NY 10011

Nutritional Regulation of Immune Function at the Extremes of Life: In Infants and in the Elderly

Ranjit Kumar Chandra, MD, FRCP(C)

Department of Pediatrics, Medicine, and Biochemistry, Memorial University of Newfoundland, St. John's, Newfoundland, Canada A1B 3V6

INTRODUCTION

There are many apparent similarities between the two ends of the age spectrum. Among other observations, both neonates and elderly have suboptimal immune responses and are susceptible to infection. When nutritional deficiency complicates the picture, impairment of immunocompetence is more marked and longer-lasting. Although nutritional regulation of host resistance has now been studied for over two decades [Chandra, 1983d], our knowledge about the contribution of nutrient imbalance to immunologic abnormalities in the perinatal period and in old age is far from complete.

The ontogenetic development of the immune system takes place in early pregnancy and midpregnancy and continues into the last trimester and the first few months after birth. If the infant is born prematurely or if he exhibits growth retardation as a result of a number of environmental factors, including maternal malnutrition or infection, immunocompetence is reduced [Chandra and Matsumura, 1979]. The impact on T-lymphocyte numbers and cell-mediated immunity is most discernible. The preterm low-birth-weight infant generally recovers its ability to mount immune response by the age of 3 months. However, the small-for-gestational-age infant may continue to show reduced cell-mediated immunity for several months and years. In laboratory animal models of intrauterine malnutrition, immune responses are impaired both in first- and second-generation offspring [Chandra, 1975a].

At the other extreme of life, clinical experience indicates that infectious disease is common in the elderly [Schneider, 1983; Stead and Lofgren, 1983]; this increased risk of infection may be attributed to the age-related chronic diseases and both iatrogenic and nosocomial factors as well as impaired resistance due to the "normal" aging process. Nutrient intake declines as a result of reduced emotional motivation, dental problems, and altered taste acuity; absorption is impaired and catabolism is exaggerated. The accumulated result of these phenomena is altered nutritional status and body composition; lean body mass is both relatively and absolutely decreased, whereas body fat is increased. Thus the question may be asked: Is declining immunity in old age due, at least in part, to undernutrition? Recent observations indicate that at least one-third of free-living elderly in Canada and the United States show evidence of nutritional deficiency; nutritional support results in improved capacity to show immune responses [Chandra et al, 1982b]. These data are of considerable importance to public health.

NUTRITION AND IMMUNOCOMPETENCE IN INFANTS

Many field studies have documented increased mortality and morbidity in infants with protein-energy malnutrition (PEM). The probability of death among young children increases progressively with deterioration in nutritional status. Most of the deaths are due to infectious illness and diarrheal illness. The attack rate, duration, and severity of infectious diseases are increased. The most cited examples are measles and diarrhea. In North American hospitals, opportunistic infections are common in undernourished patients [Chandra, 1983b, 1983d].

The thymus of malnourished infants is small and shows lymphocyte depletion [Chandra, 1980]. The corticomedullary distinction is blurred. Skin tests with common recall antigens, such as candidin, trichophytin, streptokinase-streptodornase, mumps, and purified protein derivative of tuberculin, evaluate the memory response dependent on T lymphocytes and inflammatory cells; results are generally lower in patients with protein-energy malnutrition [Harland, 1965; Chandra, 1972; Neumann et al, 1975; Puri et al, 1980]. Some studies performed with agents such as keyhole limpet hemocyanin, BCG vaccine, and 2,4 dinitrochlorobenzene have also demonstrated impairment of the primary afferent limb of delayed hypersensitivity. Lymphopenia is seen in approximately one-sixth of malnourished infants. There is a reduction in the proportion and absolute numbers of circulating thymus-dependent T lymphocytes [Bang et al, 1975].

Our recent studies [Chandra et al, 1982a; Chandra 1983a] documented a significant change in the number and function of T-cell subpopulations. T4+ helper cells are reduced to one-half of control values, whereas changes in T8+ suppressor cells are less prominent. Furthermore, in vitro immunoglobulin synthesis is reduced but is restored on the addition of control T cells. Thus a numerical functional deficiency in T helper cells was found in PEM.

The proportion of "null" cells without the conventional surface markers of T and B lymphocytes is markedly increased. The possibility that these cells may be undifferentiated T lymphocytes is suggested by a significant decrease in serum thymic hormone activity and an elevation in leukocyte terminal deoxynucleotidyl transferase [Chandra, 1979]. The addition of calf thymus extract in vitro to mononuclear cell preparations from undernourished individuals results in an increase in the number of rosetting cells.

Hypergammaglobulinemia and increase in immunoglobulin levels are common findings in PEM. This may be the result of frequent infections as well as reduction in T suppressor cell numbers and activity. Secretory IgA [Watson et al, 1978] and mucosal antibody responses are decreased. Serum levels of many complement components are reduced as a result both of decreased synthesis and increased consumption. Chemotaxis of neutrophils is delayed and there are deficits in postphagocytic metabolic bursts of oxidative and glycolytic activity. The intracellular killing of ingested bacteria is variably reduced [Selvaraj and Bhat, 1972]. The effects of the deficiencies of individual nutrients have been the subject of much recent work and have been reviewed elsewhere [Beisel, 1982; Chandra, 1983c; Chandra and Dayton, 1982].

Fetal growth retardation is associated with thymic atrophy and prolonged depression of cell-mediated immunity [Chandra, 1975b]. The number of circulating T cells is reduced and lymphocyte transformation response to mitogens is decreased. Serum levels of IgG, especially IgG_1 and IgG_3, and antibody titers are lower as a result of decreased placental transfer of immunoglobulins [Chandra, 1975c]. Serum concentrations of C3 are decreased and opsonization is suboptimal. The levels of factor B are reduced and correlate with opsonic activity. The depression of cell-mediated immunocompetence in small-for-gestational-age (SGA) low-birth-weight infants has been shown to persist for several months to years [Dutz et al, 1976; Moscatelli et al, 1976; Chandra, 1981]. In contrast, appropriate-for-gestational-age infants of comparable weight recovered their immune function by the age of 3 months. Thymic hormone activity is reduced in SGA infants and may serve as a prognostic marker [Chandra, 1981]. These prolonged immunosuppressive effects may have clinical and biological significance, particularly on frequency, severity, and duration of infection.

If malnutrition and infection are a conjugate pair handicapping the development of infants, what interventions can help? A scheme of multiple steps to deal with this problem is shown diagrammatically in Figure 1 and discussed elsewhere [Chandra, 1980].

NUTRITION AND IMMUNOCOMPETENCE IN THE ELDERLY

There are several theories of aging, perhaps as many as there are researchers. If for the moment we discount the inevitability of aging as a developmental event, as suggested by the programmed aging theory, we should consider the alternative theory that postulates that senescence results from a progressive accumulation of abnormal molecules and faulty somatic cells, the latter as a

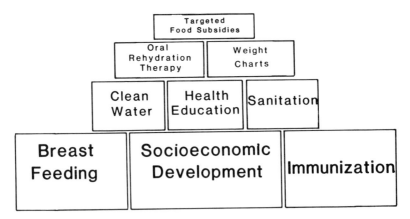

Fig. 1. Interventions to deal with malnutrition and infection. The relative importance of various steps is indicated by the size of the box and lettering. Thus, socioeconomic development, promotion of breast feeding, and implementation of effective immunization programs should be the foundations of intervention strategies.

consequence of attrition and environmental insults or of genetic errors during the synthesis of DNA, RNA, or proteins from substrates. We can entertain nutritional factors as important variables of the "wear and tear" that may not be appropriately replaced if nutritional imbalance is present.

Several reports have documented the progressive loss of immune function in old age [Antonaci et al, 1983; Sohnle et al, 1980, 1983]. Cell-mediated immunity is impaired [Kay, 1983]. This may be due in part to marked reduction in the putative thymic hormone(s). Other studies have documented alterations in nutritional status and body composition, including decreased lean body mass, loss of visceral protein, and increase in the relative proportion of body fat. These changes in body constituents may result from a variety of pathogenetic factors, such as altered taste acuity, reduced food intake, malabsorption, and the metabolic consequences of concurrent disease. To date, there are few studies that have looked concurrently at both nutrition and immunity in the elderly [DuChateau et al, 1981; Chandra et al, 1982b; Goodwin and Garry, 1983].

Among a group of 51 subjects above the age of 60 years, we found evidence of nutritional deficiencies in 21 and studied the nutritional and immunologic status of these malnourished elderly individuals before and after 8 weeks of dietary supplementation [Chandra et al, 1982b]. There was clinical (pitting edema in 6 subjects), anthropometric (reduced weight-for-height and skinfold thickness), biochemical (mean serum albumin 2.8 ± 0.6 gm/dl), and hematologic (hemoglobin less than 11.8 gm/dl in 4 subjects) evidence of malnutrition. Serum ferritin was low in 4 and plasma zinc low in 7. After 8 weeks of supplementation, there was improvement in delayed hypersensitivity response, num-

**TABLE I. Lymphocyte Stimulation Response Index
to Phytohemagglutinin**

Antigen	Elderly	Young
Candida	21 ± 6[a]	38 ± 9
Tetanus toxoid	5 ± 2	32 ± 8
Streptokinase-Streptodornase	15 ± 5	19 ± 7

[a]Results are expressed as ratio of counts per minute in cell cultures in the presence of phytohemagglutinin divided by counts in cultures without the mitogen.

**TABLE II. Effect of 50 mg Oral Zinc Supplements Daily on
Delayed-Hypersensitivity Skin Reactions in the Elderly**

Group		Before	After
Zinc therapy	n = 33	12[a]	18
Not treated	n = 34	14	13

[a]Number showing a positive response.

ber of T cells, and lymphocyte proliferation response to mitogens [Chandra et al, 1982b] and antigens (Table I).

Individual nutrient deficiencies are not uncommon in the elderly. Thus correction of these may also be expected to improve immune responses (Table II).

The age-related declines in cell-mediated immunity, T cell number, and thymic factor activity resemble to some extent those seen in protein-calorie malnutrition. Since the elderly are known to be among the most poorly nourished in industrialized countries and since changes in food intake, body composition, and protein metabolism are known to occur with advancing age, the possibility arises that altered immune status in the elderly could be ascribed in part to nutritional deficiency. The crucial test for this is to evaluate nutritional and immunologic status before and after deliberate supplementation. Our preliminary observations show that protein-calorie malnutrition was present in 41% of elderly individuals surveyed. Supplementing the diet with formula that supplied about 500 kcal extra energy intake per day and contained vitamins, minerals, and trace elements in moderate amounts resulted in improved nutritional status and immunocompetence. To date, the contribution of altered nutritional status in the elderly to deficits in their immune responses has not been adequately evaluated. Our data indicate that a causal relationship does exist between undernutrition and impaired immunity in many elderly individuals and that this is a correctable abnormality in the majority. It is not clear whether maintenance of good nutrition and improved immunocompetence will alter morbidity and longevity. Obviously, long-term prospective studies are required to answer these questions. These are urgently needed and will have enormous public health importance.

REFERENCES

Antonaci S, Jirillo E, Lucivero G, Gallitelli M, Garofalo AR, Bonomo L (1983): Humoral immune response in aged humans: Suppressor effect of monocytes on spontaneous plaque forming cell generation. Clin Exp Immunol 52:387-392.

Bang BD, Mahalanabis D, Mukerjee KL, Bang FB (1975): T and B lymphocyte rosetting in undernourished children. Proc Soc Exp Biol Med 149:199-202.

Beisel WR (1983): Single nutrients and immunity. Am J Clin Nutr 35:417-468.

Bistrian BR, Blackburn GL, Scrimshaw NS, Flatt JP (1975): Cellular immunity in semistarved states in hospitalized adults. Am J Clin Nutr 28:1148-1153.

Chandra RK (1972): Immunocompetence in undernutrition. J Pediatr 81:1194-1200.

Chandra RK (1975a): Antibody formation in first and second generation offspring of nutritionally deprived rats. Science 190:189-190.

Chandra RK (1975b): Fetal malnutrition and postnatal immunocompetence. Am J Dis Child 129:450-455.

Chandra RK (1975c): Levels of IgG subclasses, IgA, IgM and tetanus antitoxin in paired maternal and foetal sera. Findings in healthy pregnancy and placental insufficiency. In Hemmings WA (ed): "Materno-Foetal Transmission of Immunoglobulins." London: Cambridge University Press, pp 77-90.

Chandra RK (1979): T and B lymphocyte subpopulations and leukocyte terminal deoxynucleotidyl transferase in energy-protein malnutrition. Acta Paediatr Scand 68:841-845.

Chandra RK (1980): "Immunology of Nutritional Disorders." London: Arnold.

Chandra RK (1981): Serum thymic hormone activity and cell-mediated immunity in healthy neonates, preterm infants and small-for-gestation age infants. Pediatrics 67:407-411.

Chandra RK (1983a): Numerical and functional deficiency in T helper cells in protein calorie malnutrition. Clin Exp Immunol 51:126-132.

Chandra RK (1983b): The nutrition-immunity infection nexis: The enumeration and functional assessment of lymphocyte subsets in nutritional deficiency. Nutr Res 3:605-615.

Chandra RK (ed) (1983c): "Primary and Secondary Immunodeficiency Disorders." Edinburgh: Churchill-Livingstone.

Chandra RK (1983d): Nutrition, immunity and infection: Present knowledge and future directions. Lancet 1:688-691.

Chandra RK, Dayton D (1982): Trace element regulation of immunity and infection. Nutr Res 2:721-733.

Chandra RK, Matsumura T (1979): Ontogenetic development of immune system and effects of fetal growth retardation. J Perinat Med 7:279-287.

Chandra RK, Gupta S, Singh H (1982a): Inducer and suppressor T cell subsets in protein-energy malnutrition. Analysis by monoclonal antibodies. Nutr Res 2:21-26.

Chandra RK, Joshi P, Au B, Woodford G, Chandra S (1982b): Nutrition and immunocompetence of the elderly. Effect of short term nutritional supplementation on cell-mediated immunity and lymphocyte subsets. Nutr Res 2:223-232.

Duchateau J, Delepesse G, Vrijens R, Collet H (1981): Beneficial effects of oral zinc supplementation on the immne response of old people. Am J Med 70:1001-1004.

Dutz W, Rossipal E, Ghavami H, Vessel K, Kohout E, Post G (1976): Persistent cell mediated immune deficiency following infantile stress during the first 6 months of life. Eur J Pediatr 122:117-129.

Goodwin JS, Garry PJ (1983): Relationship between megadose vitamin supplementation and immunological function in a healthy elderly population. Clin Exp Immunol 51:647-653.

Harland PS (1965): Tuberculin reactions in malnourished children. Lancet 1:719-721.

Kay MMB (1983): Immunodeficiency in old age. In Chandra RK (ed): "Primary and Secondary Immunodeficiency Disorders." Edinburgh: Churchill Livingstone, pp 166-186.

Moscatelli P, Bricarelli FG, Piccinini A, Tomatis C, Dufour MA (1976): Defective immuno-competence in foetal undernutrition. Helv Paediatr Acta 31:241–247.

Neumann CG, Lawlor GJ Jr, Stiehm ER, Swenseid ME, Newton C, Herbert J, Ammann AJ, Jacob M (1975): Immunologic responses in malnourished children. Am J Clin Nutr 28:89–101.

Puri V, Misra PK, Saxena KC, Saxena PN, Saxena RP, Agarwal CG (1980): Immune status in malnutrition. Indian Pediatr 17:127–132.

Schneider EL (1983): Infectious disease in the elderly. Ann Intern Med 98:395–400.

Selvaraj RJ, Bhat KS (1972): Metabolic and bactericidal activities of leukocytes in protein-calorie malnutrition. Am J Clin Nutr 25:166–172.

Sohnle PG, Larson SE, Collins-Lech C, Guansing AR (1980): Failure of lymphokine-producing lymphocytes from aging humans to undergo activation by recall antigens. J Immunol 124:2169–2174.

Sohnle PG, Collins-Lech C, Huhta KE (1983): Kinetics of lymphokine production by lymphocytes from elderly humans. Gerontology 29:169–175.

Stead WW, Lofgren JP (1983): Does the risk of tuberculosis increase with old age? J Infect Dis 147:951–955.

Watson R, Reyes MA, McMurray DN (1978): Influences of malnutrition on the concentration of IgA, lysozyme, amylase, and aminopeptidase in children's tears. Proc Soc Exp Biol Med 157:215–218.

Malnutrition: Determinants and Consequences, pages 253–258
© 1984 Alan R. Liss, Inc., 150 Fifth Avenue, New York, NY 10011

Effects of Maternal Factors Upon the Immunologic Status of the Infant

Armond S. Goldman, MD, Randall M. Goldblum, MD,
Cutberto Garza, MD, PhD, Nancy Butte, PhD, and Buford Nichols, MD
The University of Texas Medical Branch, Galveston 77550 (A.S.G., R.M.G.) and
Baylor College of Medicine, Houston, Texas (C.G., N.B., B.N.)

INTRODUCTION

During the past several decades, considerable evidence has been uncovered concerning the influence of maternal factors upon the resistance of young mammals to infectious agents. It has been found that protective maternal factors are transferred prenatally via the placenta and amniotic fluid, or postnatally via the mammary gland. Furthermore, the routes of transfer for the factors differ in the various orders of mammals. In the Ruminantia, a large amount of immunoglobulin G (IgG), but only small quantities of other immunoglobulins, are secreted into the milk [1]. Upon ingestion, IgG is absorbed through the intestinal tract of the newborn of those species. In those animals, immunoglobulins are not transferred through the placenta. The pattern in Primates is quite different, and the differences are correlated with the acquisition of a hemocordial placenta and evolutionary changes in the mammary gland. In Primates, including Homo sapiens, a major class of immunoglobulins is conveyed to the fetus by the placenta, and a wide array of host resistance factors that appear to act locally to enhance mucosal immunity are passed to the nursing infant via the milk secretions [2,3]. In this chapter, the maternal factors that affect the immunologic status of the human infant will be reviewed.

PLACENTAL CONTRIBUTION

IgG is transported actively and passively via the placenta to the human fetus during the last 6 months of pregnancy, particularly during the last 3 months

[4]. The distribution of each of the four subclasses of this immunoglobulin in the umbilical cord blood of the full-term newborn is similar to that found in maternal serum [5]. Owing to the active transport of the protein, the concentration of the entire class of that immunoglobulin is somewhat higher in the infant's blood than in the maternal blood. No other types of immunoglobulins are passed through the human placenta. Because of the selective transfer, the paucity of antibody formation during the intrauterine period due to antigen-sheltering, and certain innate delays in the maturation of the immunologic system, the levels of the other immunoglobulin isotypes in the blood at birth are very low. The levels of transferred IgG decrease steadily until a nadir is reached at 3–4 months of age. Afterwards, the concentrations of this immunoglobulin rise in response to foreign antigens until adult levels are reached at about 8–10 years of age.

AMNIOTIC FLUID CONTRIBUTION

Components of amniotic fluid are derived from several sources including the umbilical cord, fetal urine, cervical glands of the female fetus, amniotic epithelium, and transudation from umbilical cord blood. Low levels of IgG, IgA, IgM, IgD, and lysozyme have been detected in amniotic fluid [6,7]. The origins of some of the components are undetermined, but studies of allotypic markers suggest that the IgG in human amniotic fluid is of maternal origin [8]. The role of amniotic fluid in the protection of the human fetus has not been ascertained, but it is of interest that specific antibodies against herpes viruses and other microorganisms have been found in those secretions [9].

MAMMARY GLAND CONTRIBUTION

During the extragestate period, a complex set of immunologic factors is passed to the nursing infant via the secretions of the mammary gland [2,3]. The components of the immunologic system in human milk include growth factors for the protective bacterium *Bifidobacillus bifidum*, low levels of complement proteins, proteins that avidly bind nutrients used by pathogenic microorganisms, an enzyme that lyses the cell wall of certain bacteria, antibodies directed against many enteric and respiratory pathogens, other soluble antiviral and antibacterial components, and leukocytes with special properties that are not found in their counterparts in peripheral blood.

There are seven features that characterize the immunologic system in human milk. 1) The system appears to protect mucosal surfaces by noninflammatory mechanisms [10]. 2) The concentrations of most of the components decrease as lactation proceeds. 3) Appreciable amounts of many of the factors persist throughout lactation. 4) The quantitative secretion of some of the components may be inversely related over time to the mucosal production of them by the developing infant. 5) Many of the components are relatively resistant to enzymatic digestion. 6) The components are often synergetic with each other or with host resistance factors produced by the infant. 7) The system aids in regulating the microbial flora of the intestinal tract of the breast-fed baby.

To gain a further understanding of this immunologic system, recent studies of three key soluble components and of the leukocytes in human milk will be reviewed.

Lactoferrin

In in vitro systems, lactoferrin has been found to have bacteriostatic and bactericidal properties that are due to the ability of this apoprotein to chelate ferrous iron from microorganisms such as enteric bacterial pathogens. Lactoferrin is one of the principal whey proteins in human milk. Lactoferrin in human milk is largely unsaturated and is therefore protective and refractory to enzymatic degradation. The highest concentrations of this iron-binding protein in human milk are found during the first few days of lactation [11]. The concentration of lactoferrin decreases during the first few months, but substantial concentrations (about 1 mg/ml) persist during gradual weaning at 6 months [12] and throughout partial breast feeding during the second year of lactation [13]. As much as 125–250 mg is ingested per kilogram per day by the nursing infant during the first 4 months of life [14], but the fate of this iron-binding protein in the recipient is undetermined.

Lysozyme

Lysozyme destroys certain bacteria by cleaving peptidoglycans from the cell walls of those organisms or by interacting with other components in human milk to achieve a bactericidal effect. Very little lysozyme is present in cow's milk, whereas a great deal is found in human milk throughout lactation. The pattern of the development of this protein is quite different from other immunologic components that have been found in human milk [11-13]. The mean concentration of the enzyme falls from about 80 μg/ml in colostrum to a nadir of 25–30 μg/ml at 4–6 weeks of lactation. Then the levels rise to a high of about 250 μg/ml at 6 months. Afterwards, those levels are maintained during gradual weaning at 6 months [12] and partial breast feeding in the second year of lactation [13]. Approximately 4–6 mg of lysozyme is ingested per kilogram per day by the nursing infant during the first 4 months of life [14]. Large amounts of the protein are found in the stools of the breast-fed infant [15], but the in vivo actions of lysozyme in the recipient are as yet unknown.

Immunoglobulin A

The major type of antibodies in human milk is immunoglobulin A (IgA), and the principal molecular form of that immunoglobulin throughout lactation is secretory IgA. Secretory IgA provides antibodies against a host of microbial pathogens that inhabit the intestinal tract or the respiratory system. Experimental evidence and human observations indicate that cells that produce these antibodies originate from lymphoid precursors in Peyer's patches in the intestinal tract and the submucosa of the bronchial tree [16,17]. Furthermore, these enteromammary and bronchomammary pathways are activated by hormones that are produced during lactation [18] and by specific antigens that are presented to the precursor cells in the intestinal tract or the bronchi. The highest concentrations of IgA are found in colostrum [11]. Although the level of this immunoglobulin falls in the next several weeks of lactation, significant amounts of this protein persist throughout lactation [11–13]. About 75–100 mg of IgA are ingested per kilogram per day by the nursing infant during the first 4 months of life [14]. In keeping with that finding, the low production of IgA during early life, and the resistance of this polymeric immunoglobulin to enzymatic digestion, the stools of breast-fed infants contain a great deal more secretory IgA than those of non-breast-fed ones [19].

Leukocytes of Human Milk

These cells are particularly prominent in colostrum (1.5–3.5×10^6/ml), but by 8–12 weeks they are difficult to detect [11]. Beginning with the initial studies of the immunologic properties of human milk leukocytes [20], it was evident that the cells were unusual. To begin with, many of the leukocytes, particularly the neutrophils and macrophages, were lipid-laden to a degree that interfered with their identification. The distribution of these leukocytes was also quite different from those found in peripheral blood in that lymphocytes constituted 6–10% of the total leukocytes, whereas macrophages accounted for 40–50% of the cells. Although the neutrophils and macrophages had well-developed phagocytic abilities, the microbicidal capacity of those cells was reduced [21]. A further indication of the unusual character of these cells was the discovery that they harbored about 4–5% of the IgA in human colostrum [22]. The way that these phagocytic cells sequester IgA is unknown, but recent investigations reveal that about 40% of these secretory IgA antibodies are released from the cells during phagocytosis [22]. Subsequent studies have indicated that the release is a secretory event that is initiated by transsurface membrane signals and is dependent upon microtubules [23]. Thus, it is possible that some of these phagocytic cells protect by secreting secretory IgA antibodies that neutralize pathogens or their products or interfere with the attachment of the microorganisms to epithelial surfaces.

EFFECTS OF MATERNAL NUTRITION UPON THE IMMUNOLOGIC SYSTEM IN HUMAN MILK

Two studies have recently been published regarding the effects of maternal nutrition upon the concentrations and functions of certain components of the immunologic system in human milk. In the first study [24], no alterations were found; in the second one [25] colostral levels of IgG, IgA, and C4 were decreased significantly. It would seem that more detailed studies are required to ascertain whether the degree of nutritional deficits may alter the development or function of this system. The effect of diet on milk volume is of particular concern. Recent reviews suggest that the daily milk volume produced by undernourished women is reduced by 20% as compared to more affluent populations [26]. The impact of this reduction of the net protective effect of human milk is not known.

CODA

In summary, the immunologic system of the infant is augmented during the intrauterine period by maternal factors including IgG from the placenta and amniotic fluid and during the postnatal period by a host of immunologic factors in human milk that are important in the local defense of the intestinal tract and respiratory system. In the next several years one can anticipate that a more complete understanding will develop regarding these transmitted immunologic components and the nature of their effects upon the resistance of the breast-fed infant.

ACKNOWLEDGMENTS

This work was supported in part by contracts from the National Institutes of Child Health and Human Development (DHEW NO1-HD-8-2828 and NIH-NO1-HD-22814) and by the US Department of Agriculture/ARS Children's Nutrition Research Center at Baylor College of Medicine and Texas Children's Hospital.

REFERENCES

1. Newby TJ et al (1977): The nature of the local immune system of the bovine mammary gland. J Immunol 118:461–465.
2. Goldman AS, Smith CW (1973): Host resistance factors in human milk. J Pediatr 82:1082–1090.
3. Goldman AS, Goldblum RM (1980): Anti-infective properties of human milk. Pediatr Update 1:359–365.
4. Spiegelberg HL (1974): Biological activities of immunoglobulins of different classes and subclasses. Adv Immunol 19:259–289.
5. Morell A et al (1971): Human IgG subclasses in maternal and fetal serum. Vox Sang (Basel) 21:481.
6. Cederqvist LL et al (1978): Detectability and pattern of immunoglobulins in normal amniotic fluid throughout gestation. Am J Obstet Gynecol 130:220–224.
7. Larsen B et al (1974): Muramidase and peroxidase activity of human amniotic fluid. Obstet Gynecol 44:219–223.

8. Ruoslahti E et al (1966): Origin of proteins in amniotic fluid. Nature (London) 212:841.

9. Cox D et al (1982): Antibody activity against herpes simplex virus in human amniotic fluid. Br J Obstet Gynecol 89:226–230.

10. Goldman AS, Goldblum RM (1983): An hypothesis: Anti-inflammatory properties of human milk (in preparation).

11. Goldman AS et al (1982): Immunologic factors in human milk during the first year of lactation. J Pediatr 100:563–567.

12. Goldman AS et al (1983): Immunologic components in human milk during weaning. Acta Paediatr Scand 72:133–134.

13. Goldman AS et al (1983): Immunologic components in human milk during the second year of lactation. Acta Paediatr Scand 72:461–462.

14. Butte NF et al (1984): Daily ingestion of immunologic components in human milk during the first four months of life. Acta Paediatr Scand (in press).

15. Rosenthal L, Lieberman H (1931): The role of lysozyme in the development of the intestinal flora of the newborn infant. Infect Dis 48:226.

16. Goldblum RM et al (1975): Antibody forming cells in human colostrum after oral immunization. Nature 257:797–799.

17. Fishaut M et al (1981): Bronchomammary axis in the immune response to respiratory syncytial virus. J Pediatr 99:186–191.

18. Weisz-Carrington P et al (1978): Hormonal induction of the secretory immune system in the mammary gland. Proc Natl Acad Sci USA 75:2928.

19. Michael JG et al (1971): The antimicrobial activity of human colostral antibody in the newborn. J Infect Dis 124:445.

20. Smith CW, Goldman AS (1968): The cells of human colostrum. I. *In vitro* studies of morphology and functions. Pediatr Res 2:103–109.

21. Pickering LK et al (1980): Polymorphonuclear leukocytes of human colostrum. I. Oxidative metabolism. J Infect Dis 142:165.

22. Weaver EA et al (1981): Enhanced IgA release from human colostral cells during phagocytosis. Infect Immunity 34:498–502.

23. Weaver EA et al (1984): Secretion of immunoglobulin A by human milk leukocytes initiated by surface membrane stimuli. J Immunol (in press).

24. Cruz JR et al (1982): Studies on human milk. III. Secretory IgA quantity and antibody levels against *Escherichia coli* in colostrum and milk from underprivileged and privileged mothers. Pediatr Res 16:272.

25. Miranda R et al (1983): Effect of nutritional status on immunologic substances in human colostrum and milk. Am J Clin Nutr 37:632–640.

26. Jelliffe DB, Jelliffe EFP (1978): The volume and composition of human milk in poorly nourished communities: A review. Am J Clin Nutr 31:492–515.

Malnutrition: Determinants and Consequences, pages 259–270
© *1984 Alan R. Liss, Inc., 150 Fifth Avenue, New York, NY 10011*

Infectious and Diarrheal Disease

O. Brunser, MD, G. Figueroa, RT, M. Araya, MD, PhD, and J. Espinoza, MD

Divisions of Gastroenterology (O.B., M.A., J.E.) and Microbiology (G.F.), Institute of Nutrition and Food Technology, University of Chile, Santiago 11, Chile

Children in the less-developed countries are subject to a high risk of acquiring infectious diseases. The most significant among these are acute diarrhea and respiratory infections. According to Walsh and Warren [1979], about 5–10 billion episodes of diarrhea every year affect the children of Latin America, Asia, and Africa, and from these episodes, 5–10 million children die. These numbers are very high but, as shown in Table I, which summarizes some data on mortality from acute diarrhea in the Western Hemisphere, there is an overall decline in mortality. A good example of this trend is what has happened in Chile in recent years. Infant mortality decreased from 70.5 per 1,000 newborns in 1971 to 31.9 in 1980. At the same time the mortality for gastroenteritis in the same age group decreased from 11.8 per 1,000 newborns in 1971 to 1.9 per 1,000 newborns in 1980 [AESNS, 1972/1981]. When both curves are plotted together and expressed per 1,000 live newborns, there is a striking parallelism (Fig. 1) that suggests that deaths due to gastroenteritis are an important component of infant mortality.

Data on hospitalizations for acute diarrhea in Metropolitan Santiago are shown in Table II. This shows that the incidence of acute diarrhea resulting in the need for hospitalization is low in children up to 27 days of age and that the greatest proportion of admissions occurs between 1 and 11 months of age. Acute diarrhea declines considerably among preschoolers and school-age children. Of all the hospital admissions in Metropolitan Santiago in 1975 recorded as due to infectious and parasitic diseases, almost 90% (20,713 of 23,608) were due to acute diarrhea. For the sake of comparison, it is worthwhile noting that during the same period admissions due to respiratory diseases were 19,518 [AESNS, 1976]. The low rate of hospitalization due to acute gastroenteritis

TABLE I. Number of Deaths and Rates per 100,000 Population Due to Acute Diarrhea Among Infants and Preschool Children, 1970–1979

Country	Year	Infants		Preschool children	
		No. of deaths	Rate	No. of deaths	Rate
Argentina	1970	4,561	880.5	722	38.5
	1979	2,641	463.3	420	20.0
Chile	1970	3,853	1,418.1	422	46.7
	1979	705	264.9	85	8.6
Canada	1969	95	27.5	36	2.3
	1975	66	18.4	16	1.1
Colombia	1968	9,608	1,438.2	7,022	257.0
	1975	6,788	883.9	3,486	105.0
Costa Rica	1970	845	1,509.5	271	108.1
	1979	136	195.3	24	11.2
Cuba	1979	1,313	564.7	82	8.6
	1979	237	122.7	41	4.3
Ecuador	1970	2,382	968.9	1,691	194.4
	1979	3,667	1,144.1	2,605	231.0
Guatemala	1970	3,643	1,817.8	5,749	807.6
	1979	3,934	1,311.3	3,864	424.1
Mexico	1970	37,197	1,744.2	20,464	274.0
	1979	30,806	1,258.8	11,393	127.2
Peru	1970	5,501	1,802.1	3,798	209.1
	1979	4,872	751.8	3,058	144.6
United States	1968	1,032	29.5	245	1.7
	1975	713	22.7	91	0.7
Venezuela	1970	3,673	874.7	1,373	94.2
	1979	2,836	600.8	634	38.2

among infants under one month of age and its increase between 28 days and 11 months of age suggest that some factor(s) protects the younger age group against the microbiologic contamination of the environment. It is reasonable to postulate that this protection is associated with breast feeding. The reduction in hospitalization rates observed after 1 year of age must be due to a different cause, because breast feeding is not frequent at these ages in Chile. On the other hand, the contamination of the environment in which these children live is probably not different from that to which infants are subjected. Besides, older children are more mobile and have not yet acquired proper hygienic habits and should have more opportunities to come into contact with pathogens. It seems reasonable to ascribe this decrease in diarrhea to the appearance of immunity against the most common pathogens present in the milieu. In the analysis of the factors that modify the incidence of diarrhea at these early ages, three components stand out clearly. These are: the contamination of the environment, the protection afforded by breast feeding in the case of infants, and

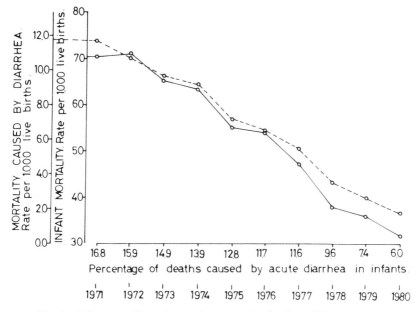

Fig. 1. Infant mortality and mortality caused by diarrhea, Chile, 1971–1980.

TABLE II. Hospital Admissions for Infectious and Parasitic and for Respiratory Diseases by Age Group, Metropolitan Santiago, Chile, 1975

Age group	Infectious and parasitic diseases	Acute diarrhea	Respiratory diseases
0–28 days	2,478		1,275
28 days–11 months	23,608	20,713	19,518
1–4 years	8,606		22,667
5–9 years	4,441		9,990
10–14 years	4,520		4,902
0–15 years	43,741		58,440

Source: National Health Service.

the appearance of specific immunity. Closely related to the latter is the adequacy of nutritional status. The discussion that follows reviews succinctly these four factors.

Unpublished longitudinal studies, carried out by us in different areas of Metropolitan Santiago for 9 months, showed that in a group of 168 families that included 1,105 individuals, the monthly incidence of morbidity due to diarrhea was 2.4 per 100 individuals for the whole group, 6.6 for children under 7 years, and 9.3 for children less than 2 years of age. In the same group, the monthly incidence of diarrhea was estimated to be 1.6 episodes per child and per year for infants under 6 months of age. Between 6 and 11 months, this rate increased to 2.8 [Brunser et al, 1982]. Again, these last numbers are indicative of the protective role of maternal milk. This is further supported by our observation that when carriage of bacterial enteropathogens is investigated in a comparable group of infants, the same rate is observed among the bottle-fed and the breast-fed. Nevertheless, those who receive maternal milk develop less diarrhea [Figueroa et al, 1983]. This has also been reported for cholera [Glass et al, 1983].

The intense microbiologic contamination of the environment means that it is easy for enteropathogens to gain access to the digestive tract through food and water or by close contact with sick individuals or carriers that shed pathogenic agents. We have attempted to gain insight into the forms of dissemination of pathogenic bacteria by studying the contamination of certain foodstuffs, and the hands, nails, nipples, and areolae of nursing mothers in Santiago. These were cultured for fecal coliforms, mesophilic aerobic counts, and the presence of enteropathogens. The proportion of positive cultures among these sources varied but in general they were considered to be high. Thus, 26% of samples from nipples of lactating mothers were positive for fecal coliforms or *Staphylococcus aureus*. The former were grown from 60% of formula bottles and close to 46% of hand imprints. The percentage of fecal contamination among greens and other vegetables was practically 100%. Studies among subjects of high socioeconomic level also disclosed considerable fecal contamination of hands and of greens and other vegetables ready to be served despite ample availability of drinking water and proper knowledge about its use and general hygienic norms [Araya et al, 1982]. The gross contamination of the environment with enteropathogens means that there are many opportunities for pathogens to populate the lumen of the gut and to produce either acute diarrhea, the carrier state, or another condition called chronic environmental enteropathy. The latter begins early in life and is characterized by mild to moderate, nonspecific changes of the small intestinal mucosal architecture (some blunting and increased basophilia of the cytoplasm of the cells at the tip of villi, and increased cellularity of the lamina propria, mainly with lymphocytes and plasma cells). The bacterial population of the lumen of the upper segments of the small intestine is increased, with a greater variety of species detected, including anaerobes. The transport capacity of the mucosa is impaired, with decreased absorption of glucose, vitamin B_{12}, and D-xylose. Fecal excretion of nitrogen and fat is increased [Scrimshaw et al, 1983]. Espinoza [1982] demonstrated that fecal losses of fat and nitrogen increase more than expected when fiber from natural sources is included in the diet in moderate amounts. The increased cellularity of the lamina propria, including the numerous lymphocytes observed among the epithelial cells of the villi, probably represents evidence of the stimulation of the local immune system by the altered lumenal flora or its products. It may also result from defects in the barrier function of the mucosa. The morphologic changes revert to normal when individuals move to sanitary environments [Scrimshaw et al, 1983].

As previously stated, maternal milk has properties that prevent acute infectious diarrhea while at the same time does not appear to protect against the passage of bacteria along the gut [Figueroa et al, 1983; Glass et al, 1983]. These special properties stem from the cells and the specific and nonspecific antimicrobial factors they contain. Colostrum and early milk include large numbers of cells, up to 10 million per milliliter; these are macrophages, immunocompetent T and B lymphocytes, null cells, and neutrophils [Sahni and Chandra, 1983]. The number of cells decreases in later stages of breast feeding, when mature milk is produced. B and T lymphocytes in milk originate, at least in part, from the gut-associated (GALT) or the bronchial-associated (BALT) lymphoid tissue. For the lymphocytes originating from the intestinal lamina propria a cycle has been described. B or T lymphocytes are primed in the mucosa of the gut by antigens present in the lumen. They migrate to the mesenteric lymph nodes, and through the lymph vessels and the thoracic duct they finally reach the systemic circulation. Some of them home back to the lamina propria of the intestine, which they reach as fully mature plasma cells or T cells. Some of the lymphocytes in the circulation become lodged in the acini of the mammary gland, completing the other leg of this migration, the so-called enteromammary cycle [Kleinman and Walker, 1979]. This means that mature immunocytes, producing specific antibodies, will be present in the maternal gut and in the milk that will reach the intestinal lumen of the infant. Through the enteromammary cycle infants may acquire some cellular immunity [Ogra et al, 1977], by means of transfer of maternal T cells or under the influence of some lymphocyte-derived products in the milk. The factors that regulate the appearance of these cells in the milk are not well understood.

Oral administration of nonpathogenic strains of *Escherichia coli* to lactating women is associated with the rapid appearance in the milk of antibodies against somatic antigens of the same strain of bacteria [Carlsson et al, 1976]. This has been confirmed by other authors not only for nonpathogens but also for pathogenic bacteria, against which it affords protection [Dluholucký et al, 1980]. This defense appears to be dependent, at least in part, on the presence of antibodies against one or more bacterial antigens and their toxins [Glass et al, 1983]. The secretory immunoglobulin A (sIgA) secreted by the mammary gland is resistant to the proteolytic activity of the enzymes of the gastrointestinal tract. This resistance is conferred by the dimeric state of sIgA, in which two IgA units are joined together by a junction piece (J), while a secretory component (SC) molecule probably induces conformational changes in the dimer that allow it to be transported across membranes and into the intestinal lumen, and to resist digestion [Tomasi and Bienenstock, 1968]. In addition to sIgA, the mammary gland secretes IgM by an active process that also may involve the secretory component as in the small intestinal mucosa. Milk IgG, instead, has probably transudated passively from the maternal blood. Under normal conditions the concentrations of sIgA and sIgM decrease from 2–4 mg per milliliter of the former and 3 mg of the latter in the first days of lactation to about one-fourth those values by the second or third month. This may be due to dilution in the increased volumes of milk produced [Chandra, 1978; Chandra, 1979]. Malnourished mothers secrete decreased amounts of IgG, IgA, and the fourth component of the complement (C4), but concentration of other fractions remains essentially unchanged. Furthermore, some specific antibodies maintain levels comparable to the normals. All this suggests that the effect of malnutrition upon the mammary gland is highly selective [Miranda et al, 1983]. Another characteristic of human milk is that its relatively low protein content confers on it a rather restricted buffering capacity. The high lactose content (about 7 gm/dl) and the relative lactase deficiency of the absorptive epithelium at birth leave a portion of the sugar undigested and this serves as substrate for an anaerobic, autochthonous flora, whose main representatives are the Bifidobacteria. These thrive in the low lumenal pH that results from the fermentation of carbohydrate, and in turn help maintain an environment that is resistant to colonization by most enteropathogens [Gyorgi, 1958]. The autochthonous microflora does not induce an immune response in the host but, by a variety of mechanisms, it constitutes one of the main defense mechanisms against invasion either of the lumen or the bloodstream by potentially dangerous bacteria [Berg and Garlington, 1979]. These defense mechanisms by the resident microbiota operate in all age groups.

The presence of an antigen in the lumen of the intestine triggers an immune response. The foreign substance is incorporated into the lamina propria of the mucosa after translocation in small quantities across the absorption epithelium. This may involve some receptors in the plasma membrane, or specialized cells in Peyer's patches [Owen and Jones, 1974]. Although antigenic sampling probably occurs at any place in the intestinal surface, some areas seem to be specialized: Peyer's patches have in their surface differentiated cells, the M cells, that phagocytize and process antigens for transfer to the large, lymphoblastic cells in the medullary portion of the patches [Owen and Jones, 1974]. It has also been shown that some species of *Escherichia coli* first attach to these cells during the early phases of intestinal colonization [Inman and Cantey, 1983].

Whatever the mechanisms of penetration, which may be specific for different antigens, they are processed by the cellular components of the lamina propria probably by the same mechanisms that operate in other parts in the body:

The antigen is processed by macrophages and presented to the T cells, which in turn activate the B cells that transform into plasma cells. T lymphocytes are also responsible for the maturation and functional control of IgA-producing B cells in the lamina propria of the intestinal mucosa. B lymphocytes, each one of them producing one class of immunoglobulin, return as mature immunocytes to the lamina propria, IgA-synthesizing cells predominating. The migratory cycle of the lymphocytes means that although the priming contact with the antigen may have occurred in a rather restricted area of the gut, the blood-borne return ensures the seeding of the lamina propria of the whole length of the organ with committed immunocytes. The mucosal immunocytes synthesize specific antibodies. The predominant type of immunoglobulin present in biologic fluids is sIgA. Its concentration in intestinal fluid is about 0.2–0.3 mg/ml, although higher and lower values have been reported. For IgM, the concentration may be about 0.01 mg/ml, and for IgE it is in the vicinity of 40–45 ng/ml. The concentration of IgG is lower than that of IgM and probably is close to 7 μg/ml [Plaut and Keonil, 1969]. By the use of the immunofluorescence technique it is possible to demonstrate that the majority of plasma cells in the lamina propria of the healthy human small intestine synthesize IgA, whereas IgM-synthesizing cells are less frequent and very few produce IgG [Brantzaeg and Baklien, 1976]. It is not known what proportion of the immunoglobulins that eventually reach the lumen of the small intestine are formed locally and what proportion transudates from the plasma. The available evidence suggests that, as in other tissues, most of the IgG originates in the plasma.

The study of the pathways followed by immunoglobulins during their secretion across the intestinal epithelium has revealed that complex mechanisms are involved. These have been reported by Brandtzaeg and co-workers and Brown and co-workers [Brantzaeg, 1975, 1976; Brown et al, 1976, 1977]. Apparently most of the secretion takes place in the crypts of Lieberkühn, the mature absorptive cells playing a lesser role. Most of the IgA is located along the basal and lateral membranes of the epithelial cells and in the supranuclear cytoplasm Because the IgA seen in the lateral membranes is not extracted by repeated saline washes, it is likely that it is not free in the intercellular spaces but is linked to some membrane fraction. Goblet and enteroendocrine cells do not contain this immunoglobulin. IgM is found in the mucosa in a pattern comparable to that of IgA. However, the intensity with which it stains is much less than that of IgA. IgG is very seldom observed in the absorptive epithelium. Surprisingly, some IgG is seen in goblet cells, in the interstitium of the crypts, and in the pericryptal connective tissue. Very few cells staining for IgE are detected in the lamina propria.

Ultrastructural studies using peroxidase-labeled antibodies demonstrated that the three immunoglobulins were present in the perinuclear cisterna, the endoplasmic reticulum, and the Golgi apparatus of plasma cells. In the epithelium of the crypts of Lieberkühn, IgA and IgM were found in the outer aspect of the basal and lateral plasma membranes. Neither of the two immunoglobulins was detected in the intercellular space of the epithelium beyond the zonula occludens, which means that they do not leak into the lumen but that they are mobilized by complex mechanisms. Immunoglobulins were not found in the microvillar plasma membrane of these cells but instead appeared concentrated in the mucous layer overlying it. They were detected in pinocytotic vesicles originating or emptying at the basal and lateral plasma membranes and in vesicles at the base of the brush border, between microvilli.

Numerous immunoglobulin-containing vesicles were observed in the supranuclear portions of the cytoplasm. The distribution of SC in the epithelium did not match exactly that of the immunoglobulins, as some of it was also detected in the nuclear envelope, in the rough endoplasmic reticulum, and in Golgi sacculi and cisternae. This suggests that SC is being synthesized in the enterocytes and that it plays a role in the translocation of the immunoglobulins across the plasma membranes. SC was also detected in coated vesicles and coated pinocytotic pits, which are engaged in transport of macromolecules by absorptive endocytosis. Therefore, although the membrane location of immunoglobulins is comparable to that of SC, the latter has a peculiar intracellular location that probably reflects its synthesis in the crypt epithelium. It is quite possible that the SC acts as a receptor for immunoglobulins A and M and that it may be a transmembrane protein that is divided into smaller fragments at the time of secretion. During this process one of these fragments remains with the immunoglobulin molecule [Bienenstock and Befus, 1983].

The synthesis of SC may be regulated by the amounts of IgA that are presented to the membranes. The presence of SC, in turn, probably controls the amounts of sIgA ultimately formed. Thus, synthesis of each of these substances may be one of the factors that regulates the amounts of the other that are formed. SC is synthesized intracellularly independently of the synthesis of IgA. IgA synthesis in plasma cells of the lamina propria is, in turn, independent of SC synthesis. Patients deficient in IgA have high levels of SC, indicating some form of mutual regulation. SC is not synthesized by the other cell types in the gut epithelium: goblet cells, enteroendocrine cells, or lymphocytes. It is not known whether monomeric IgA can be internalized into the cytoplasm of enterocytes without being previously bound to SC. The presence of the J chain, a polypeptide that joins monomeric (7S) IgA to form dimeric (11S) IgA, is necessary for linkage with SC. Pentameric IgM (19S) also binds to SC for transport across the epithelium [Brantzaeg, 1975]. The chemical nature of this bonding may not be the same as for IgA. sIgM is not as resistant to digestion as sIgA. The mechanisms used for transport of IgA and IgM are not shared by IgG transport.

Being complex antigenic mosaics, enteropathogens elicit the production of more than one antibody. It has been demonstrated that these antibodies may act synergistically to inhibit bacterial colonization of the gut [Glass et al, 1983]. How do secretory antibodies act? One of the mechanisms proposed is the exclusion of antigens through the formation of antigen-antibody complexes that are either blocked from entering the absorptive cells or, if they enter the cytoplasm, are digested by the acid hydrolases of lysosomes [Walker and Isselbacher, 1974]. Another possible role of immune reactions in the surface of the absorptive epithelium is to induce the discharge of goblet cells, which results in the formation of a barrier that prevents further contact of the antigen with the brush border. This may liberate false receptors into the lumenal milieu, and may provide bulk for efficient peristaltic sweeping [Walker et al, 1977]. Fubara and Freter [1973] have presented evidence indicating that sIgA blocks bacterial adherence to the mucosal surface, a basic step in colonization and the genesis of diarrheal disease. This is further supported by observations that there is an inverse relationship between the geometric mean of serum antibody titers to heat-labile toxin (LT) and the occurrence of diarrhea due to LT-producing *Escherichia coli* in a group of susceptible individuals. Besides antibodies against toxins, antibodies against the fimbriae or pili, or colonization factor antigens may be of importance in preventing diarrhea in humans. In pigs, antibodies against K88, K99, asnd 987P fimbriae prevent the appearance of diarrhea due to the homologous strains of *E coli* that produces LT [Morgan et al, 1978]. The availability of pure preparations of human and animal fimbrial antigens and their utilization in the production of specific antibodies provides an opportunity to obtain vaccines against diarrhea caused by *E coli*.

Acquisition of immunity against enteropathogens requires a normally operating immune system. It has been repeatedly demonstrated that individuals who have inborn or acquired immune deficiencies show increased susceptibility to infection, even by opportunistic organisms that normally do not colonize healthy individuals [Hartong et al, 1979; Saulsbury et al, 1980]. The most frequent cause of immune deficiency is malnutrition. Medical practitioners and public health specialists of the less-developed countries have long been aware of the fact that infectious diseases are more frequent, more severe, and more long-lasting in malnourished individuals. On the other hand, in most instances, an infectious episode appears as the cause of death while the underlying malnutrition remains unrecorded. Cellular immunity is impaired in malnutrition: Delayed cutaneous hypersensitivity reactions are blunted or suppressed; the number of circulating T lymphocytes and their response to mitogens is decreased [Chandra, 1980]. Other components of the cellular immune responses have also been shown to be defective in protein-energy malnutrition. These are some of the soluble mediators of reactivity to mitogens, the mixed lymphocyte responses, etc [Chandra, 1980]. Inflammatory responses may be altered not only because of alterations in T lymphocytes but also because other cellular elements such as macrophages or eosinophils may also be altered. Immunoglobulin concentrations are frequently normal in malnourished infants, although in some that are severely marasmic IgG levels may be decreased [Newman et al, 1975]. sIgA responses are reduced [Chandra, 1979; Golden et al, 1978; Gross and Newberne, 1980]. This may be a consequence of reduced numbers of sIgA-synthesizing plasma cells. Deficiencies of zinc, vitamin A, iron, lipoprotein factors, etc are also known to decrese the humoral responses. In view of the previous discussion about the importance of local immunity to the protection against enteropathogens, the relevance of this defect in malnutrition becomes evident. Another characteristic of malnourished individuals is the reduction in the number of intraepithelial lymphocytes in the intestinal mucosa, mainly of the T line. This may be a manifestation of thymic atrophy [Martins Campos et al, 1979]. As these lymphocytes may play an important role in the acquisition or expression of local immune responses, this defect may result in impaired responses to enteropathogens. The altered immune status in the intestinal mucosa in malnutrition is supported by the finding that the type of microorganisms recovered from malnourished individuals resembles those found in immunodeficient states [Sahni and Chandra, 1983]. Although immune defects may be important in allowing colonization of the gut surface, the increased fecal losses of water and electrolytes are the immediate cause of death in acute diarrhea.

Children of high socioeconomic strata, who live in a more sanitary environment, and whose anthropometric parameters were normal, had 2.8 episodes of diarrhea per month per 100 individuals. A group who were studied contemporaneously and were comparable in age and sex but were of the lower socioeconomic strata of Chilean society and suffered mild degrees of malnutrition (Araya et al, unpublished data, 1983) had 7.4 episodes. In a group of infants hospitalized in Santiago for acute diarrhea, those with weight deficits after rehydration had longer-lasting episodes than those of a matched group with normal weight-for-age (Araya et al, unpublished data, 1983).

The knowledge gained in recent years about the etiology of acute diarrhea, its pathogenic and defensive mechanisms, including the immunologic aspects, raises the possibility of better forms of prevention and treatment for the vulnerable groups. Control of diarrheal disease is a difficult, complex task. In the short term, vaccines developed on the basis of our increased knowledge about immunity in diarrhea may come to represent one of the most powerful tools. However, the ultimate goals remain the improvement of the nutritional status and educational levels of the population, and improvement of the quality of the environment.

REFERENCES

AESNS (1972/1981): "Anuarios Estadísticos del Servicio Nacional de Salud, Chile 1972 y 1981." Santiago, Chile: Imprenta del Ministerio de Salud, Servicio Nacional de Salud.

AESNS (1976): "Anuarios Estadísticos del Servicio Nacional de Salud, Chile, 1976." Santiago, Chile: Imprenta del Ministerio de Salud, Servicio Nacional de Salud.

Araya M, Espinoza J, Figueroa G, Montesinos N, Brunser O (1982): "Markers" of contamination in individuals and their environment in different socioeconomic levels. In "Proceedings of the XX Annual Meeting of the Latin American Society for Pediatric Research, Lima, Perú. Ciba Chemical Company, p 26.

Berg RD, Garlington AW (1979): Translocation of certain indigenous bacteria from the gastrointestinal tract to the mesenteric lymph nodes and other organs in a gnotobiotic mouse model. Infect Immun 23:403–411.

Bienenstock J, Befus AD (1983): Some thoughts on the biological role of immunoglobulin A. Gastroenterology 84:178–185.

Brantzaeg P (1975): Human secretory immunoglobulin M. An immunochemical and immunohistochemical study. Immunology 29:559–570.

Braentzeg P (1976): Complex formation between secretory component and human immunoglobulins related to their content of J. chain. Scand J Immunol 5:411–419.

Brantzaeg P, Baklien K (1976): Immunohistochemical studies of the formation and epithelial transport of immunoglobulins in normal and diseased human intestinal mucosa. Scand J Gastroenterol 11(Suppl 36):5–45.

Brown WR, Isobe Y, Nakane PK (1976): Studies on translocation of immunoglobulins across intestinal epithelium. II. Immunoelectromicroscopic localization of immunoglobulins and secretory component in human intestinal mucosa. Gastroenterology 71:985–995.

Brown WR, Isobe K, Nakane PK, Pacini B (1977): Studies on translocation of immunoglobulins across intestinal epithelium. IV. Evidence for binding of IgA and IgM to secretory component in intestinal epithelium. Gastroenterology 73:1333–1339.

Brunser O, Araya M, Espinoza J, Figueroa G, Spencer E, Montesinos N (1982): Changes in environment and their reflection upon microbial contamination and acute diarrhea. Report of Project 3P-80-0083 submitted to International Development Research Centre, Ottawa, Canada.

Carlsson B, Ahlstedt S, Hanson LA, Lidin-Janson G, Lindblad BS, Sultana R (1976): Escherichia coli O antibody in milk from healthy Swedish mothers and mothers from a very low socioeconomic group of a developing country. Acta Paediatr Scand 65:417–424.

Chandra RK (1978): Immunological aspects of human milk. Nutr Rev 36:265–272.

Chandra RK (1979): Nutritional deficiency and susceptibility to infection. Bull WHO 57:167–177.

Chandra RK (1980): Cell-mediated immunity in nutritional imbalance. Fed Proc 39:3088–3092.

Chandra RK, Au B, Woodford G, Hyam P (1977): Iron status, immunocompetence and susceptibility to infection. Ciba Found Symp 51:249–268.

Dluholucký S, Sirágy P, Dolezel P, Svac J, Bolgác A (1980): Antimicrobial activity of colostrum after administering killed Escherichia coli O 111 vaccine orally to expectant mothers. Arch Dis Child 55:458–460.

Espinoza J, Araya M, Krause S, Egaña JI, Barrera G, Pacheco I, Brunser O (1982): Fiber and fecal nutrient loss in environmental enteropathy (abstract). Fed Proc 41:712.

Figueroa G, Troncoso M, Araya M, Espinoza J, Brunser O (1983): Enteropathogen carriage in healthy individuals living in a poorly sanitized area. J Hygiene (Cambridge) (in press).

Fubara ES, Freter R (1973): Protection against enteric bacterial infection by secretory IgA antibodies. J Immunol 111:395–403.

Galls RI, Svennerholm AM, Stoll BJ, Khan MR, Hossain KMB, Hug MI, Holmgren J (1983): Protection against cholera in breast-fed children by antibodies in breast milk. N Engl J Med 308:1389–1392.

Golden MHN, Golden B, Harland PSE, Jackson AA (1978): Zinc and immunocompetence in protein-energy malnutrition. Lancet 1:1126–1128.

Gross RL, Newberne PM (1980): Role of nutrition in immunologic function. Physiol Rev 60: 188–302.

Gyorgi P (1958): N-containing saccharides in human milk. In "Ciba Foundation Symposium on the Chemistry and Biology of Mucopolysaccharides." London: Churchill pp 140–154.

Hartong WA, Gourley WK, Arvanitakis C (1979): Giardiasis: Clinical spectrum and functional-structural abnormalities of the small intestinal mucosa. Gastroenterology 77:61–69.

Inman LR, Cantey JR (1983): Specific adherence of Escherichia coli (Strain RDEC-1) to membranous (M) cells of the Peyer's patch in Escherichia coli diarrhea in the rabbit. J Clin Invest 71:1–8.

Kleinman R, Walker WA (1979): Enteromammary immune system. Important new concept in breast milk host defense. Digest Dis Sci 24:876–882.

Martins Campos JV, Neto UF, Patricio FRS, Wheba J, Carvalho AA, Shiner M (1979): Jejunal mucosa in marasmic children. Clinical, pathological, and fine structural evaluation of the effect of protein-energy malnutrition and environmental contamination. Am J Clin Nutr 32: 1575–1591.

Miranda R, Saravia NG, Ackerman R, Murphy N, Berman S, McMurray DN (1983): Effect of maternal nutritional status on immunologic substances in human colostrum and milk. Am J Clin Nutr 37:632–640.

Morgan RL, Isaacson RE, Moon HW, Bronton CC, To CC (1978): Immunization of suckling pigs against enterotoxigenic Escherichia coli-induced diarrheal disease by vaccinating dams with purified 987 or K99 pili: Protection correlates with pilus homology of vaccine and challenge. Infect Immun 22:771–777.

Newman, CG, Lawlor GJ, Stiehm ER, Swendseid ME, Newton C, Herbert V, Ammann AJ, Jacob M (1975): Immunologic responses in malnourished children. Am J Clin Nutr 28:89–104.

Ogra SS, Weintraub D, Ogra PL (1977): Immunological aspects of human colostrum and milk. III. Fate and absorption of cellular and soluble components in the gastrointestinal tract of the newborn. J Immunol 119:245–248.

Owen RL, Jones AL (1974): Epithelial cell specialization within human Peyer's patches: An ultrastructural study of intestinal lymphoid follicles. Gastroenterology 66:189–203.

Plaut AG, Keonil P (1969): Immunoglobulins in human small intestinal fluid. Gastroenterology 56:522–530.

Sahni S, Chandra RK (1983): Malnutrition and susceptibility to diarrhea. With special reference to the antiinfective properties of breast milk. In Chen L, Scrimshaw NS (eds): "Diarrhea and Malnutrition. Interactions, Mechanisms, and Interventions." New York: Plenum, pp 99–109.

Scrimshaw NS, Brunser O, Keusch G, Molla A, Ozalp I, Torún B (1983): Diarrhea and nutrient requirements. In Chen L, Scrimshaw NS (eds): "Diarrhea and Malnutrition. Interactions, Mechanisms and Interventions." New York: Plenum, pp 269–286.

Saulsbury FT, Winkelstein JA, Yolken RH (1980): Chronic rotavirus infection in immunodeficiency. J Pediatr 97:61–65.

Tomasi TB, Bienenstock J (1968): Secretory immunoglobulins. Adv Immunol 9:1–96.

Walker WA, Isselbacher JJ (1974): Uptake and transport of macromolecules by the intestine: Possible role in clinical disorders. Gastroenterology 67:531–550.

Walker WA, Wu M, Block KJ (1977): Stimulation by immune complexes of mucus release from goblet cells of the rat small intestine. Science 197:370–372.

Walsh JA, Warren KS (1979): Selective primary health care: An interim strategy for disease control in developing countries. N Engl J Med 301:967–974.

DETERMINANTS OF AN INDIVIDUAL'S FOOD INTAKE

Malnutrition: Determinants and Consequences, pages 273–283
© 1984 Alan R. Liss, Inc., 150 Fifth Avenue, New York, NY 10011

Cultural Determinants of Food Selection

Juan José Hurtado V., MD, MA
Puesto de Socorro de San Juan Sacatepequez, Guatemala, and Bethel College, North Newton, Kansas 67117

INTRODUCTION

The effects of nutrient intake on the growth patterns and health of human beings have been clearly established, but there has been less systematic attention to the food behavior of the individual. The complexity of human behavior in relation to food is widely recognized; interest in the topic and a growing recognition of its importance can be inferred from the great amount of research, and the importance of the publications on the sociocultural aspects of food, community nutrition, and the development of foodways. The reader who wishes to explore the literature on this subject will find very useful bibliographies compiled by Wilson [1973], Arnott [1975], and Montgomery [1977].

"Foodways" is defined as the human population's adaptation to the environment through uniform and diverse activities related to food selection, food procurement, food distribution, food manipulation, food storage, food consumption, and the disposal of uneaten food [Bass et al, 1979]. "Foodways" have been called "food habits" by nutritionists [Burgess and Dean, 1962] and represent the nonnutritional aspects of food [Kandel et al, 1980].

To understand how a person responds to the environment in matters related to food selection and consumption, it is important to realize that food behavior is a part of the culture, and it has to be explored within the cultural context. Human beings are both physical products of a long line of evolution and embodiments of unique behavior patterns or designs for living called culture. Herein "culture" is to be understood as "a set of learned ways of thinking and acting that characterizes any decision making human group" [Beals et al, 1977:28].

Cultural patterns include all the ways of thinking and behaving of a particular group of people; these ways of living result in a distinctive set of customs, which includes customs related to food. The following statement by Bennett illustrates this cultural approach: "Men utilize and exploit the natural environment only to the extent allowed them by their customs and traditions. Between human beings and foodstuffs in the natural environment there exists a cultural screen, which modifies and controls the selection of available food" [Bennett et al, 1942:647].

Nutrition and nutritional conditions depend on both biologic and cultural factors; the consequences of food selection and food intake are biologic, but the nature of food selection and intake is influenced by social, political, and cultural processes. Anthropology has both a biology and a social science component; these two components unite only in the study of the distant evolutionary past, and there are very few areas where they have been conjoined in the study of living populations. The study of nutrition offers the most adequate ground for the integration of biologic and social aspects of people's food behavior.

It is only recently that the study of people's food behavior has taken a place alongside studies of the physical and chemical aspects of nutrition. There is a growing interest among anthropologists working in the area of nutrition and food behavior in shaping research strategies and conceptual units that allow them to link their data with the data of biochemical and biomedical research [Pelto and Jerome, 1978; Jerome et al, 1980; Ritenbaugh, 1982]. Nutrition scientists are becoming more aware of the importance of people's food behavior as they turn their attention to the challenge of applying biochemical knowledge to the solution of human nutritional problems.

It is my purpose in this paper to extract from the data gathered in the *municipio* of San Juan Sacatepequez, Guatemala, information that will provide a broad base for understanding the complex influence of culture on patterning food selection in a traditional society.

THE RESEARCH

On February 4, 1976, at 3:00 A.M., Guatemala was struck by an earthquake that measured 7.5 on the Richter scale, and lasted 33 seconds. Over 25,000 people were killed, 75,000 were severely injured, and more than a million were left homeless as their houses collapsed [Ferraté and Arimany, 1982]. San Juan Sacatepequez, the administrative center of the municipality of the same name in the Department of Guatemala, and the villages of the *municipio* were almost leveled. The "Puesto de Socorro de San Juan Sacatepequez," a private, nonprofit organization, was formed on February 6 to help one of the most damaged communities in the Guatemalan highlands. A 6-week emergency program was implemented. The principle that intervention programs should take local culture into account [Manners, 1968] was strictly followed, in order to avoid cultural disruption. Along with the concern over cultural appropriateness, there were concerns with what is called in the literature "appropriate technology" [Goulet, 1975; Baker, 1976] and with local participation in the planning and execution of the assistance program [Foster, 1978].

Two aims motivated the study of food habits of the Mayacakchikel population of San Juan Sacatepequez, both of an immediate practical nature. First, the "Puesto de Socorro" medical and paramedical personnel were interested in implementing a nutrition program that potentially involved changes in the dietary habits of some of the inhabitants of the *municipio*. Second, the Indian people served during the 6-week disaster assistance program requested the implementation of a primary-care health program on a long-term basis.

The study was an attempt to collect the data relevant to ideas about food, food habits, and their relationship to medical beliefs and practices. Different methods were used, including the usual ethnographic ones of both formal and informal interviews, and participant observation; many case studies and medical histories were collected. After several months of data collection there was enough material to allow formulation of questionnaires focusing on the areas of food, disease, and medicines. Since we were attempting to change food habits, it was most important to know why certain foods are preferred. We tried to get at the attitudes or influential factors in food preferences; motivational studies were carried out along different lines.

We found, as medical people working in nutrition with limited funds and resources, that field observation was a reliable method of obtaining information on food habits. For learning the medical beliefs (ideas) and practices, group discussion was very useful. The essence of the method is a lengthy conversation around the main topic, with the leader asking no direct questions, but always encouraging people to express their personal views about the subject under study; you learn from every interview, and you direct subsequent discussions so as to obtain more of the kind of information you want. The tape recording of the conversation can be analyzed afterwards.

The socioeconomic characteristics of the people were examined for each family, the variables under study being arranged in four classes — land and animal resources, housing material, sanitary facilities, and education and cultural features. The procedure was a simplified version of that of Arroyave et al [1970].

Since the author had firsthand medical experience in the area (1949–1951), and had studied the *municipio* intensively [Hurtado, 1970], research benefitted from previous background knowledge of the culture.

THEORETICAL CONSIDERATIONS

The theoretical orientation already discussed here and elsewhere [Hurtado, 1970, 1973; Hurtado and Glavis, 1978] and the practical issues drawn from it, will be used as a guide for a brief analysis of some of the data gathered over a

6-year period in the "Puesto de Socorro" in San Juan Sacatepequez.

The main hypotheses are the following. 1) The distribution of available food within the family is determined by the cultural pattern; 2) food habits are preserved in the old members of the family; and 3) food habits are preserved and perpetuated in the new members a) through attitudes toward and concepts of health and disease, b) through the transmission of traditional ideas regarding food values, and c) through ideas about the foods that are necessary and suitable for people at different ages and physiologic states.

CURRENT DIETARY PATTERN OF INDIAN FAMILIES

Of the several hundred foods listed in the Central American Food Composition Table [Flores et al, 1960], consumption of about 130 was observed. Table I gives the relative frequency of foods most commonly consumed; these frequencies do not bear a relation to quantity consumed or to nutritional value.

The dietary survey revealed that the existing diet consists of a single staple. Maize prepared in several ways is the basic food; *tortillas* constitute the largest portion of a meal. Black beans, served four times a week, are the second most important food in the diet and, with coffee and chile, supplement the diet. Coffee is consumed at each meal. Poor families mix coffee with corn well toasted on the clay griddle, and this mixture is boiled in water sweetened with unrefined brown sugar (*panela*). Vegetables are served no more than three or four times a week, and some of them no more than once; among these *macuy*

TABLE I. Relative Frequency of Foods in the Diet
of the Indian People of San Juan Sacatepequez

Tortillas	13.06
Beans	12.73
Coffee	8.50
Chile	8.25
Unrefined sugar	8.00
Güisquil	7.20
Tomato	6.90
Black nightshade	5.20
Rice	4.00
Eggs	3.20
Onion head	2.29
Beef	2.50
Other foods	18.17

Figures show percentages of instances in which particular foods were recorded in 97 dietary surveys. Frequencies do not bear a relation to amounts ingested.

(black nightshade), squash, *güisquil*, radishes, chile peppers, tomatoes, onions, *parsil*, and garlic are the most common. A variety of green wild plants (low-prestige food) are frequently consumed. There is a variety of fruits, but on the whole their consumption is not great. Whenever funds allow, eggs, meat, fish, refined sugar, and white bread are bought, mainly for special occasions.

Some few items considered by many as a novelty, such as edible starches, potato chips, corn chips, and the like, do not contribute significantly to the local diet. Carbonated beverages — a kind of prestige food — are a significant drain on the village economy, since they are purchased at the equivalent cost of one bottle of carbonated beverage per two pounds of corn or a half pound or less of black beans.

The importance of maize, a "cultural superfood" [Jelliffe, 1967], is easily appreciated if the following facts are considered: First, it is grown wherever Indian people live, since they are inclined to fear that if they do not grow maize, they may go against God's will and they may go hungry. In San Juan Sacatepequez, as in the rest of the country, there is a scarcity of land for Indians. The land frequently does not yield enough corn to meet the food requirements of the family; nevertheless, people derive a degree of psychologic security from growing even a little. Second, the average Indian, according to our field experience, eats a little over a pound of corn daily; and Mata [1978] reported that in the same cakchikel area of the Guatemalan highlands an average family of five — parents and three children under 10 years of age — consumes approximately 1,600 pounds of maize a year. Maize is the dominant staple, the main source of calories and proteins [Mata, 1978]. Its production and preparation occupy a major part of the community worktime, both agricultural and domestic. It has a semidivine status, and its cultivation is interwoven with several ritual ceremonies [Hurtado, 1970].

The outstanding characteristics of the diet are the relatively few foods that are consumed, the contributions of a few to most of the bulk, and the predominance of protein of vegetal origin.

FOOD CLASSIFICATION AND DISEASE

As in other areas in Guatemala [Adams, 1952; Adams and Rubel, 1967; Cosminsky, 1972, 1975; Douglas, 1969; Gillin, 1951; Gonzales, 1964, 1969; Neunswander and Souder, 1977; Woods, 1968], it was clear that in San Juan Sacatepequez foods were classified within the contrasting categories of hot and cold. Evidence also suggested that other categories such as light/heavy, weak/strong, and food/*alimento* were used.

Our principal interest in the hot and cold classification was that it is used to describe particular properties of a) body states, b) environmental conditions,

TABLE II. Hot-Cold Classification of the Most Frequently Consumed Foods

Food	Hot	Cold	*Regular*	Unknown
Tortillas	70	1	20	9
Beans	76	10	10	3
Coffee	95	2	2	1
Chile	95	2	0	3
Unrefined sugar	74	5	11	9
Güisquil	26	12	53	8
Tomato	21	12	54	12
Black nightshade	4	12	51	16
Rice	24	30	35	11
Eggs	47	12	32	8
Onion head	35	18	36	11
Beef	64	10	22	5

Expressed in percentage, N = 97.

and c) foods and herbs. Here we will illustrate the function of the hot/cold belief complex in native ways of selecting food as it is related to efforts to avoid and cure illness. Table II shows the classification of the most frequently consumed foods as hot, cold, or *regular*; people use their cakchikel words for hot and cold, but for the intermediate category, *regular*, a Spanish word, is used. The informants explained that it is "neither hot nor cold," it "does not harm" or "does not cause illness."

The normal healthy body is conceptualized as being in a state of balance between hot and cold; the concept of balance is similar to that described by several writers [Logan, 1973; Foster, 1976; Neunswander and Souder, 1977; Hurtado and Glavis, 1978]. This state is maintained by the careful balancing of the body (internal) and environmental (external) conditions.

Some temporary states such as menstruation, pregnancy, postpartum, and inebriation are characterized by the lack of balance and are classified as "hot." This explains why menstruation, pregnancy, and postpartum lactation call for particular and carefully selected diets. The body assumes the property which is passed on to the blood and the milk of a lactating woman, which explains why for many people weaning is mandatory if menses reappear or if a new pregnancy occurs.

Males spend most of their working time under the sun. Both the activity and the sun are considered heat-producing; also some activities that involve work near the fire, such as making vegetal charcoal, brick burning, or use of lime kilns, are considered to be heat-producing tasks. Housewives also perform heat-producing tasks, eg, cooking. In addition, their bodies frequently are in a hot state because of menstruation, pregnancy, and lactation. In order to maintain a proper balance of body temperature (health), it is important to combine foods judiciously, mixing an appropriate amount of hot and cold foods at the

TABLE III. Hot-Cold Classification of Disease Treatment

Condition of the patient	Treatment
Runny nose Colds Bronchitis (COLD)	Hot medicines, eg, chocolate or cocoa butter, cooked mint with cinnamon or cinnamon concoctions. External applications of hot substances on the thorax or other body areas. The patient is not expected to bathe and is kept bundled up to avoid exposure to cold. Nutrition: Hot foods are highly recommended, and cold foods are prohibited.
"Hot" diarrhea (feces with mucus and blood) (HOT)	Cold medicines. External application of a paste of cold herbs on the abdomen or other body areas. Nutrition: Cold foods are highly recommended, and hot foods are prohibited.
Muscular aches Arthritic pains Rheumatism (COLD)	Hot medicines, local application of hot medicinal plants. Avoidance of cold water, cold foods, and cold medicines.

same meal in order to avoid the potentially harmful effects of an excess of hot or cold in the body. In doing this, they probably are using the principle of "neutralization" as it was called by Hardwood [1971:1156].

Some of the following examples will illustrate this: Pork (cold) is usually served in the form of *tamales*, which are prepared with corn dough (hot), cinnamon, cloves, garlic (all hot). Fish (cold) is cooked with oregano, cumin, chile, and pepper (all hot); white beans (cold) are cooked with cumin, chile, and cloves (all hot). Fowl, mutton, and beef (all hot) are cooked with cold herbs, onion, and *parsil*; these meats are served almost always with cold foods such as wild greens, rice, cabbage, and tomatoes.

Cold foods are considered hazardous to health, and for this reason such foods as fruits, most corn drinks, fresh corn on the cob, rice, vegetables, fish, and meat are eaten at mealtime in small amounts; these foods have to be added to hot foods, which serve to balance the cold ones.

In case of illness the ideal for curing is to regain the lost balance; hot foods and medicinal herbs are prescribed for cold diseases and vice versa. Ideally the hot/cold classification of a disease determines the choice of food, external conditions, and medicines; Table III illustrates the behavioral, nutritional, and other therapeutic expectations.

The information we gathered has been applied in very practical and concrete ways. When prescribing diets, the medical personnel at the "Puesto de Socorro" have been very careful to balance hot with cold foods, and to choose the most adequate diet within the conceptual framework of the culture.

The problem of increasing the nutritional value of the diet was approached in three ways: a) by the enrichment of common foods with Incaparina, a high-protein vegetable mixture, and Protema's textured soya, b) by the wiser use of already available foodstuffs, and c) by the introduction of new and unfamiliar foods like the product of INCAP, Incaparina [Bressani and Scrimshaw, 1961], and the textured soya (Protema's), both marketed and sold by private industry. To promote these foods within the conceptual framework of the culture, each was recommended as a food not too "hot" or "cold," not too "weak" or "strong," not "heavy," and above all an *alimento*, a food that "fills the stomach, goes directly to the bloodstream to all the body, and gives strength."

BREAST FEEDING AND WEANING PRACTICES

In San Juan Sacatepequez, breast feeding is initiated shortly after birth and continued for months until the introduction of liquid and solid supplementary foods, which marks the start of a long period of weaning. The strong beliefs that nursing is a wholly natural function and that breast feeding is the best for a child are the factors conducive to prolonged lactation, which often extends into the second or third year of life. The weaning process begins at the time when supplementary foods, fluids, and *atoles* (gruels) are given to the child on a regular basis. The most common supplemental food is water added either with brown unrefined sugar or refined sugar, and gruels made of oatmeal, corn, or different starches. Some people attending the nutrition program used the high-protein vegetable mixture already mentioned. Very few children receive supplementary foods within the first semester of life, but most of them do in the second one. The second and third years of life mark the time when *tortillas* begin to have a predominant part in their everyday diet; at 3 years of age the diet is similar to that of adults.

Many foods are thought to be unsuitable for infants. There are systematic ideas that are part of the local concepts of physiology; some of them are related to the characterization of children's digestion as "immature" and the idea of the general "weak" status of infants. These ideas are conducive to the belief that several "heavy" or "strong" foods are unsuitable for an "immature and weak stomach," and will cause vomiting, diarrhea, colic, and other gastrointestinal ailments. These kinds of ideas are the background for the resistance to the introduction of supplemental foods at weaning time.

In San Juan Sacatepequez, as in other areas of Guatemala [Mata, 1978], diarrhea is a major cause of morbidity and mortality, particularly in the course of transition from breast feeding to the adult diet. The term "weaning diarrhea" has been used to describe this condition [Gordon et al, 1963; Scrimshaw et al, 1959, 1968; Morley, 1973]. If a child develops any kind of upset when a supplementary food is being started, the illness is attributed to that particular food, which is avoided in the future. In digestive upsets, purging is very common. Castor oil is the most popular purgative and leads to a chronic gastroenteritis, which may affect dietary intake. The onset of protein-energy malnutrition is often related in this way to the introduction of new foods in the diet. In general a child who develops diarrhea is likely to go through severe food intake restrictions, and usually almost all foods are thought to be harmful; a liquid diet is prescribed—gruels and sugar water, which are classified as suitable "light" foods.

CONCLUSIONS

The aim of the study was to collect data relevant to food beliefs, foodways, and their relationship to medical beliefs and practices. Nevertheless, from the analysis of data concerning the socioeconomic characteristics of the people studied, it became apparent that the economic situation is a potent factor in determining what food is available and therefore what food is selected.

Availability plays a primary role in determining food selection, and the specific items consumed by the San Juan people have been limited to what were available to them. The availability of food has depended upon the purchasing power of the family as well as their capacity to produce their own food supplies. The influence of poverty on purchasing capacity is not widely documented in Guatemala, but there is evidence in several communities where longitudinal growth studies, food consumption, and cost of living data are available that the people eat less well and are poorer than at midcentury. Their capacity to produce their own food supplies is a major factor, with population increase putting more pressure on the land. These trends involve sensitive political issues that ultimately can profoundly influence such basic cultural patterns as foodways.

REFERENCES

Adams RN (1952): "Un análisis de las creencias y prácticas médicas en un pueblo indigena de Guatemala." Publicación especial del Instituto Indigenista Nacional No. 17. Guatemala: Editorial del Ministerio de Educación Pública.

Adams RN, Rubel AJ (1967): Sickness and social relations. In Wanchope R, Nash M (eds): "Handbook of Middle American Indians." Austin: University of Texas Press, pp 333–355.

Arnott ML (ed) (1975): "Gastronomy: The Anthropology of Food and Food Habits." The Hague: Mouton.

Arroyave G, Mendez A, Ascoli W (1970): Relación entre algunos indices bioquímicos del estado nutricional y nivel sociocultural de las familias en el area "rural" de Centro América. Arch Latinoam Nutr 20:195–216.

Baker R (1976): Innovation, technology transfer, and nomadic pastoral societies. In Glanz MH (ed): "The Politics of Natural Disaster." New York: Praeger.

Bass MA, Wakefield L, Kolasa K (1979): "Community, Nutrition, and Individual Food Behavior." Minneapolis: Burgess.

Beals RL, Hoijer H, Beals AR (1977): "An Introduction to Anthropology." 5th Ed. New York: MacMillan.

Bennett JW, Smith HL, Passim H (1942): Food and culture in southern Illinois: A preliminary report. Am Soc Rev 7:645–660.

Bressani R, Scrimshaw NS (1961): The development of INCAP vegetable mixtures. I. Basic animal studies. In "Progress in Meeting Protein Needs of Infants and Preschool Children." Washington, DC: National Academy of Sciences–National Research Council, Publication No. 483, pp 35–48.

Burgess A, Dean RFA (eds) (1962): "Malnutrition and Food Habits." London: Tavistock Publications, Chapt 2, pp 9–17.

Cosminsky S (1972): Decision-making and medical care in a Guatemalan Indian community. PhD Dissertation. Brandeis University.

Cosminsky S (1975): Changing food and medical beliefs and practice in a Guatemalan community. Ecol Food Nutr 4:183–191.

Douglas W (1969): Illness and curing in Santiago Atitlán. PhD Dissertation. Stanford University.

Ferraté LA, Arimany L (1982): Geographic distribution of housing loss and human casualties following the 1976 Guatemalan earthquake. In Bates F (ed): "Recovery, Change and Development: A Longitudinal Study of the 1976 Guatemalan Earthquake." Final Report Vol 2. Athens: University of Georgia, Chapt 13, pp 708–730.

Flores M, Flores Z, García B, Gularte Y (1960): "Tabla de Composición de Alimentos de Centro América y Panamá." Guatemala: INCAP.

Foster GM (1976): Disease etiologies in non-western medical systems. Am Anthropol 78:773–782.

Foster GM (1978): Medical anthropology and international health planning. In Logan MH, Hunt EE (eds): "Health and the Human Condition: Perspectives on Medical Anthropology." Belmont, California: Wadsworth, pp 301–313.

Gillin J (1951): "The Culture of Security in San Carlos." Middle American Research Institute Publication, No. 16. New Orleans: Tulane University Press.

Gonzales NS (1964): Beliefs and practices concerning medicine and nutrition among lower-class urban Guatemalans. Am J Pub Health 54:1726–1734.

Gonzales NS (1969): Beliefs and practices concerning medicine and nutrition among lower-class urban Guatemalans. In Lynch LR (ed): "The Cross-Cultural Approach to Health Behavior." Rutherford, NJ: Fairleigh Dickinson University Press.

Gordon JE, Chitkara ID, Wyon JB (1963): Weanling diarrhea. Am J Med Sci 245:345–377.

Goulet D (1975): The paradox of technology transfer. Bull Atomic Sci 21:39–46.

Hardwood A (1971): The hot and cold theory of disease: Implications for treatment of Puerto Rican patients. JAMA 216:1153–1158.

Hurtado JJ (1970): Ethnographic data from Cruz Blanca, an Indian village in the Guatemalan central highlands. MA Thesis. Lawrence: University of Kansas.

Hurtado JJ (1973): Algunas ideas para un modelo estructural de las creencias en relación con la enfermedad en el altiplano de Guatemala. Guatemala Indígena 8(1):77–22.

Hurtado JJ, Glavis J (1978): The traditional "hot-cold" classification of food as determinant of nutritional practices among indigenous Guatemalans in five highland communities. Paper presented at the IX International Congress of Nutrition, Rio de Janeiro.

Jelliffe DB (1967): Parallel food classification in developing and industrialized countries. Am J Clin Nutr 20:279–281.

Jerome NW, Pelto GH, Kandel RF (1980): An ecological approach to nutritional anthropology. In Jerome NW, Kandel RF, Pelto GH (eds): "Nutritional Anthropology." New York: Redgrave, pp 13–45.

Kandel RF, Jerome NW, Pelto GH (1980): Introduction. In Jerome NW, Kandel RF, Pelto GH (eds): "Nutritional Anthropology." New York: Redgrave, pp 1–11.

Logan M (1973): Humoral medicine in Guatemala and peasant acceptance of modern medicine. Hum Organ 32:385–395.

Manners RA (1968): Functionalism, realpolitik, and anthropology in underdeveloped areas. In Manners RA, Kaplan (eds): "Theory in Anthropology." Chicago: Aldine.

Mata LJ (1978): "The Children of Santa María Cauqué: A Prospective Field Study of Health and Growth." Cambridge: MIT Press, Chapt 11, pp 228–253.

Montgomery E (1977): Anthropological contributions to the study of food related cultural variability. In Margen S (ed): "Progress in Human Nutrition." Westport, Conn: Avi.

Morley D (1973): "Paediatric Priorities in the Developing World." London: Butterworth.

Neunswander HL, Souder SD (1977): The hot-cold, wet-dry syndrome among the Quiche of Joyabaj: Two alternative cognitive models. In Neunswander HL, Arnold DE (eds): "Cognitive Studies of Southern Mesoamerica." Summer Institute of Linguistics. Dallas: Academic Publications.

Pelto GH, Jerome NW (1978): Intracultural diversity and nutritional anthropology. In Logan MH, Hunt EE (eds): "Health and the Human Condition: Perspectives on Medical Anthropology." Belmont, California: Wadsworth, pp 322–328.

Ritenbaugh CK (1982): New approaches to old problems: Interactions of culture and nutrition. In Chrisman N, Maretzki T (1982): "Clinically Applied Anthropology." Dordrecht, Holland: Reidel, pp 141–178.

Scrimshaw NS, Taylor CE, Gordon JE (1959): Interactions of nutrition and infection. Am J Med Sci 237:367–403.

Scrimshaw NS, Taylor CE, Gordon JE (1968): Interactions of nutrition and infection. WHO Geneva Monograph Series, No. 57.

Wilson CS (1973): Food habits: A selected annotated bibliography. J Nutr Ed 5(Suppl 1):39–72.

Woods CM (1968): Medicine and culture change in San Lucas Toliman: A highland Guatemalan community. PhD Dissertation. Stanford University.

Malnutrition: Determinants and Consequences, pages 285–293
© 1984 Alan R. Liss, Inc., 150 Fifth Avenue, New York, NY 10011

Intrahousehold Food Distribution Patterns

Gretel H. Pelto, PhD

Department of Nutritional Sciences, University of Connecticut, Storrs, Connecticut 06268

INTRODUCTION

Intrahousehold food distribution is becoming a matter of increasing interest to nutritionists and others concerned with the causes of malnutrition. It has long been recognized that malnourished children are often found in households where their siblings approach normal height and weight. There is tacit recognition of the problem by administrators of intervention programs, who expect "leakage" of supplemental foods from "targeted" individuals to other family members. These phenomena point to intrahousehold food distribution patterns as a potentially important component of nutritional epidemiology. Thus, an individual's intake is not only affected by factors that influence household food *availability* and *food selection* (including food preferences) but also by factors that influence intrahousehold food distribution or allocation.

The terms *allocation* and *distribution* are not intended to convey an image of conscious, deliberate decision making, but are used to indicate a process by which household members acquire food from the family supply. Some of it is served; some of it is given casually; and some of it is taken. The extent to which resource allocation is deliberately controlled and rationalized will undoubtedly vary from one culture to another and within cultures and may or may not be related to equity in distribution.

PATTERNS OF DISTRIBUTION: TYPES OF EVIDENCE

Although intrahousehold distribution has received implicit recognition, there has been very little systematic study of the process. Nutritional epidemiology has tended to focus either on individual food intake or on household food consumption. When consumption is measured at the household level, adequacy is estimated either as a per capita average (total household intake divided by number of persons) or as a percentage of total household requirement based on the age/sex structure of the household. While both methods give a rough indicator of food availability, they are subject to considerable error as estimates of individual intake.

Our present knowledge of distribution patterns comes from several sources: 1) ethnographic data describing cultural expectations and normative practices, 2) morbidity, anthropometric, and dietary data analyzed comparatively by age and sex classifications, and 3) household nutrition studies in which intake of all family members is measured.

Unfortunately, the third type of evidence is rare, and many of our assumptions about distribution patterns are based on the first two categories, which are indirect data sources, at best. Furthermore, one suspects that distribution patterns are most likely to be described (by whatever method) in situations where there is marked inequity. The cultural anthropologist, for example, is more likely to describe "exotic" food prescriptions and proscriptions than to report their absence. Similarly, the epidemiologist and nutritionist are more likely to be concerned about age and sex differences, and to examine intrahousehold consumption, when the cultural milieu or clinical experience gives rise to a suspicion of inequality. Thus, the available evidence may be weighted in the direction of inequitable distribution patterns. This possibility, plus the lack of systematic data, means that generalizations must be approached with great caution.

ETHNOGRAPHIC PERSPECTIVES ON INTRAHOUSEHOLD DISTRIBUTION

In Tamilnad, India, many women avoid fish during pregnancy for fear that its consumption will cause an abortion [Ferro-Luzzi, 1973]. Chagga men in Tanzania avoid green vegetables, sugar cane, and mangoes [Swantz, 1975]; these same foods are withheld from children in West Malaysia [McKay, 1971]. In central Mexico many newly delivered mothers eat chicken and drink a locally fermented beer, *pulque*, to increase their milk supply [CRSP, 1982]. Throughout the world there are cultural prescriptions and proscriptions of food that serve to differentiate "women's food" from "men's food" or "children's food" from "adult food." Often food beliefs are based on cultural theories of disease causation or concepts about the nature of pregnancy, lactation, growth, and development. In some societies food beliefs are reinforced by religious sanctions; in others they are purely secular.

When cultural principles or "rules" identify types of individuals or classes of events with food prescriptions and proscriptions, they serve, in effect, to channel food distribution within households. For example, the Chagga proscription against a male's consumption of green vegetables presumably means that only the women and children of a household will eat them. The operational logistics of this type of rule has interesting implications for consumption patterns.

In addition to cultural prescriptions and proscriptions, another aspect of cultural dynamics that may affect intrahousehold food distribution is the matter of the social value of food. Virtually all societies assign differential value to the foods that make up the local diet. Animal protein foods tend to be most highly regarded in nonvegetarian societies. This cultural fact, alone, does not predict differential distribution within households. However, in societies in which the social value of individuals (or types of individuals) is strongly demarcated, the congruence of social value with food value is likely to affect intrahousehold food distribution. Distribution patterns in which the male household head receives meat while other household members do not, and patterns in which the male head receives the choicest and largest portions of meat, are the classic examples of this process.

The ethnographic literature provides us with insights about the cultural mechanisms of intrahousehold distribution. It also provides data the interpretation of which is often problematic. As summarized by Rosenberg [1980], there are many societies in which food beliefs discriminate against women. There are also many societies in which discriminatory beliefs are *not* found. When food restriction beliefs occur, their force in actual practice appears to be highly variable. For example, Laderman [1979] reports that the majority of women in her Malay village sample did not follow pregnancy food restrictions. On the other hand, in a Chagga village, a disease outbreak traced to contaminated meat was confined to men, which suggested that a cultural rule restricting meat consumption to males was operative [Swantz, 1975]. Thus, the identification of cultural beliefs that purportedly affect intrahousehold distribution can be regarded as suggestive but not definitive.

Ethnographic data suggest that, in some societies, intrahousehold distribution directs a disproportionate share of calories and protein to men. In some, young children are particularly favored; in others they are disadvantaged. Some traditional societies direct extra food to adolescents in connection with puberty and marriage preparation. In all societies, modernization and urbanization are undoubtedly having profound effects on the nature of these beliefs and practices, so that distribution processes are becoming increasingly fluid.

EPIDEMIOLOGIC PERSPECTIVES

The suggestion that sex differentials in mortality are a reflection of intrahousehold food distribution is based on a set of propositions linking food intake to nutritional status to immune system functioning to mortality [Chen et al, 1981]. In countries where malnutrition is a significant contributing cause of mortality, it appears reasonable to regard mortality profiles as indirect indicators of food distribution patterns as well as general indicators of food availability. However, for many developing countries, reporting procedures are incomplete and irregular, so that caution must be exercised in interpretation.

Sharp contrasts in death rates by sex have been reported for India and Bangladesh [WDR, 1980]. For example, in Matlab, Bangladesh, female mortality exceeded that of males at all ages from 1 to 44 years, the greatest differential occurring in the 1–5 years age group, when mortality from infectious disease-malnutrition interaction is greatest [Chen et al, 1981].

Data on anthropometric status and clinical symptoms of malnutrition show sex differentials in a number of countries. In the Matlab study, three times as many girls as boys showed severe deficits in weight-for-age. Other parts of India and Bangladesh report similar statistics. Sex differentials in anthropometry have also been reported for Latin America, but appear to be marked only in very young children [Scofield, 1979:83].

Special interpretive problems occur when we shift our focus from sex differentials to age differentials in anthropometry as a reflection of distribution patterns. It is well known that in situations of food scarcity, infants and young children are at considerable risk of growth deficit. Individual deviations from growth standards based on well-nourished populations depend not only on food intake but on other factors, particularly disease experience. Also, there are behavioral adaptations to low intake that reduce requirements. These complex adjustments (and changes in age cohort composition through death) make it difficult to interpret anthropometric data, by age group, in relation to household distribution. For example, if children between 2 and 4 years of age show a greater deficit in weight-for-age than children in the age group 4–6 years, this may not reflect differences in access to family food resources but, rather, differences in disease experience, differences in adjustment to low energy intake, or both.

Mean values summarizing dietary data on individuals, analyzed by age and sex categories, are more directly indicative of intrahousehold distribution. However, they are not an exact reflection for two reasons: 1) Only a portion of an individual's intake is within the household, so sex and age differentials in "per capita household studies" may be partially the result of differential access to food outside of the household supply. Typically, studies of individual intake do not identify the source of food. 2) In any study, some (usually unknown) portion of the sample does not live in households that contain both adult males and females. In many societies female-headed households are less well off economically, so that as the proportion of women in female-headed households in a sample increases, the average differential in favor of men also increases.

In view of the morbidity and anthropometric data, it is not surprising that dietary data from South Asia show substantial sex differentials. Data from Mexico provide an illustrative case for the Western Hemisphere. An examination of selected nutrients for a sample from the state of Tlaxcala showed that intake of males, relative to requirement, exceeded that of females for all nutrients examined. Although pregnant and lactating women increased their intake, it was not sufficient to meet their increased needs, particularly for calcium, iron, and ascorbic acid [Martinez et al, 1977].

The Tlaxcala data are particularly interesting because of the parallel patterns of male and female intake. For the nutrients in which males' intakes exceeded requirement, females' intakes also exceeded requirement, except for iron. This suggests that men and women are not eating differently, but rather that men are simply eating more of the basic foods in the typical diet.

INTRAHOUSEHOLD FOOD DISTRIBUTION STUDIES

The foregoing materials suggest that intrahousehold distribution patterns in *some* societies are associated with inadequate nutrient intake of females as contrasted with males, and of children as contrasted with adults. However, indirect studies such as these do not demonstrate that differences in morbidity, anthropometry, or average intake are the result of inequities in intrahousehold distribution. Thus, those few studies that have actually measured household food flow provide uniquely important data.

Chen and colleagues, in the Matlab, Bangladesh study, compared household members' intake over a 3-month period, finding that "per capita male food intake consistently exceeded that of females in all age groups," with caloric differentials increasing steadily with age [Chen et al, 1981:60]. Protein intake differentials paralleled calorie differences closely, which suggested that males were not getting more high-quality protein foods.

In the Philippines, Valenzuela and colleagues [1977] examined household members' intake and analyzed the data in terms of a nutrient adequacy ratio, comparing all intake to that of the mother. In caloric intake the male household head received a greater share of calories (relative to need) than did children of any age. For most age divisions male children received more than female children. With the exception of adolescent girls, children received proportionately more protein than did either fathers or mothers, although the differential between husband and wife in protein intake also increased compared to the differential in caloric intake. Fathers and preschoolers consumed considerably more ascorbic acid than did mothers, whereas school-age children and adolescents received considerably less, which suggested differential consumption of foods rich in vitamin C. For most nutrients males of all ages consumed more than females; however, for some nutrients the differences were small. Of interest is the fact that in this sample preschool children were obtaining a considerably greater proportion of their requirement than were adolescents. This latter finding may reflect, at least in part, greater food consumption by adolescents away from home.

Preschool children also appeared to be better off than schoolchildren in a rural sample studied by Pérez and colleagues in Mexico [1970]. While total family intake averaged 92% of caloric requirement, school-age children averaged only 68%, compared to 73% for preschoolers. In a large urban sample, where the family average was 99% among low-income households, the gap between school-age and preschool children disappeared, but all children did less well than the family average, with children averaging 93% of recommended caloric intake.

In another Bangladesh study of intrahousehold distribution, Chaudury [1983] found that male intake of protein and calories exceeded female intake for all age groups. However, when intake is expressed as a percentage of requirement, the sex disparity is reversed, the females apparently obtaining a *greater* share of scarce household food than males. The significant exception to this generalization was for ages 15–30, in which males' intakes relative to requirement exceeded females'. Chaudury calculated caloric requirements not in terms of generalized age/sex guidelines, but on a formula based on BMR and theoretical energy expenditure for various levels of activity. Activity records were used to estimate actual energy expenditure of individuals.

On one hand, the methodological refinement introduced by Chaudury is vitally important for understanding the nature of intrahousehold distribution. However, when body weight is used as a component of the estimate of both BMR and of caloric requirement for activity, thin or underweight people will, by definition, have a significantly lower requirement. Thus, if females are thinner than males, reflecting differential food access, they *will appear to be better off* than they actually are. Intrahousehold food distribution patterns have to be assessed in conjunction with anthropometric data as well as activity level in order to obtain a fuller picture of the nutritional aspects of distribution.

METHODOLOGICAL AND THEORETICAL ISSUES

From the foregoing review, a number of methodological and theoretical questions that need to be addressed in future work on intrahousehold distribution become apparent. First, there are methodological concerns:

1. *The need for studies that examine intake of individual family members in relation to total household intake.* As noted above, many present ideas about intake are based on indirect data rather than on studies of food flow. As a result, there are many opinions and a great deal of anecdotal evidence, but relatively little strong data to show how distribution patterns vary in relation to

food scarcity, cultural setting, family organization, type of food procurement system, and other factors that can be hypothesized to affect distribution patterns. Furthermore, there are almost no data on the distribution of food, per se, as contrasted with nutrients, so that equity in issues of quantity versus quality is difficult to assess with present information.

2. *The need to examine total intake of household members, both within and away from home.* Studies that focus only on household consumption run the risk of underestimating the intake of individuals who eat substantial amounts away from the house. As consumption outside the home increases, the individual's share of household food *may* decline. When this occurs the apparent inequity in that individual's share of the household food supply may be a reflection of his or her greater access to food outside the household. Without data on total intake, the interpretation of the household study is quite difficult, and one may easily come to false conclusions.

3. *The need to assess intake in relation to requirement.* The analysis of intake in simple, quantitative terms, without reference to requirements, can lead to serious interpretive distortion. However, estimates of requirement are not so readily accomplished. What is needed are estimates that take into account the individual's current nutritional status and disease experience, in addition to the usual assessment of requirements for activity and growth. In other words, the assessment of intrahousehold distribution must be made in such a manner that it is not confounded by the effects of past inequity.

Turning, now, to some theoretical issues, the *description* of distribution patterns is an important initial step in the application of nutritional epidemiology to contemporary problems of malnutrition. However, beyond simply documenting the nature of food flow within households, it is important to understand the underlying reasons for the observed patterns.

From the perspective of earlier anthropological theory, patterns of food distribution and related cultural beliefs are the precipitates of past history. In this framework, food distribution represents a traditional practice, handed down from one generation to the next, and subject to change either through general processes of modernization or through the directed change of education programs.

More recent theorists, especially those who argue from the perspective of cultural ecology, have developed models in which cultural traditions are examined in terms of their *adaptive advantages*. Thus, one asks: "What are the real or perceived consequences of inequities in intrahousehold distribution that might affect the long-term survival of the social unit? Do the sacrifices of some houschold members insure the continuing productive capacity of others? Are the conditions that made these patterns adaptive in the past still operative?" The consequences of adaptive practices are not necessarily apparent to the people who maintain them, but from the perspective of cultural ecology, they are to be understood as behaviors that maximize the long-term productivity of the family unit.

Adaptation theory can also be used to analyze the development and maintenance of *maladaptive practices*. Alland [1970] and others have suggested that when the feedback loop from behavior to perception of consequences is very attenuated, it is difficult for corrections and adjustment to take place. Child feeding may be just such an area. Intrahousehold distribution that places children at a disadvantage may not be perceived as problematic because the effects are subtle; slowed growth and poor appetite associated with undernutrition may not be readily recognized. The positive changes in feeding behavior that accompany nutrition programs that utilize growth monitoring by mothers lends some support to this idea [Morley and Woodland, 1979].

Yet another perspective, which has gained prominence recently, focuses attention on differential decision-making power and male dominance. In this model, sex and age differentials in food distribution are based on exploitation and discrimination or, alternatively, on inherent biological characteristics. The latter view, reflecting the perspective of sociobiology, would suggest that patterns of inequality are very difficult to change, imbedded as they are in biological reality. On the other hand, an analysis of inequity that focuses on contemporary socioeconomic and cultural dynamics should, theoretically, be less intractable to programs of change.

The significance of intrahousehold distribution patterns for programs in nutrition and for general development efforts has been ably and eloquently outlined by Carloni [1981] and Rogers [1983]. They have also provided valuable suggestions for the description and analysis of intrahousehold distribution. To these formulations we would add that the several competing theoretical models outlined above — with their different implications for program development — suggest that more research is also needed on the underlying causes. It is very likely that different aspects of these explanatory models have different force and relevance in different cultures and socioeconomic contexts.

For the future, we suggest a dual strategy of work: 1) basic research, with carefully constructed hypotheses, which will lead to a better understanding of the underlying dynamics of household resource utilization and food distribution; and 2) the development of information-gathering protocols that can be readily used, in conjunction with other aspects of "needs assessment," to identify the nature and extent of maldistribution in particular settings where health and nutrition program activities are being undertaken.

The second activity can be an immediately applicable component of public health nutrition. The first can contribute to the formulation of broader perspectives on social change and development planning.

REFERENCES

Alland AN (1970): "Adaptation in Cultural Evolution: An Approach to Medical Anthropology." New York: Columbia University Press.

Carloni AS (1981): Sex disparities in the distribution of food within rural households. Food Nutr Bull 7:3–12.

Chaudury RH (1983): Determinants of intra-familial distribution of food and nutrient intake in a rural area of Bangladesh. Unpublished paper. International Food and Nutrition Program. Cambridge: Massachusetts Institute of Technology.

Chen LC, Huq E, D'Souza S (1981): Sex bias in the family allocation of food and health care in rural Bangladesh. Pop Dev Rev 7:55–70.

CRSP (1982): "Coordinated Research Support Program on Intake and Function: Mexico, 1982. Preliminary Report." Mexico City: INNSZ, and Storrs, CT: Department of Nutritional Sciences, University of Connecticut.

Ferro-Luzzi GE (1973): Food avoidances of pregnant women in Tamilnad. Ecol Food Nutr 2: 259–266.

Laderman CC (1979): "Conceptions and Preconceptions: Child Birth and Nutrition in Rural Malaysia." PhD Dissertation. New York: Columbia University.

Martínez C, Madrigal H, González O, García S (1977): Modificaciones dietéticas en las mujeres embarazadas y lactantes del medio rural. Cuad Nutr 2:83–89.

McKay DA (1971): Food, illness and folk medicines: Insights from Ulu Trengganu, West Malaysia. Ecol Food Nutr 1:67–72.

Morley D, Woodland M (1979): "See How They Grow — Monitoring Child Growth for Appropriate Health Care in Developing Countries." New York: Oxford University Press.

Pérez CH, Chávez AV, Madrigal H (1970): Recopilación sobre el consumo de nutrientes en diferentes zonas de México. Arch Latinam Nutr 20:361–380.

Rogers BL (1983): The internal dynamics of households: A critical factor in development policy. Unpublished paper. Medford, MA: Tufts University School of Nutrition.

Rosenberg EM (1980): Demographic effects of sex-differential nutrition. In Jerome NW, Kandel RF, Pelto GH (eds): "Nutritional Anthropology." South Salem, NY: Redgrave.

Scofield S (1979): "Development and the Problems of Village Nutrition." Institute of Development Studies, Sussex. London: Croom Helm.

Swantz M-L (1975): "Socio-economic Causes of Malnutrition in Moshi District." Research Paper No. 38, Bureau of Resource Assessment and Land Use Planning. Dar es Salaam: University of Dar es Salaam.

Valenzuela (1977): quoted in Evenson RE, Popkin BM, King-Quizon E (1979): Nutrition, work and demographic behavior in rural Philippine households: a synopsis of several Laguna household studies. Center Discussion Paper No. 308. New Haven, CT: Yale University Economic Growth Center.

WDR (1980): "World Development Report, 1980." Washington, DC: World Bank.

Malnutrition: Determinants and Consequences, pages 295–303
© 1984 Alan R. Liss, Inc., 150 Fifth Avenue, New York, NY 10011

Physiologic Determinants of Food Intake

Mark I. Friedman

Monell Chemical Senses Center, Philadelphia, Pennsylvania 19104

Research on the physiologic determinants of food intake is currently going through a period of transition. For many years, from the late 1940s until the late 1970s, research was guided in large part by theories that were based on a neurologic model consisting of brain centers in the hypothalamus for hunger and satiety. In recent years, however, the emphasis has shifted away from central mechanisms toward an examination of gastrointestinal and metabolic factors that control food intake. This change in perspective has occurred for several reasons (for a review see Friedman and Stricker [1976]).

First, the neuroanatomical basis of the hypothalamic model became more obscure. Methods used to pinpoint hunger and satiety centers were found to be less precise and specific than was originally thought. As more sophisticated anatomical methods were developed, hypothalamic "centers" quickly became "systems," which then were lost in the forebrain in one direction and in the hindbrain in the other. Second, the functions of these centers or systems became more obscure. Brain regions that were originally thought to control satiety now appear to be more directly involved in the neuroendocrine control of metabolism, whereas those believed to underlie the appearance of hunger now seem to be associated with more global functions related to arousal and sensorimotor integration. Third, in light of these developments, it became more apparent that in order to understand the role and function of the brain in the control of food intake, it would first be necessary to understand the peripheral inputs into the central nervous system that monitor and relay information concerning nutritional status.

Periods of transition in science are usually characterized by dissolution and disorder and this field of research, having departed from a conceptual framework that integrated research for many years, is no exception. However, such times can also provide an opportunity for new insights and breakthroughs; in many ways what we are currently experiencing may be the lull before the storm. A great many physiologic factors have been and continue to be examined for their role in the control of food intake. In this chapter I will focus on three of these and will then, in an attempt at some synthesis, discuss how two of them may act together in the control of food intake.

GASTRIC DISTENTION

Prior to the advent of the hypothalamic model, theories of hunger emphasized gastric factors [Cannon and Washburn, 1912]. Gastric "hunger" pangs were thought to be the stimulus for eating, whereas gastric fill was thought to be the signal for satiety. That gastric pangs are not necessary for the appearance of hunger has long been recognized. With respect to gastric fill, early experiments showed that distention of the stomach with an inflated balloon or nonnutritive bulk suppressed food intake in hungry animals [Share et al, 1952]. However, these experiments did not clarify whether these effects were due to gastric distress, since the degree of fill was often excessive, or whether normal distention of the stomach by ingested food played a role in satiety. Recent experiments [Deutsch, 1978; Deutsch et al, 1978] have circumvented these problems and have shown quite clearly that stomach distention can signal satiety.

In these studies with rats, an inflatable cuff is fitted around the pylorus, which when inflated prevents gastric emptying. Also, rats are implanted with a gastric fistula connected to an overflow valve which drains stomach contents when normal distention levels are exceeded. In this way the effects of normal gastric distention, independent of postgastric effects, can be examined. Animals are trained to consume their daily ration of food in a 6-hour period and then tested with and without the cuff inflated.

Figure 1 shows results from one of these experiments in which milk intake was measured after food or water deprivation. When the cuff was inflated, rats consumed the same amount of milk as they did when tested without the cuff inflated, despite the absence of postgastric consequences. This suggests that gastric fill alone is a sufficient cue for satiety. On the other hand, when rats were allowed to drink milk after water deprivation they increased their intake markedly when no milk was allowed to leave the stomach (cuff on). This finding indicates that inflation of the cuff does not in itself limit milk intake and suggests that controls for thirst are dependent on postgastric events.

Although these elegant studies demonstrate that gastric fill may signal satiety, it is not clear to what extent distention cues are used under more normal conditions. The restricted feeding schedule used in these experiments may maximize the use of gastric feedback, since it requires animals to consume a

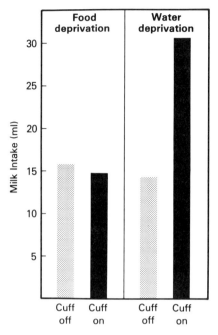

Fig. 1. Milk intake following food or water deprivation in rats with inflatable pyloric cuffs and gastric fistulas. With the cuff inflated (cuff on) milk does not escape from the stomach and drains through the fistula when normal limits of intragastric pressure are exceeded. After Deutsch et al [1978], with permission.

large amount of food in a short period of time. In addition, it is not known whether the effects are specific to liquid, as opposed to solid, diets. That gastric fill is not a critical factor in the control of food intake is indicated by the fact that rats with experimental diabetes are hyperphagic despite extreme and chronic gastric distention (Friedman, unpublished observations). It would thus appear that while gastric fill may provide a signal for satiety, this feedback operates in the service of other metabolic signals. That is, animals may learn to fill their stomachs in relation to the metabolic payoff associated with a particular food. The question then is not whether gastric distention provides a signal, but rather what this type of feedback contributes to the control of food intake.

CHOLECYSTOKININ (CCK)

The possibility that the gut hormone CCK may also serve as a satiety hormone has received a great deal of attention in recent years [Mueller and Hsiao,

1978]. Evidence for this action of CCK stems largely from the observation that injection of the hormone or its terminal octapeptide reduces food intake in hungry animals. Other evidence relies on the observation that the pattern of behavior following administration of CCK is similar to that seen following eating to satiation. The latter observation, however, is not convincing since the occurrence of sleep was the primary indication of satiety. Sedative effects of CCK injection have been reported [Fara et al, 1969] and it is thus unclear whether animals sleep after CCK treatment because they are satiated or whether they eat less because they are somnolent.

Reductions in food intake that may be observed after injections of drugs or large doses of endogenous hormones such as CCK are difficult to interpret since the decrease may simply be due to malaise. Although earlier experiments appeared to rule out malaise as a cause of reduced food intake after CCK administration [Holt et al, 1974], these studies did not provide a sensitive test for illness. When such a test is performed, it becomes apparent that injections of CCK can make animals sick. As shown in Figure 2, when consumption of a flavored solution is paired with injection of CCK and rats are given a choice between that solution and another that has not been associated with hormone injection, they quickly learn to avoid the solution paired with CCK treatment [Deutsch and Hardy, 1977].

Other experiments with rhesus monkeys have shown that CCK injections reduce food intake only when the stomach is already filled [Moran and McHugh, 1982]. These findings, taken together with reports of nausea, abdominal cramping, and feelings of sickness in humans after CCK injection [Sturdevant and Goetz, 1976; Kissileff et al, 1981], indicate that reductions in food intake after CCK treatment is due to gastrointestinal distress and not satiety. Other experiments showing that rats habituate to the effects of repeated or chronic CCK administration [Mineka and Snowdon, 1978; Crawley and Beinfeld, 1983] suggest that CCK is not a physiologic stimulus for satiety.

HEPATIC CONTROLS

Russek [1963, 1981] was the first to suggest a role for the liver in the control of food intake. Although this idea did not receive much attention for several years during the heyday of research on hypothalamic controls, it has recently gained wider interest. The location of the liver as well as its central role in the flux of metabolic fuels make it a likely place to monitor the consequences of ingestion as well as alterations in metabolism associated with fed and fasted states [Friedman and Stricker, 1976]. These changes in hepatic function may be communicated to the central nervous system via sensory nerves [Sawchenko and Friedman, 1979] or through the generation of humoral signals, although currently there is no evidence for the latter.

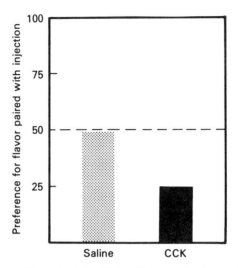

Fig. 2.   Preference for a flavored solution that had been previously paired with an injection of saline or CCK. In preference tests, rats were given a choice between the solution paired with injection and another flavored solution that was not. Values are percentage of total intake in two-bottle test from solution paired with injection. Fifty percent reflects no preference; less than fifty percent reflects an aversion. After Deutsch and Hardy [1977], with permission.

At present, much of the evidence for a hepatic mechanism in food intake control stems from studies comparing the satiating effects of portal vein and systemic injections of glucose (for a review see Sawchenko and Friedman [1979]). Many experiments have shown that portal infusions are more effective; however, inasmuch as few of these studies provided independent confirmation that these infusions had a differential effect on liver, this evidence is largely circumstantial. Another approach to the problem has taken advantage of the fact that various metabolic fuels may be used by some tissues but not others.

In these studies [Friedman et al, 1976; Stricker et al, 1977], hunger was elicited in rats by injection of insulin and the effects on food intake of intravenous infusions of fructose and ketone bodies were examined. The results showed that infusions of fructose, which is not an adequate cerebral fuel but is readily utilized by liver, prevented insulin-induced eating, whereas infusions of β-hydroxybutyrate, which is oxidized by brain but not appreciably by liver, were not effective. The differential effect of these substrates on brain was confirmed by measurement of the adrenomedullary discharge of catecholamines, which also occurs during insulin-induced hypoglycemia and is known to be mediated by cerebral receptors [Cannon et al, 1924]. Fructose failed to prevent this response, whereas β-hydroxybutyrate blocked it.

In order to obtain independent verification that fructose was acting in the liver to prevent insulin-induced eating, additional studies were performed in which the effects of the hexose were examined in rats with selective hepatic denervation [Friedman, 1980; Friedman and Granneman, 1983]. In these experiments, the hepatic branch of the vagus nerve was cut because this nerve had been shown previously to convey information about hepatic metabolism to the brain [Niijima, 1969]. The results (Fig. 3) showed that whereas fructose infusions reduced eating in intact rats, they were ineffective in rats with hepatic vagotomies. Although it is not clear from these experiments whether the effect of nerve section was due to interruption of sensory signals from the liver or due to alterations in hepatic metabolism resulting from interruption of efferent nerves from the brain, this finding demonstrates that fructose was acting in the liver to inhibit food intake. Taken together with the effects of portal vein infusions, it would appear that the provision of utilizable fuels to the liver may signal satiety. However, while there is an increase in the hepatic fuel supply following a meal, it is not yet clear whether such a feedback signal is in fact utilized under more normal circumstances.

INTERACTION BETWEEN CONTROLS

Although we may be able to isolate various controls of food intake under experimental conditions, it is likely that a range of feedback signals from the mouth, stomach, intestines, and liver are used under normal circumstances. Therefore, it will ultimately be necessary to determine the degree to which these various signals contribute to the control of intake. The problem is complicated by the possibility that signals from one source may modify signals from other sites. Such an interaction may be the case between gastric and hepatic controls of intake. In experiments with James Granneman, we have obtained evidence for a hepatic control of gastric function that appears very similar to that which controls food intake [Granneman and Friedman, 1980]. As shown in Figure 4, intravenous infusions of fructose prevent gastric acid secretion elicited during insulin-induced hypoglycemia. As with insulin-induced eating, this inhibition by fructose is eliminated by hepatic vagotomy.

These findings indicate that a similar hepatic mechanism controls food intake and gastric function. If the influence of liver metabolism on gastric activity we and others (see, for example, Kadekaro et al [1975]) have observed reflects a role for the liver in gastric emptying, then it is possible that feedback signals from the liver may exert their effect on food intake partly through changes in gastric fill. In turn, as emptying of nutrients from the stomach is altered, this would modify signals that are generated by the liver in response to changes in the supply of metabolic fuels. Thus, it seems possible that coordination between gastric and hepatic mechanisms may serve both to control

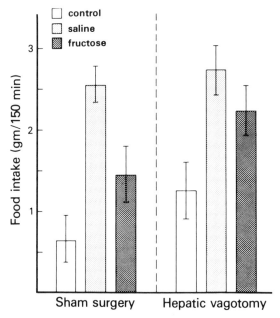

Fig. 3. Effects of intravenous infusion of fructose on food intake elicited by injection of insulin in rats with and without hepatic vagus nerve section. Rats received either no insulin or infusion (control) or insulin followed by either a saline or fructose infusion. After Friedman [1980], with permission.

emptying of nutrients from the stomach and to control the provision of nutrients to the stomach by the act of eating.

CONCLUSIONS

Understanding of the physiologic determinants of food intake is important not only from the point of view of understanding a basic biobehavioral system, but also with respect to what it may contribute to the development of treatments for eating disorders. It is critical that those in this research area begin thinking more broadly about how various mechanisms act in concert to control intake and, in a period of change in the field, not to be tempted by simple explanations and the lure of a magic bullet approach. It is equally important for those not directly involved in this research to demand more from us in the field and not passively accept single-factor explanations. The ultimate test of our knowledge will undoubtedly come from those researchers who deal with problems of anorexia and obesity on a daily basis. Our success will be measured by their success in the clinic.

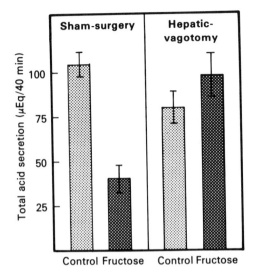

Fig. 4. Effects of intravenous infusion of fructose on gastric acid secretion elicited by injection of insulin in anesthetized rats with or without hepatic vagus nerve section. Rats received either an infusion of mannitol (control) or fructose. After Granneman and Friedman [1980], with permission.

REFERENCES

Cannon WB, Washburn AL (1912): An explanation of hunger. Am J Physiol 29:444–454.

Cannon WB, McIver MA, Bliss SW (1924): Studies on the conditions of activity in endocrine glands. XIII. A sympathetic and adrenal mechanism for mobilizing sugar in hypoglycemia. Am J Physiol 69:46–60.

Crawley JN, Beinfeld MC (1983): Rapid development of tolerance to the behavioural actions of cholecystokinin. Nature 302:703–706.

Deutsch JA (1978): The stomach in food satiation and the regulation of appetite. Prog Neurobiol 10:135–153.

Deutsch JA, Hardy WT (1977): Cholecystokinin produces bait shyness in rats. Nature 266:196.

Deutsch JA, Young WG, Kalogeris TJ (1978): The stomach signals satiety. Science 201:165–167.

Fara JW, Rubinstein EH, Sonnenschein RR (1969): Visceral and behavioral responses to intraduodenal fat. Science 166:110–111.

Friedman MI (1980): Hepatic-cerebral interactions in insulin-induced eating and gastric acid secretion. Brain Res Bull 5:63–68.

Friedman MI, Granneman J (1983): Food intake and peripheral factors after recovery from insulin-induced hypoglycemia. Am J Physiol 244:R374–R382.

Friedman MI, Stricker EM (1976): The physiological psychology of hunger: A physiological perspective. Psychol Rev 83:409–431.

Friedman MI, Rowland N, Saller C, Stricker EM (1976): Different receptors initiate adrenal secretion and hunger during hypoglycemia (abstract). Neurosci Abstr 2:299.

Granneman J, Friedman MI (1980): Hepatic modulation of insulin-induced gastric acid secretion and EMG activity in rats. Am J Physiol 238:R346–R352.

Holt J, Antin J, Gibbs J, Young RC, Smith GP (1974): Cholecystokinin does not produce bait shyness in rats. Physiol Behav 12:497–498.

Kadekaro M, Timo-Iaria C, Vincentini M de LM (1977): Control of gastric secretion by the central nervous system. In Brooks FP, Evans PW (eds): "Nerves and the Gut." Thorofare, NJ: Slack, pp 372–429.

Kissileff HR, Pi-Sunyer FX, Thornton J, Smith GP (1981): C-terminal octapeptide of cholecystokinin decreases food intake in man. Am J Clin Nutr 34:154–160.

Mueller K, Hsiao S (1978): Current status of cholecystokinin as a short-term satiety hormone. Neurosci Biobehav Rev 2:79–87.

Mineka S, Snowdon CT (1978): Inconsistency and possible habituation of CCK-induced satiety. Physiol Behav 21:65–72.

Moran TH, McHugh PR (1982): Cholecystokinin suppresses food intake by inhibiting gastric emptying. Am J Physiol 242:R491–R497.

Niijima A (1969): Afferent discharges from glucoreceptors in the liver of the guinea pig. Ann NY Acad Sci 157:690–700.

Russek M (1963): Participation of hepatic glucoreceptors in the control of food intake. Nature 197:79–80.

Russek M (1981): Current status of the hepatostatic theory of food intake control. Appetite 2:137–143.

Sawchenko PE, Friedman MI (1979): Sensory functions of the liver — A review. Am J Physiol 236:R5–R20.

Share I, Martyniuk E, Grossman MI (1952): Effect of prolonged intragastric feeding on oral intake in dogs. Am J Physiol 169:229–235.

Stricker EM, Rowland N, Saller C, Friedman MI (1977): Homeostasis during hypoglycemia: Central control of adrenal secretion and peripheral control of feeding. Science 196:79–81.

Sturdevant RA, Goetz H (1976): Cholecystokinin both stimulates and inhibits human food intake. Nature 261:714–715.

Malnutrition: Determinants and Consequences, pages 305–314
© *1984 Alan R. Liss, Inc., 150 Fifth Avenue, New York, NY 10011*

Anorexia Nervosa, Bulimia, Cachexia, and Food Intake

Paul E. Garfinkel, MD, FRCP(C) and David M. Garner, PhD
Department of Psychiatry, University of Toronto and Toronto General
Hospital, Toronto, Ontario, Canada M5G 1L7

Reports of individuals with anorexia nervosa date back several hundred
years [Morton, 1694], but it has only been in the past 100 years that anorexia
nervosa has been systematically described in the medical literature [Gull, 1868;
Lasegue, 1873]. This chapter will review recent developments in understanding
anorexia nervosa by contrasting what Gull originally wrote about the disorder
with what we know today in three areas: the clinical picture, pathogenesis, and
treatment.

CLINICAL PICTURE

Gull [1868, 1874/1964] provided an excellent clinical description of the syndrome. He described it as a morbid loss of appetite and wasting illness with a
particular age (adolescent) and sex (female) distribution; but he also recognized that it occurred in males. He recorded most of the symptoms: hiding
food, vomiting, hyperactivity, and amenorrhea. He indicated that some patients have periods of gorging (bulimia). He differentiated anorexia nervosa
from physical causes of emaciation and observed the syndrome's variable
course.

There have been at least six areas of clarification regarding the clinical picture since Gull first wrote on the subject. These involve improvement in the
understanding of 1) the importance of the drive for thinness; 2) enteroceptive
awareness; 3) the psychologic experiences of patients; 4) differentiation of
subtypes of the syndrome; 5) the effects of starvation on thinking, feeling,
and behavior; and 6) changes in hypothalamic-pituitary function that occur
with the syndrome.

The Drive for Thinness

Bruch [1973] and more recently others (see Garfinkel and Garner [1982] for a review) have described the relentless pursuit of thinness and exaggerated dread of weight gain and fat, in spite of emaciation, to be central to the disorder. The drive for thinness is related to a belief that the body feels too large, regardless of what the person weighs. The anorexic patient offers no explanation for this, except that she will feel better if she is thinner. Many of the behaviors typical of the disorder that were described clearly by Gull (hiding foods, vomiting, misuse of laxatives, hyperactivity) may be understood in terms of their purpose: to reduce body size. In spite of the progressive and severe weight loss, many anorexic women are unaware of, or deny, their emaciation and seem unconcerned about their objective poor health and unattractive appearance. The disturbance in body image may reach delusional proportions manifested by the denial of weight loss, the persistent belief that one part of the body is too large, or an extreme degree of self-loathing focused on all or a particular part of the body [Garner and Garfinkel, 1981].

Hunger Awareness

While Gull [1868] emphasized the loss of appetite in the disorder and for this reason chose the name "anorexia," most patients maintain a normal awareness of hunger, but are terrified of giving in to the impulse to eat [Garfinkel, 1974]. By contrast, the perception of satiety may be distorted. Many patients report severe bloating, nausea, and distention even after consuming small amounts of food. In addition, they do not feel satisfied after eating but feel guilty for having given in and fear being unable to stop. Recent studies [Dubois et al, 1979; Russell et al, 1983] have demonstrated delayed gastric emptying, which may contribute to these altered satiety feelings.

Psychological Experiences

The fundamental psychopathology in anorexia nervosa relates to the individual's intense need to maintain her sense of self-worth through undue self-control in the area of weight control. This fear of loss of personal control has been linked to underlying feelings of helplessness [Bruch, 1973] and to a sense of personal mistrust [Selvini Palazzoli, 1974]; rather than experiencing pleasure from their bodies, anorexic women fear the body as if it were something that must be artificially, rather than naturally, controlled. Because of these feelings about themselves, these patients often fear the demands of maturity and the increased independence that this requires. Two other areas of psychologic experience are also important. The first relates to a cognitive style that has been termed "dichotomous" (all or nothing) [Garner and Bemis, 1982]; anorexic patients typically cannot see "grey areas." They fear one pound of extra weight will become 100 pounds. This all-or-nothing thinking applies to their eating and weight but also to other areas as well—exercising, studying, and even their evaluations of people or situations in extreme good or bad terms. The second area relates to the regulation of self-worth; as a group anorexic patients are extremely sensitive to the influence of others for maintaining a sense of worth. They are extremely eager to conform to external standards and for this reason, fueled by their dichotomous thinking style, a particular cultural look or an image can be carried to a pathologic extreme.

Subtypes: Bulimics versus Restricters

Important differences have recently been described between patients who are periodically bulimic and those who are consistent dietary restricters [Garfinkel et al, 1980; Casper et al, 1980]. Bulimia is eating large quantities of food with a sense of loss of control; this is followed by self-deprecation and efforts to lose weight. The bulimics differ in a number of respects; they have generally weighed more before the illness and more commonly have been obese; they also come from families in which obesity is more common. They are the individuals who are much more likely to induce vomiting and misuse laxatives in their attempts to control their weight. They are an impulsive group. This is evident not only in their eating behavior but in other areas as well: They frequently have problems with alcohol or street drugs; they may have extreme mood fluctuations, and compared to restricters they more frequently attempt self-mutilation and suicide. They tend to be involved in social and sexual relationships although these are often perceived as unpleasant and degrading. The bulimic group of anorexics have been shown to have a chronic course and a less favorable outcome [Garfinkel et al, 1977; Garfinkel and Garner, 1982]. They are much more likely to have complications; the most frequent serious ones are 1) hypokalemia from diarrhea and vomiting, 2) suicide attempts due to their impulsivity, and 3) various gastrointestinal changes, ranging from parotitis and esophagitis to gastric dilatation and perforation.

Effects of Starvation

Since the publication of the Minnesota studies on starvation [Keys et al, 1950] there has been an accumulation of information on the effects of chronic semistarvation on thinking, feeling, and behavior. Features that at times have been considered to be specific to anorexia nervosa are now known to be general effects of starvation. For example, starving people experience many food-related symptoms: they are preoccupied with food and may dream of food; they "dawdle" over meals and display food fads; some are hungrier after they have eaten and a few have episodes of bulimia. Cognitively, they display poor concentration and indecisiveness. Their moods are characterized by irritability, anxiety, and lability. Sleep may become fragmented. Social withdrawal and a narrowing of interests are common. Libido decreases. Gastric emptying is markedly reduced. Knowledge of the effects of starvation has been important in helping to explain why anorexia nervosa frequently develops into a self-perpetuating problem: when the anorexic patient experiences these starvation effects she feels more out of control and then increases her dieting to enhance her sense of personal control and worth.

Hypothalamic-Pituitary Function

Amenorrhea is a prominent feature in anorexia nervosa and was first related by Gull [1874/1964] to starvation. However, after Simmonds [1914] described pituitary insufficiency there followed a 25-year period of confusion between the two disorders; many anorexics were likely misdiagnosed as having a primary pituitary disorder. Studies of the last 15 years have significantly clarified the factors related to the disordered hypothalamic-pituitary functioning that occurs.

The neuroendocrine changes are due to several factors: a) Some are the direct result of caloric deprivation; these include elevated levels of fasting plasma growth hormone (GH) and reverse triiodothyronine (T3) and reduced levels of T3. These changes revert to normal prior to any significant weight restoration. b) Weight loss is responsible for other changes; reduced levels of luteinizing hormone (LH), LH responsivity to provocative tests, and amenorrhea are all most closely, but not exclusively, determined by body weight and body fat. Reduced catecholaminergic functioning is also closely tied to body weight [Johnson et al, 1983]. c) Some of the changes in endocrine functioning are due to the thyroid's conservation response, which in turn is the result of starvation. Changes in both adrenal steroid and testosterone metabolism are partially due to the changes in T3. d) Some neurohumoral changes are not fully understood at present. Incomplete GH responses to provocative tests, and excessive cortisol production [Walsh et al, 1978] that is out of proportion to the degree of emaciation, are examples of these changes. The patient's emotional distress, depression, sleep disturbance, and hyperactivity may play a role in explaining these abnormalities. This subject has been more fully reviewed elsewhere [Brown et al, 1983].

PATHOGENESIS

Gull [1868] first described the disorder as apepsia hysterica but he changed the name to anorexia nervosa since he felt that there was a lack of appetite that was due to a "morbid mental state" [Gull, 1874/1964]. The term nervosa was added to emphasize the presumed central origin. Gull dropped the name hysterica because hysterical disorders were then thought to occur in females only and anorexia nervosa was known to occur in males.

Knowledge of the pathogenesis has advanced considerably in the past 20 years. Today many would consider anorexia nervosa to be a multisource disorder with risk factors in the individual, the family, and the culture. These have in common an interaction that produces dieting to enhance one's sense of self-control and self-worth. However, as weight further reduces, starvation and other factors supervene and a self-perpetuating cycle may develop. Various risk factors will be briefly described here; they have been more completely discussed elsewhere [Garfinkel and Garner, 1982].

Cultural Factors

A cultural component of the pathogenesis is suggested by epidemiologic data related to the illness: while it was once considered to be rare, recent studies have documented a prevalence in one serious case in 100–150 adolescent girls [Nylander, 1971; Crisp et al, 1976]. Anorexia nervosa has increased in frequency in the past 15 years and this increase has been in females only [Jones et al, 1980]. About 95% of cases are females. While once limited to the upper and middle class of a particular age [12–25], there is evidence that as it has become more common it has become more equally distributed through all the social classes and now occurs more often in women over 25 [Garfinkel and Garner, 1982].

There is some evidence to link two cultural factors to the pathogenesis. These are 1) the idealization of the thin female form and 2) pressures on women to achieve, often for others rather than for oneself. Garner et al [1980] have documented an increased emphasis on idealization of a smaller body size and dieting in women beginning in the late 1960s. Garner and Garfinkel [1980] hypothesized that if pressures to be slim were a risk factor to the illness, anorexia nervosa would be more common in women who by career choice had to be slim. They found an increased prevalence of the disorder in dance and modeling students. Moreover, the frequency of anorexia nervosa developing within dance settings varied greatly; anorexia nervosa was almost twice as common in those dance settings that were intensely achievement- and performance-oriented.

Familial Factors

Investigators studying the families in which anorexia nervosa occurs have emphasized that they are a heterogeneous group [Garfinkel et al, in press], but certain risk factors may be present: 1) Some illnesses are overrepresented in families with an anorexic member: depression, alcoholism, and anorexia nervosa are all more common than one would expect [Hudson et al, 1983; Garfinkel and Garner, 1982]. Whether the presence of these illnesses conveys a risk of anorexia nervosa because of shared genetic features, biologic vulnerability, or psychologic factors is not known. 2) There have been few empirical studies of the psychologic characteristics of anorexics' parents. Two recent studies have documented an increase in obsessionality or conscientiousness in fathers of anorexics [Crisp et al, 1974; Garfinkel et al, in press]. This finding might be important, especially in view of the cultural role of heightened expectations of achievement and in view of the anorexics' strong need to please others. 3) There has been much clinical reporting of familial interaction patterns [Minuchin et al, 1978; Selvini Palazzoli, 1974], but few studies have empirically examined these patterns. Garfinkel et al [in press] recently compared families with an anorexic member in both Canada and Ireland, and social class matched controls in each country. They found that, in both countries, the families with an anorexic individual perceived more problems in areas of performance expectations, role adaptability, style of communication, and expression of feelings. While this finding may be important, at present we do not know if it is entirely due to having a chronically ill family member or whether it is part of the pathogenesis.

Individual Factors

Not everyone with these familial and cultural risk factors develops the disorder; factors within the individual are important.

1. Difficulties in emotional separation and functioning autonomously have been noted by many [Garfinkel and Garner, 1982]. There are many reasons why an individual may not be capable of living independently — including a variety of psychologic issues that impede the development of a sense of personal identity. Such individuals fail to develop a sense of mastery or control over their lives; rather they have a sense of personal helplessness, and dieting may then be used as an isolated area of personal control.

2. Difficulties in self-perception are common and are closely linked to this sense of helplessness. Experimentally they have been studied for the past 10 years in terms of both body image and recognition of inner feelings (see Garner and Garfinkel [1981] for a review). If an individual has little awareness of inner states or of changes in one's body, it is hard to rely on oneself or to feel comfort in one's body; rather the body feels foreign.

3. Obesity may play a role, particularly for the bulimic group [Garfinkel et al, 1980]. An individual who has been obese may be extremely aware of past humiliations that she attributes to her obesity. This may serve as a potent factor in predisposing to relentless dieting especially if the person's self-worth is largely determined by appearance.

4. Personality characteristics are important as they relate to the regulation of self-worth. Anorexics are generally individuals whose self-esteem is closely bound to external standards for performance and appearance. Expectations are less internally derived but are tied to pleasing others, and self-esteem can be related to an image.

5. A further risk factor may relate to conceptual development, but it has received less study to date. Bruch [1979] has suggested that anorexics remain fixed at earlier levels of cognitive functioning. There are a variety of clinical correlates of this, including the anorexics' "all or nothing" style of thinking.

There are likely other important risk factors to the illness [Garfinkel and Garner, 1982] but they have not been clarified.

While these risk factors in the individual, the family, and the culture tell us why this illness has been "chosen," they do not determine when it occurs. Different initiating factors precipitate the illness; these are not specific to anorexia nervosa but are similar to the precipitating factors that precede other illnesses. Factors that sustain the illness may be very different from the predisposing or initiating factors. Common sustaining factors include the presence of the starvation syndrome, relying on vomiting as a means of controlling weight, the familial relationships that change with the illness, the person's social and vocational skills, and others [Garfinkel and Garner, 1982].

TREATMENT

Gull recognized that the illness could be fatal and felt that this clinical point had to guide all treatment. He observed that the family had no control over the situation and that the patient had to be separated from family and friends; someone else had to assume control. He also recognized that food must be given according to the physician's instructions: "The inclination of the patient must be in no way consulted." He noticed that many other medical attendants would say "Let her do as she likes, don't force foods." Gull himself had earlier thought that this was reasonable advice but he learned from experience the danger in doing so.

The principles of treatment today are based on an understanding of the pathogenesis and progression of the disorder: 1) The starvation effects must be reversed if the patient is to benefit meaningfully from psychotherapy. 2) The patient must always be dealt with openly and honestly and with particular attention to her disordered self-esteem, even though much of her overt behavior may appear to be stubbornly defiant or mistrusting. 3) Psychotherapies must be directed at the specific predisposing and perpetuating factors operating in any individual to prevent recurrences and to minimize sequelae. 4) A relationship-type of psychotherapy with a slowly evolving sense of trust is a useful context for facilitating the preceding techniques.

People with anorexia nervosa feel out of control, and are mistrustful, both of themselves and others. The management of the anorexic patient must begin with an emphasis on developing a working alliance and mutual trust. This occurs through the demonstration of a patient, yet firm, noncritical approach, through consistency and a sensitivity to the varied needs of the individual. An initial weight goal must be set. This is one that the patient can maintain without undue dieting and that allows for the restoration of normal hormone production and cognitive functioning. In general, this weight is about 90% of average for age and height. Many patients can gain weight out of the hospital with regular weighing, support, and guidance, and the initiation of psychotherapy, but about half require in-hospital treatment.

The in-hospital methods of restoring weight vary. We have utilized bed rest, emotional support, and a gradually increasing caloric intake. Often a patient is allowed out of bed for increasing times as her weight is being restored. If necessary, a small dose of a short-acting benzodiazepine or a sedating neuroleptic may reduce the person's anxiety about inactivity and having to eat.

Use of this approach means that tube-feeding, intravenous feeding and more formal behavioral modification plans are seldom necessary. The goals and method of weight restoration must be clearly understood by all staff or conflicts ensue. Dietary management to reverse the starvation syndrome is important. Dietary education must be provided to dispel myths about food, and to place the patient on a well-balanced diet. Initially she should ingest only about 1,500 calories per day but this can be increased over 2 weeks. When patients are eating about 3,000 calories, with reduced activity a steady weight gain occurs.

During the hospital stay, individual and often family psychotherapies are initiated. They must begin to focus on the psychologic problems relating to the individual's sense of helplessness, confusion of inner feelings, and conflicts with control and autonomy. Psychotherapy must be flexible but it generally involves education (about one's body, the illness, and starvation); reality-oriented feedback (regarding the distorted beliefs and perceptions); encouragement for accurate recognition of affects and their appropriate expression. Enhancing self-esteem, independent of weight or an image, becomes important. The patient's learning to trust herself comes later. There are few conditions that generate such panic, anger, and guilt in parents as seeing their starved child refuse to eat. The parents and siblings of the anorexic often need to be included in psychotherapy.

This treatment emphasizes flexibility. Treatment must be directed to the specific problems of the individual patient; but two issues must regularly be addressed: 1) The patient must regain weight; one cannot profit from a psychotherapy when starvation exists. 2) There should be an ongoing psychotherapy to deal with the risk factors and to allow the sense of autonomy to emerge. Using this type of continued flexible approach to treatment likely has reduced both the mortality and morbidity due to anorexia nervosa. While one-third of the patients still have a chronic illness, as many as half may completely recover with adequate attention to physical and psychologic needs.

REFERENCES

Brown GM, Garfinkel PE, Grof E, Cleghorn JM, Brown P (1983): A critical appraisal of neuroendocrine approaches to psychiatric disorder. In Mueller EE, MacLeod RM (eds): "Neuroendocrine Perspectives, Vol 2." Amsterdam, New York: Elsevier, pp 329–364.

Bruch H (1973): "Eating Disorders: Obesity, Anorexia Nervosa and the Person Within." New York, Basic Books.

Bruch H (1979): Anorexia Nervosa. In Wurtman RJ, Wurtman JJ (eds): "Nutrition and the Brain, 3." New York: Raven, pp 101–115.

Casper RC, Eckert ED, Halmi KA, Goldberg SC, Davis JM (1980): Bulimia, its incidence and clinical importance in patients with anorexia nervosa. Arch Gen Psychiatry 37:1030–1034.

Crisp AH, Harding B, McGuiness B (1974): Anorexia nervosa. Psychoneurotic characteristics of parents: Relationship to prognosis. A quantitative study. J Psychosom Res 18:167–173.

Crisp AH, Palmer RL, Kalucy RS (1976): How common is anorexia nervosa? A prevalence study. Br J Psychiatry, 218:549–554.

Dubois A, Gross HA, Ebert MH, Castell DO (1979): Altered gastric emptying and secretion in primary anorexia. Gastroenterology 77:319–323.

Garfinkel PE (1974): Perception of Hunger and Satiety in Anorexia Nervosa. Psychsom Med 4:309–315.

Garfinkel PE, Garner DM (1982): "Anorexia Nervosa: A Multidimensional Perspective." New York: Brunner-Mazel.

Garfinkel PE, Moldofsky H, Garner DM (1977): Prognosis in anorexia nervosa as influenced by clinical features, treatment and self-perception. Can Med Assoc J 117:1041–1045.

Garfinkel PE, Moldofsky H, Garner DM (1980): The heterogeneity of anorexia nervosa: Bulimia as a distinct subgroup. Arch Gen Psychiatry 37:1036–1040.

Garfinkel PE, Garner DM, Rose J, Darby PL, Brades JS, O'Hanlon J, Walsh N (in press): A comparison of characteristics in the families of patients with anorexia nervosa and normal controls. Psychol Med.

Garner DM, Bemis K (1982): A Cognitive-behavioral approach to anorexia nervosa. Cog Ther Res 6:1–27.

Garner DM, Garfinkel PE (1980): Socio-cultural factors in the development of anorexia nervosa. Psychol Med 10:647–656.

Garner DM, Garfinkel PE (1981): Body image in Anorexia Nervosa: Measurement, Theory and Implications. Int J Psychiat Med 12:263–284.

Garner DM, Garfinkel PE, Schwartz D, Thompson M (1980): Cultural Expectations of thinness in women. Psych Rep 47:483–491.

Gull WW (1868): The Address in medicine delivered before the annual meeting of the BMA at Oxford. Lancet 2:171.

Gull WW (1874/1964): Anorexia Nervosa. Trans Clin Soc (Lond) 7:22–28. Reprinted in Kaufman RM, Heiman M (eds): "Evolution of Psychosomatic Concepts. Anorexia Nervosa: A Paradigm." New York: International Universities Press.

Hudson JI, Pope Jr H, Jonas JM, Yungelun-Todd D (1983): Family history study of anorexia nervosa and bulimia. Br J Psychiatry 142:133–138.

Johnson JL, Leiter LA, Burrow GN, Garfinkel PE, Anderson GJ (1983): Excretion of urinary catecholamine metabolites in anorexia nervosa: Effect of body composition and energy intake. Federation of American Societies for Experimental Biology.

Jones DJ, Fox MM, Babigan HM, Hutton HE (1980): Epidemiology of anorexia nervosa in Munroe County, New York, 1960–1976. Psychosom Med 42:551–558.

Keys A, Brozek J, Henschel A, Michelson O, Taylor HL (1950): "The Biology of Human Starvation." Minneapolis: University of Minnesota Press, Vol. 1.

Lasegue CA (1873): De l'anorexie hysterique. Arch Gen de Med 385. Reprinted in Kaufman RM, Herman M (eds): "Evolution of Psychsomatic Concepts of Anorexia Nervosa: A Paradigm." New York: International Universities Press.

Minuchin S, Rosman BL, Baker L (1978): "Psychosomatic Families: Anorexia Nervosa in Context." Cambridge, MA: Harvard University Press.

Morton R (1694): "Phthisiologica: Or a Treatise of Consumptions." London: S. Smith and B. Walford.

Nylander I (1971): The feeling of being fat and dieting in a school population: Epidemiologic interview investigation. Acta Sociomed Scand. 3:17-26.

Russell D, Freedman ML, Feighlin DHI, Jeejeebhoy KN, Swinson RP, Garfinkel PE (1983): Delayed gastric emptying in anorexia nervosa — Improvement with Domperidone. Am J Psychiatry 140:1235-1236.

Selvini Palazzoli M (1974): "Anorexia Nervosa." London: Chaucer Publishing Co.

Simmonds M (1914): Veber embolische Prozesse in der Hypophysis. Arch Pathol Anat 217:226-239.

Walsh BT, Katz JL, Levin J, Kream J, Fukushima DK, Hellman LD, Weiner H, Zumoff B (1978): Adrenal activity in anorexia nervosa. Psychosom Med 40:499-506.

Malnutrition: Determinants and Consequences, pages 315–324
© l984 Alan R. Liss, Inc., 150 Fifth Avenue, New York, NY 10011

Psychosocial Factors and Food Intake

Alexander R. Lucas, MD

Section of Child and Adolescent Psychiatry, Mayo Clinic and Mayo
Foundation, Rochester, Minnesota 55905

Eating behavior is multidetermined, based on biologic, psychologic, and social influences (Fig. 1). Eating and drinking are among the most basic of biologic requirements, along with the need for air, warmth, and shelter. Some sources of energy and essential chemicals are required by all living organisms from the simplest cells to the most complex animals. Food requirements become increasingly complicated with the complexity of the animal. Biologic *need*, expressed through *hunger*, underlies all eating behavior. There are complex physiologic mechanisms originating centrally in the nervous system and peripherally in the body that mediate, monitor, and direct hunger, taste, and satiety. The human, as an omnivorous animal, eats a wide variety of food substances. The basic nutritional requirements can be met by almost endless varieties of foodstuffs, varying with geographic distribution, availability, economics, and cuisine.

Food *preference* is based on innate factors and acquired taste. It dictates *appetite* for and selection of particular foods and combinations. Visual as well as gustatory factors play a role in this process. Individual psychologic and family patterns lead to *habit*, a major determinant of eating behavior. Social patterns, based on cultural and religious beliefs and practices, lead to *custom* in eating behavior. Habit and custom can shape and alter food preference. These three factors, preference, habit, and custom, may override hunger and satiation to result in eating patterns that deviate from the demands of biologic need. Some of these deviations are not undesirable. Indeed, they are a hallmark of civilization. Some become ritualized and others are identified as ethnic characteristics. Aberrations in individual thought processes and family patterns, however, can alter eating behavior in extreme and idiosyncratic ways as manifested by fads, phobias, and obsessions.

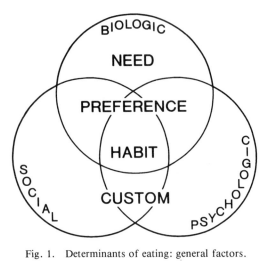

Fig. 1. Determinants of eating: general factors.

BIOLOGIC FACTORS

One cannot consider psychosocial factors and food intake without taking into account the biologic ones. All are so intertwined. The biologic factors have been extensively studied. Despite many physiologic studies the complex mechanisms that control hunger and satiety are still not fully understood. The mechanism clearly is not a simple one based on a single parameter such as blood sugar, but depends on the interaction of peripheral and central mechanisms [Mayer, 1980]. In most animals and humans the mechanism works marvelously, permitting growth and weight gain during the developmental phase and maintaining weight within narrow limits during the adult stage. Even special future needs are anticipated, such as seasonal variation in the availability of food, and impending famine. While this control mechanism usually works well, many people have trouble controlling their weight. This continues to be an important problem in western societies. The desire to lose weight has stimulated a huge popular literature and the weight control industry. There continues to be a search for medications to control appetite, for ways to alter eating behavior, and for means to change the thinking associated with eating.

Rozin [1976] has pointed out that food selection requires a *sensory* system to recognize food and an *internal detector system* to provide the motivation to eat (Fig. 2). For primitive organisms with limited food choices the system is simple and requires only the chemical sensor to recognize a specific food, and the motivational system to eat when there is a nutritional need. In omnivorous animals genetically determined specific receptor systems have been identified for sodium, water, and oxygen. A similar system is probably present for energy balance. Sugar preference is seen among primates. Rats and humans also

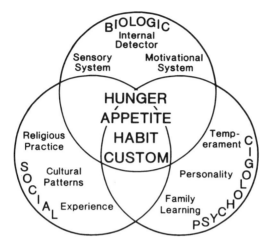

Fig. 2.   Determinants of eating: specific factors.

have a poison avoidance system related to the bitter taste of toxic alkaloids and glycosides. There are genetically determined taste sensitivities that differ greatly among individuals [Williams, 1956]. They contribute to food preferences and dislikes. Individuals with metabolic defects must avoid certain nutrients such as sugar or specific amino acids. To what extent individual nutritional needs differ among normal persons, and whether these needs dictate their food choice, remain open questions.

PSYCHOLOGIC FACTORS

Psychologic factors in the individual come to bear upon food choices and habit formation in eating patterns. Family and broader social and cultural patterns, however, set the stage on which the individual characteristics can assert themselves.

There is no compelling evidence that the first foods experienced in life become imprinted to form the basis for future preferences [Rozin, 1976]. In fact, as a rule, in mammals and many human societies, milk is not consumed after weaning. Innate differences are observed among children in their eating patterns, as in other areas of their behavior [Thomas et al, 1964]. Some are *temperamentally* good, predictable eaters from infancy on, and adapt easily to new foods, while others are fussy, irregular, and picky eaters who reject new foods.

Parental attitudes and the psychologic makeup of the child interact in establishing family attitudes and expectations around eating. These may be casual or rigid, and lay the psychologic foundation for comfort around eating or for future eating problems. A relationship between eating and emotions has long been recognized. Food plays a central role in bonding between mother and infant. Disturbances in the parent-child relationship are often reflected in feeding difficulties. *Family eating patterns* are often conveyed to the offspring to form the basis of lifelong habits. This is most conspicuous in obesity when overfeeding of infants and family example are factors. At the other extreme, neglect and emotional detachment lead to deprivation syndromes with profound implications for children's physical and intellectual development as seen in malnutrition [Galler et al, 1983]. Clinically there are a number of conditions, including failure to thrive, rumination, and pica, in which the quality of the emotional relationship with the parent has been implicated.

Parents can be overly conscientious about assuring the optimum diet (Fig. 3). In our society the notorious "food that is good for you" raises the specter of horror for many children. When parents place excessive value on satisfactory eating, and see food refusal as rejection of their love, oppositional syndromes may develop and eating can become a powerful weapon at the disposal of the child. Years ago, the pediatrician Clara Davis demonstrated that young children will make nutritionally sound choices when given great latitude in selecting their own food from an available variety without adult direction [Davis, 1933]. Hilde Bruch described a parental attitude that may lead to serious eating disturbances in the child's later life. It occurs in infants who are well cared-for in every detail, but with everything done according to the parents' decision without regard for the child's initiative [Bruch, 1978].

SOCIAL FACTORS

Social and *cultural factors* are fundamental determinants of eating behavior. Humans are a product of their cultural as well as their family experiences. Social groups that developed under various geographic and climatic conditions were led by necessity and invention to eat what nature provided and what they were able to hunt, catch, and produce. This varied from the agrarian societies of the tropics to the ocean-dependent societies of the permafrost region. In between were the hunting and agricultural societies of the temperate continental regions and the Polynesian societies fortunate enough to be able to harvest the plentiful yield of the islands and warm oceans. Many societies had to labor hard and long hours to produce their daily bread, and many were frequently confronted by the disasters of drought, crop failure, and famine.

Humans developed their characteristic food selection patterns by passing through several phylogenetic sequences [Rozin, 1976]. Primordial man was omnivorous, with the emphasis mainly on plants, but the diet included some meat, as in the present diet of baboons and chimpanzees. This was the era of the hunter-gatherer. With the invasion of the savannah the human became

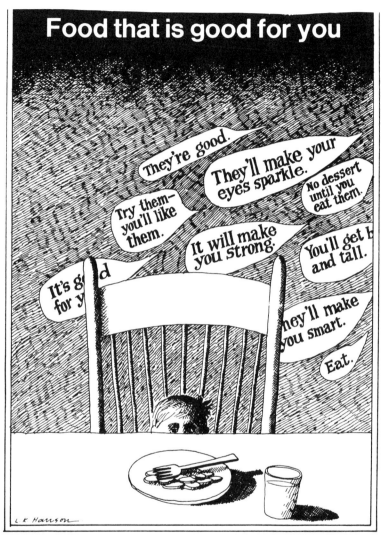

Fig. 3.   Parental attitudes and diet. From the Minneapolis *Star and Tribune*, with permission.

more carnivorous. The era of meat eating was thought to have lasted for some hundreds of thousands of years when man was primarily a carnivorous species until the agricultural revolution, 7,000–10,000 years ago. Along with the cultivation of edible plants came the domestication of animals and the beginning of our present pattern of wide-ranging omnivorous appetites.

Location, climate, and man's ingenuity limited the availability and variety of foodstuffs. Local mores and religious beliefs further directed patterns of food choices and preparation, limiting and rationing the available food to individuals in the society. Beliefs based on rational or irrational thinking established practices and rules to govern the procurement, production, distribution, and consumption of food in societies.

Peoples of primitive cultures engaged in many special practices around eating [Frazer, 1959]. The acts of eating and drinking were often imbued with special dangers. In regions as remote from each other as Africa, Sumatra, and Fiji it was believed that evil spirits could enter the body, and the soul might escape from the mouth while taking nourishment. North and South American hunters and fishers believed that the characteristics of animals they ate would be transmitted to them. Thus, those who fed on venison would be swifter than those who lived on the flesh of the bear or domestic cattle. Similar beliefs in Africa attributed courage to those who ate the hearts of lions.

Taboos regarding food were widespread among primitive societies. Certain animals and plants were avoided as dangerous and fatal. Frazer thought these prohibitions were superstitious fancies, but some may well have had their origins in unfortunate experiences transmitted by word of mouth for generations. Kings and priests had even more stringent food restrictions either to protect them from poisoning or to nourish them more lavishly. Some cultural beliefs are based on superstition, but others on the folk wisdom of many generations. An example was the widespread practice of eating certain mushrooms in a region of the Bohemian Forest. Folklore pointed out that the species *Boletus edulis* allegedly prevented cancer. Scientific studies have confirmed that the mushroom yielded a tumor-inhibiting substance [Lucas, 1959].

Food rituals and prohibitions have persisted in enlightened societies to modern times in the form of *religious practices*. The sacramental use of bread and wine in the Christian church, the avoidance of meat on holy days by Catholics, the prohibition of meat and animal products by Hindus, and the prohibition of pork by Jews and Mohammedans are examples.

INTERACTION OF THE FACTORS

No single one of these factors in the biologic, psychologic, and social realm acts by itself as a sole determinant of eating behavior. All are necessary. Their relative strength varies in different situations. Each factor influences and modifies the effect of the others.

Food selection in humans is dictated by two systems that operate interdependently [Rozin, 1976]. The first is a specific system for recognizing foods, which has its biologic basis deep in the mammalian heritage, and guides food selection. The second is an open-ended system based on learning, from experience, what to eat and what not to eat. Lau et al [1983] emphasized the multiplicity of factors affecting food selection including genetic, early experience facilitated by the mother, and the psychologic meaning of food. Rozin [1976] further pointed out that omnivores eat a variety of foods; the range of diet makes both poisoning and specific nutritional deficiencies likely possibilities. He emphasized that omnivores are subject to conflicting reactions to food, both serving important survival purposes. *Neophobia*, or the suspicion and avoidance of new foods, sees new foods as all potentially dangerous. This principle assures continuation of the consumption of familiar food that supplies necessary nutrients and energy, and it assures against poisoning by unfamiliar, untried foods.

Neophilia, or the desire to try new foods, provides the possibility of trying and discovering new sources of energy, particularly important when there is lack of previously available major food sources, but it carries with it the risk of poisoning. Rozin believes that omnivores maintain an ambivalent, highly emotionally charged reaction to new foods, and see them as potentially dangerous but also as potentially new sources of nutrition. This is manifested by an initial strong, often violent avoidance of new foods, followed by a cautious sampling of them.

A CASE HISTORY

A child born half a century ago in Central Europe was nursed by his mother but did not develop a special attachment to warm milk. Food was plentiful and the diet well-balanced. He was taught to eat at least a spoonful of every food, even those he disliked, and to finish everything on his plate. It was considered sinful to waste any food because his parents lived in a world where deprivation and food shortages were commonplace. He hated vegetables and developed a preference for sweets, perhaps partially on a biologic basis and partly because of the exposure in his family. As a child he was somewhat frail and thin, and not considered a good eater. His father, a scientist with a concern for nutrition and an intuitive sense for child psychology, developed a game for the children called "Sp-Sp-Sp": *Speziale-Speise-Spiel* (special food game), which involved a list of foods that the children rated on a three-point scale. The cuisine was a mixture of Austrian, Hungarian, Bohemian, and Bavarian influences. With his mother's culinary skills and his father's continued interest, he thrived and grew. Although the home was nominally Protestant, meat was never served on Good Friday or Christmas Eve because of the mother's early Roman Catholic upbringing. With the outbreak of World War II, the family emigrated to the United States. On shipboard they were appalled by the wasteful American practice of dumping trays full of day-old baked goods overboard to be devoured by scavenger fish and seagulls. The move to a new land required dietary readjustments. Among the most difficult was the acceptance of white "cottony" bread. It was incomprehensible why American children who ate this

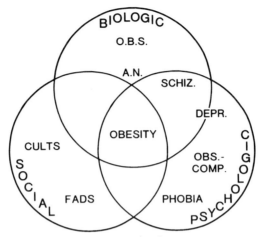

Fig. 4. Abnormal eating patterns.

bread often refused the crust, which seemed hardly any firmer than the rest of the bread. Salted butter and the combination of salt and sugar in many foods was at first objectionable. Rare meat served at friends' homes was considered barbaric. The mother was unable to duplicate European baked goods because of differences in the flour and other ingredients. Adaptation to new foods came quickly, however, for the preadolescent boy and his siblings. Some changes were highly pleasant — such as the plentiful availability of ice cream, which had been a rare luxury in prewar Europe. With maturation to adulthood taste preferences changed and culinary horizons expanded. Fish and other seafoods rarely experienced in childhood became an acquired taste. Certain consistencies — such as that of barley soup, once nauseating at European school lunches — became acceptable. Strange and exotic foods that formerly went untasted have taken on interest. Yet, there is still a distant and nostalgic longing for Central European cuisine — crips well-done pork roast, Bohemian potato pancakes and dumplings, and grandmother's special vanilla crescent Christmas cookies. The bread — large, round loaves fresh out of the corner baker's oven; still warm, the crisp, heavy crust sprinkled with flour — is incomparable. Aging and illness has caused some necessary diet adjustments. Elevated serum cholesterol levels impose difficult diet restrictions especially in regard to eating out. Minimizing salt in the diet has been surprisingly easy and has not imposed a hardship, even though he preferred salt as a child. It has led to an interesting experimentation with herbs and spices that have served to make foods more interesting and flavorful.

ABNORMAL EATING PATTERNS

Individuals and groups often engage in faddism and cultism that involve their eating patterns (Fig. 4). Fads and cultish patterns are deviations from us-

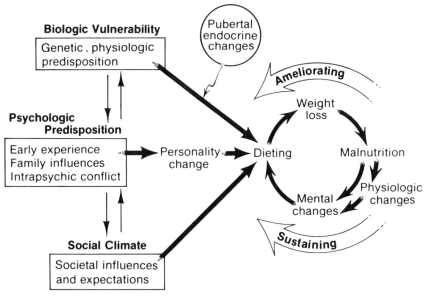

Fig. 5. Multifactoral influences in anorexia nervosa. From Lucas [1981], with permission.

ual practices that are not based on scientific fact. They may be useless or harmful practices. Some individuals with psychiatric disturbances such as phobias, obsessive-compulsive neuroses, depressive illness, and schizophrenia, as well as with organic cerebral illness, manifest severe aberrations in their eating behavior as part of their illness [Mayer, 1976]. In schizophrenia there may be delusions about the content of food, which leads to self-starvation. Obsessive-compulsive rituals can lead to the avoidance of certain foods or interfere with the eating process. Conversely, rituals can be developed in an attempt to avoid eating, when there is the underlying fear of food or of becoming fat. In severe depression there is loss of appetite that leads to weight loss. Milder forms of depression may lead to increased eating and weight gain. Certain emotional states such as boredom, loneliness, and anger may lead, in some individuals, to increased eating.

The complex interaction of biologic, psychologic, and social influences is exemplified in the causes and perpetuation of the eating disorder anorexia nervosa (Fig. 5) [Lucas, 1981]. Factors stemming from these three spheres have greater or lesser influences in each individual and lead to the process of personality change, dieting, and a vicious cycle involving weight loss, malnutrition, and physical and mental changes. The cycle is perpetuated by factors that facilitate the process, whereas others impede or arrest the process, permitting recovery from the illness.

Changing eating patterns is a vexing challenge to nutritionists, physicians, and public health workers who treat individuals with eating disorders, who are involved in public health care of malnourished populations, or who plan preventive programs of nutrition education aimed at reducing obesity, heart disease, hypertension, and stroke. Kolasa [1981] observed that it would be naive to think that food behavior can be changed directly or quickly through nutrition education She stated that since food behavior is deeply embedded in culture, its change is governed by the same gradual forces that shape cultural changes. Those working with individuals who have eating disorders are equally aware that biologic and psychologic forces are impediments to change.

While in all three spheres there are elements resistant to the change that we, as nutritional reformers, deem healthy, there are protective and restorative forces in each individual that have evolved through time. They are perhaps difficult to improve upon over the short term.

CONCLUSIONS

Multiple biologic, psychologic, and social influences operate as the determinants of food intake in health and in disease states. Because of the complexities inherent in these factors and their interaction, changing individual and societal eating patterns is a gradual process, not easily accomplished through exhortation, treatment, or legislation.

REFERENCES

Bruch H (1978): Anorexia nervosa. Nutrition Today 13:14–18.

Davis CM (1933): A practical application of some lessons of the self-selection of diet study to the feeding of children in hospitals. Am J Dis Child 46:743–750.

Frazer JG (1959): Gaster TH (ed): "The New Golden Bough." New York: Criterion Books.

Galler JR, Ramsey F, Solimano G, Lowell WE, Mason E (1983): The influence of early malnutrition on subsequent behavioral development. I. Degree of impairment of intellectual performance. J Am Acad Child Psychiatry 22:8–15.

Kolasa KM (1981): Nutrition education and changing behavior. In Selvey N, White PL (eds): "Nutrition in the 1980s." New York: Alan R. Liss, pp 415–422.

Lau D, Krondl M, Coleman P (1983): Factors affecting food selection (in press).

Lucas AR (1981): Toward the understanding of anorexia nervosa as a disease entity. Mayo Clin Proc 56:254–264.

Lucas EH (1959): The role of folklore in discovery and rediscovery of plant drugs. Centennial Rev 3:173–188.

Mayer J (1980): Physiology of hunger and satiety. In Goodhart RS, Shils ME (eds): "Modern Nutrition in Health and Disease." 6th Ed. Philadelphia: Lea & Febiger, pp 560–577.

Meyer J-E (1976): Psychopathology and eating disorders. In Silverstone T (ed): "Appetite and Food Intake." Berlin: Dahlem, pp 355–368.

Rozin P (1976): Psychobiological and cultural determinants of food choice. In Silverstone T (ed): "Appetite and Food Intake." Berlin: Dahlem, pp 285–312.

Thomas A, Chess S, Birch HG, Hertzig ME, Korn S (1964): "Behavioral Individuality in Early Childhood." New York: New York University Press.

Williams RJ (1956): "Biochemical Individuality." New York: Wiley, pp 127–130.

IMPEDIMENTS TO THE INCREASED USE OF TECHNOLOGY

Malnutrition: Determinants and Consequences, pages 327–335
© *1984 Alan R. Liss, Inc., 150 Fifth Avenue, New York, NY 10011*

Preharvest and Postharvest Losses of Crops

Malcolm C. Bourne

New York State Agricultural Experiment Station, and Institute of Food Science, Cornell University, Geneva, New York 14456

INTRODUCTION

The incidence of malnutrition is widespread in the Western Hemisphere. A survey taken in 1972–1974 showed that 15% of the population of Latin America, amounting to 46 million people, have a daily food intake that provides less than the critical level of 1.2 times the Basic Metabolic Rate [FAO, 1977a].

Nutrition surveys generally show that most of the undernourished suffer from multiple nutritional deficiencies. Increasing the intake of one or two nutrients will do little to improve the state of health. What is needed is more of almost every nutrient, that is, more food. The problem is how to increase food consumption among people who may already be spending more than 50% of their income on food. The poverty–malnutrition–poor health–inability to work energetically nexus is a vicious cycle of many interconnected elements that seems almost impossible to break. This chapter will show how the reduction of food losses can be a powerful weapon in breaking the vicious cycle.

One of the tragedies of this unfortunate situation is that large quantities of good food that have already been produced are never consumed by people. These are known as food losses, and they represent a loss of valuable nutrients and money to people who are undernourished and poor.

The harvest and postharvest sectors are sometimes combined into what is known as the postproduction or postmaturity system [Bourne, 1977].

Many activities are required to convert the mature agricultural product in the field into a form suitable for human consumption and to deliver it to the bowl of the consumer on time. There are many opportunities for food to be lost in the harvest and postharvest system. It is beginning to be realized that it is a waste of effort to increase food production if the increase does not reach the stomach, where the utilization of its nutritional value begins and the pleasant feeling of satiety is induced. Food must not only be produced, it must be delivered to the ultimate consumer in an acceptable form if it is to fulfill its nutritional destiny [Bourne, 1977].

World attention was focused on the problem of food losses in September 1975 when the United Nations General Assembly passed the following resolution: "The further reduction of post harvest food losses in developing countries should be taken as a matter of priority, with a view to reaching at least a 50% reduction by 1985. All countries and competent international organizations should cooperate financially and technically in the effort to achieve this objective."

This resolution has drawn the attention of the highest levels of governments and donor organizations around the world to the problem of food losses and the potential contribution that reducing these losses can make to the improvement of the nutritional status of the poor. The resolution is realistic; it recognizes that food losses will never be reduced to zero but calls for efforts to reduce sharply the high levels of loss that presently occur.

MAGNITUDE OF LOSSES

The magnitude of losses is highly variable. Quoted data are sometimes unreliable because the amount of loss has been estimated rather than measured. Sometimes the problem is dramatized by citing "worst case" figures that only apply to a limited quantity of the crop. Nevertheless, conservative estimates indicate that more than 100 million tons of cereal grains and legumes are lost each year in developing countries [NAS, 1978]. This is sufficient to provide the minimum energy requirements of about 300 million people.

Table I shows typical loss figures for rice and legumes in several Latin American countries. Losses are higher than 10% in most countries. Similar loss figures are found for other cereal crops.

Table II shows typical percentage loss figures for a number of staple and perishable foods in Colombia, and also the actual weight loss and the dollar value of the lost food. The losses range from 5.1% for maize to 31.7% for oranges. More than 1.1 million tons of good food worth more than US$233 million is lost in Colombia each year.

Most other tropical countries in this hemisphere do not have as complete data as does Colombia. Nevertheless, the limited figures that are available from these countries indicate that their losses follow a pattern similar to that in Colombia [FPRD, 1981, IICA, 1977].

FACTORS AFFECTING LOSSES

A number of factors can cause losses or affect the rate at which they occur. The major factors are listed below.

TABLE I. Typical Food Losses in Latin America

Country	Food	Loss (%)
Belize	Rice	20–30
Belize	Legumes	20–50
Bolivia	Rice	16
Brazil	Rice	1–30
Brazil	Legumes	15–25
Costa Rica	Legumes	24
Dominican Republic	Rice	6.5
Honduras	Legumes	20–50
Nicaragua	Legumes	10–35
Paraguay	Legumes	15

Data from FAO [1977b] and NAS [1978].

TABLE II. Postharvest Losses of Major Foods in Colombia

Product	Loss Percentage of total product	Loss Weight (1,000 tons)	Loss Value[a] (US$1,000)
Bananas	15.0	120	12,000
Beans	7.3	5	6,200
Carrots	19.8	30	6,100
Cassava	9.5	198	46,300
Maize	5.1	44	13,500
Oranges	31.7	70	10,000
Pineapples	22.0	23	5,400
Plantains	9.2	206	29,900
Potatoes	12.1	250	42,700
Rice	4.6	88	35,900
Soybeans	7.0	10	3,900
Tomatoes	25.7	63	21,300
Wheat	5.2	2	400
Total		1,109	$233,200

Data from Valdes [1981] and Buckle et al [1978].
[a]Based on 1979 prices and exchange rate of US$1.00 = Col$44.00.

Harvest Problems

Rain or humid weather at harvest time makes grain vulnerable to the growth of mold. Birds and field rodents may consume a mature crop before it is harvested. Rough handling of fruits, vegetables, roots, and tubers causes bruising and breaks the skin, opening the way for invasion of the underlying tissue by rotting organisms [FAO, 1981].

Inherent Stability

Stable foods such as cereal grains can be stored in good condition for several years if handled properly. Perishable foods such as fruits and vegetables and fats and oils have an inherent shelf life of 1 week to several months under good conditions. Highly perishable foods such as raw milk, fish, meat and poultry have an inherent life of hours or a few days before they spoil and become unfit for human consumption. Perishable foods can be transformed into more stable forms by refrigeration, pasteurization, canning, freezing, dehydration, and chemical preservatives. However, these technologies increase the cost severalfold and usually raise the price beyond the purchasing power of the poor. Higher losses can be expected in perishable foods than in stable foods.

Environment

High ambient temperatures accelerate the rate of losses in foods. For example, insects grow and reproduce more quickly as the temperature increases from 15°C to 35°C. The physiologic life processes that continue in horticultural crops after harvest, and the growth of rotting organisms on these crops both occur more rapidly as the temperature rises.

Figure 1 shows the mean monthly temperature at four locations. The high ambient temperature throughout the year in Panama (27–28°C) makes it difficult to maintain the quality of food held in common storage. The lower temperature in Bogota (14–15°C) renders the problem of food storage less severe than Panama, and in Medellin (21–22°C) the extent of the problem can be expected to be intermediate between that of Bogota and Panama. From this temperature pattern it can be predicted that, other factors being equal, Panama would suffer more food losses than Medellin, and both would suffer more loss than Bogota. In contrast, Cipoletti, with its seasonal temperature variation, could be expected to suffer moderately high losses from December through February, when the temperature is above 20°C, and low losses from May through September, when the temperature is below 10°C.

Relative humidity (RH) is another environmental factor that affects losses. A low relative humidity in storage facilities minimizes the risk of damage by mold growth on cereal grains and other dry foods.

Figure 2 shows the mean monthly relative humidity at four locations. Dry foods are likely to mold if stored in an atmosphere with the relative humidity above 70%. The horizontal line drawn at 70% RH divides the relative humidity range into mold-prone and mold-free zones. Cuidad Juarez should have little problem with mold spoilage because the relative humidity is below 70% all year. San Carlos de Bariloche should have little problem with mold from October through March, when the RH is below 70%, and some mold problem from April through September, when the RH is above 70%. Paramaribo can be expected to have mold problems all year long, because the RH is always

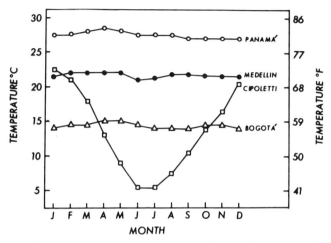

Fig. 1.   Mean monthly temperature in Bogota, Cipoletti, Medellin, and Panama.

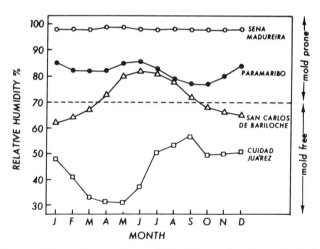

Fig. 2.   Mean monthly relative humidity in Cuidad Juarez, San Carlos de Bariloche, Paramaribo, and Sena Madureira. Mold growth is likely to occur when the relative humidity surrounding the food is above 70%.

above 70%. Sena Madureira, with its RH of 98% can be expected to have very severe problems with mold spoilage throughout the year.

Sanitation

The amount of consumption and damage to stored food by insects, rodents, and microbes depends on the size of the pest population. These pests increase exponentially. A high initial infestation of these pests in stored food increases losses. Sanitation and good housekeeping can aid by keeping the initial population size down and so decrease losses. This is done primarily by denying shelter to rodents where they can nest and breed, eliminating places where insects can hide, keeping new grain separated from old grain, thoroughly cleaning food stores as soon as they are empty, and promptly removing waste food material from the proximity of the store.

Time

The longer food is stored the greater opportunity there is for every kind of loss to occur. For example, losses caused by insects in properly dried grain are generally low for the first few months after harvest but become higher after 5–6 months of storage and may be very high shortly before the next harvest season.

FOOD LOSS CONTROL

Table III summarizes the methods of control for each cause of loss in each class of food.

The next major task is to reduce the well-known sciences of food preservation to technologies that are cost-effective, simple and safe to use, and appropriate to local conditions. The science of food preservation is universal, but the technology for applying it must be site-specific. Recommendations for improved technologies are based sometimes on practices in developed countries that often do not work well in another location, where climatic conditions, marketing practices, and availability and cost of equipment, services, and labor are different.

IMPLICATIONS FOR NUTRITION

In isolated villages that depend upon one annual crop, the food in the store is often exhausted before the next harvest season. This period of food shortage, known as the "hungry season" coincides with the period of high energy need for land preparation and planting. Reduction of food losses could help overcome seasonal food shortages by extending the stored food supply to the next harvest. In addition, the farmer would no longer need to buy expensive food brought into the village nor go into debt at high interest rates to buy food.

All food has monetary value. Stored food is the major asset of most subsistence farmers; it is their equivalent of money in the bank. Losses in stored food are serious economic losses. Thus, reduction of food losses can improve both the nutritional and economic status of a subsistence farm family.

TABLE III. Causes of Loss and Control of Loss in Foods

Commodity	Major causes of loss	Methods for reducing loss
Grains, cereal legumes	Fungi	Adequate drying, prompt drying, dry stores
	Insects	Good sanitation, use of insecticides and fumigants, gas-tight stores
	Rodents	Good housekeeping, rodent-proof stores, baits, traps, fumigation
	Inefficient handling and processing	Better equipment, maintenance of equipment, knowledgeable management
Fruits and vegetables	Bruising	Gentle harvesting and handling, protective packaging to maintain intact skin
	Rotting by bacteria and fungi	Good sanitation, cool storage, use of fungicides
	Senescence	Cool storage, prompt marketing, processing into stable forms
	Wilting	Maintenance of high-humidity surroundings
Roots and tubers	Rotting by bacteria and fungi	Maintenance of intact skin, promotion of suberization and wound cork formation, good sanitation, cool storage, application of fungicides
	Sprouting	Cool storage, application of anti-sprout agents
	Bruising	Gentle harvesting and handling, protective packaging
	Senescence	Prompt marketing, cool storage, processing into stable forms
	Insects	Good sanitation, use of insecticides
Fresh fish, meat, poultry, milk	Bacterial spoilage	Refrigeration, good sanitation, pasteurization, processing into stable forms
Dry fish	Insects	Good sanitation, use of insecticides
	Fungi	Adequate drying, prompt drying

From Bourne [1981], with permission.

The general trend in price that occurs as food moves from the producer to the consumer is shown schematically in Figure 3. Part of the cost in the price trend is the cost of losses of food. If these losses could be reduced, the possibility exists of lowering the price to the consumer without lowering the price paid to the farmer or reducing the margins charged by the middleman. Without losses, the consumer has the potential for buying more food for the same amount of money.

Although one cannot predict just who will gain how much in this situation without empirical within-country research, it is clear that there should be gains to producers, middlemen, or consumers, or all three. The only losers would be

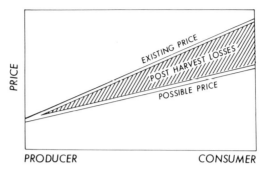

Fig. 3. Simple schematic representation of the general trend in price of food as it moves to the consumer, and the potential savings that can accrue from reducing food losses. From UNEP [1983], with permission.

the "stealthy thieves," the rodents, insects, and microbes that spoil our food. Figure 3 is a simple model of the potential savings that can come from the reduction of postharvest losses. It needs to be pointed out that human nature and economic forces being what they are, this picture will not always hold. Nevertheless, the potential for savings throughout all sectors of the economy does exist, including the possibility for providing more food for the same cost to the poor. This is why reduction of food losses can be a powerful weapon in breaking the poverty–malnutrition–poor health cycle.

IMPLEMENTATION PROBLEMS

Most countries that have a food loss program started it in response to the 1975 UN resolution and spent the first few years organizing and funding activities, assembling trained personnel, and gathering loss data on the foods important to their country. Many countries are still in this phase. Some countries have not yet begun.

Some major problems are the following:

1. Lack of reliable data on magnitude of losses, causes of losses, and economic aspects for loss reduction programs specific for each country or region.

2. Shortage of financial resources for building good storage structures and for efficient equipment for food-processing operations such as milling cereals.

3. Shortage of people with training in the care and storage of foods, and shortage of good instructional materials.

4. The need for site-specific adaptive research to develop improved technology that is compatible with other segments of the food storage and distribution system, is cost-effective, and uses inputs that are readily available. The

subsistence farmer in a developing country usually follows close to optimal procedures to preserve his food supply, given the constraints and limited resources available to him. It takes time to develop new technology that is really effective. It takes more time to teach people how to use the new technology and get them to accept it.

The focus of interest on food loss reduction is less than 10 years old. It is too soon to make a judgment about the effectiveness of programs that are still in the development stage. We know that high losses can be reduced, and we expect both the nutritional and economic status of the poor to improve as greater attention is given to caring for food after it has been produced.

REFERENCES

Bourne MC (1977): "Post Harvest Food Losses – The Neglected Dimension in Increasing the World Food Supply." International Agriculture Monograph No. 53. Ithaca, New York: Cornell University.

Bourne MC (1981): The world problem of post harvest food losses. Industry Environ 4(1):3-5.

Buckle TS, Silva MC, Mendoza LC, Zapata LE (1978): "Estudio Preliminar de Algunos Casos de Perdidas de Alimentos Post-Cosecha en Colombia." Anales del Tercero Seminario Avanzado de Technologia de Alimentos. Bogota: Ministerio de Agricultura.

FAO (1977a): "The Fourth World Food Survey." Food and Nutrition Series No. 10. Rome: Food and Agriculture Organization.

FAO (1977b): "Analysis of an FAO Survey of Post Harvest Losses in Developing Countries." AGPP Misc./27. Rome: Food and Agriculture Organization.

FAO (1981): "Food Loss Prevention in Perishable Crops." Agricultural Services Bulletin No. 43. Rome: Food and Agriculture Organization.

FPRD (1981): "Report of Post Harvest Losses Consultative Meeting Caribbean" (2 vols). London: Food Production and Rural Development Division, Commonwealth Secretariat.

IICA (1977): "Proceedings of a Seminar on Reduction of Post Harvest Food Losses of Agricultural Products in the Caribbean and Central America" (5 vols). Santo Domingo, Dominican Republic: Inter-American Institute for Cooperation in Agriculture.

NAS (1978): "Post Harvest Food Losses in Developing Countries." Washington, CD: US National Academy of Sciences.

UNEP (1983): "Guidelines for Post Harvest Food Loss Reduction Activities." United Nations Environment Programme. Paris: Industry and Environment Programme.

Valdes H (1981): An attempt to evaluate post harvest losses in Colombia. Industry Environ 4(1): 19-21.

Malnutrition: Determinants and Consequences, pages 337–345
© *1984 Alan R. Liss, Inc., 150 Fifth Avenue, New York, NY 10011*

Decisions About Agricultural Uses of Land

Sylvan H. Wittwer, PhD

Agricultural Experiment Station and Department of Horticulture, College of Agriculture and Natural Resources, Michigan State University, East Lansing, Michigan 48824

INTRODUCTION

The topic of decision making in regard to the agricultural uses of land in the United States and elsewhere is unusually timely. Today in the summer of 1983, farmers and governments in much of the Western Hemisphere are plagued with unprecedented overproduction, surpluses, and low food prices. In the United States years of bumper crops have produced a nationwide surplus of 5 billion bushels of corn and wheat. With this as a background US farmers, responding to the Payment in Kind (PIK) program, have idled an estimated 83 million acres or almost one-fourth the cultivated land area. We have less land devoted to crop production than at any time during the past 75 years [Batie and Healy, 1983].

The sixfold to sevenfold growth in agricultural output of the United States during the past century has been accomplished without a consistent increase in land devoted to food, feed, and fiber production (Fig. 1).

This massive land diversion (retirement) program is unparalleled in history. If coupled with adverse spring weather and delayed plantings and a summer drought, it could within one season spell near disaster and result in a complete reversal of food supplies, surplus, and prices. Today over a hundred nations rely on North American grain [Brown, 1981]. The uncertainties of weather and climate still constitute the first determinant and most unpredictable factor in the stability of food production and the output of our land resources.

Agricultural land use has always been dynamic. Uses change in response to prices, domestic and international markets, the vicissitudes of climate, and land-owner preferences [NAS, 1982]. Governmental policies resulting in expo-

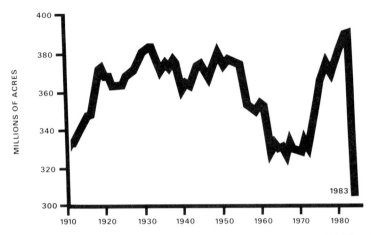

Fig. 1.   Cropland in the United States in actual production from 1910 to 1983. There is no consistent trend. Peaks were reached in the early 1930s, the 1950s, and again in 1981 and 1982. The Payment in Kind (PIK) program for 1983 has resulted in the lowest level in 73 years. Data derived from the US Department of Agriculture.

nential increases in agricultural exports have dramatically affected land use during the past decade. A remarkable transition from mixed crop-livestock systems to cash-cropping has occurred in US agriculture and in other Western Hemisphere countries (Canada, Argentina, Brazil) during the past two decades. The precipitous rise in the production of corn, soybeans, wheat, and sorghum has exacerbated problems of soil erosion, sedimentation, and runoff. One estimate of soil erosion in the US corn belt is that two bushels of topsoil are lost for each bushel of corn harvested. It is further reported that 90% of the land used for row crops and small grains in the United States is largely untouched by soil conservation practices and that erosion today is worse than it was during the dust bowl of the 1930s. Environmental policies also affect agricultural output and are leading to greater diversification and more intensive land use. The extensive land areas set aside from cropping in 1983 provide an unprecedented opportunity for US farmers, and those in other Western Hemisphere nations, to plant soil-improving cover crops and thus reduce soil erosion, water runoff, and sedimentation.

Land use decisions have been and continue to be serious constraints for agriculture. It is reported that over 2 million acres of prime agricultural land in the United States are taken out of production each year [NAS, 1982]. Irreversible land use and soil erosion have resulted in the permanent removal of land from crop production [CAST, 1982; Eckholm, 1976; Larson et al, 1983; Schultz, 1982]. Furthermore, it is generally accepted that increases of 10–15% in crop land in addition to substantial increases in the productivity of currently farmed land will be required to support the expected world population increase and its demands by the year 2030 [Johnson and Wittwer, 1983].

LAND AS A RESOURCE

Land as a resource for food production comes first. Paramount in importance to future global habitability is the productivity of the land. It is the land that makes the predominant contributions to food and fiber production and other renewable resources. As far as food is concerned most calories and 95% of the protein consumed by people are derived from the land. The 20 crops that stand between humankind and starvation are products of the soil [Wittwer, 1981].

Dependable production is just as important as the magnitude of output. More stable yields of crops that provide directly or indirectly over 95% of the food people consume should be the most sought-after goal of humanity. Production uncertainty — prompted by uncertainties of climate and pestilence — is coupled with market instabilities. During the 1970s, world food production went through one full cycle — from surplus to shortage and back to surplus. Two phenomena — total agricultural output and dependability of production, both primarily crop-dependent and land-dependent — are critical to the future of all people of the earth.

Accurate assessment of land resources leaves much to be desired [NASA, 1983]. The ability to classify and quantify accurately changes in land use either by ground observations or from satellites needs dramatic improvement. The widely quoted figure of 2 million acres of prime agricultural land in the United States being annually taken out of production is likely in error by over 50%. Global estimates for clearing of closed canopy forests range from 7 to 30 million acres per year. Deforestation may be twice some of the current estimates. Important for tomorrow's agriculture will be the monitoring, through advanced remote sensing techniques, of changes in land cover and characteristics of water and energy and in mineral resources and reserves, and the biogeochemical cycles of the atmosphere, the land, and the water that affect life-supporting systems.

Land use is undergoing constant change. Between 1967 and 1975, 66 million acres of cropland in the United States was converted to other uses; at the same time over 40 million acres in other uses was converted to cropland [NAS, 1982].

Many factors are diverting prime agricultural land to other uses [Batie and Healy, 1983]. Industry competes for farmland both in acres and a labor force withdrawn from farms. Federal highway programs coupled with urban and industrial development are taking their toll. Massive water reclamation projects, while increasing in some instances irrigated agriculture, have flooded other vast areas of cropland and made some adjacent areas useless for farming. Residential developments of rural areas is resulting in irreversible use of much prime agricultural land.

Finally, cropland may be increasingly claimed for the production of energy, in realms ranging from coal mining to the production of fuels from crops or their residues [Brown, 1980; Hodgson, 1980]. The potential for dramatic increases in the productivity of forest lands and demand for forest products [Bingham, 1980; Johnson and Wittwer, 1983] will place additional constraints on decisions for agricultural uses of land.

CURRENT STATUS AND PROJECTIONS

One may summarize land resource issues for the Western Hemisphere as follows. Soil erosion continues unabated globally. After 45 years of a soil conservation program and expenditures of $16–18 billions, no more than 25–35% of the US farmlands are under approved conservation practices. Topsoil continues to be lost at an enormous rate. This soil pollutes lakes, streams, and estuaries and vokes additional regulatory actions. The situation, coupled with deforestation, is even worse in many tropical countries [Eckholm, 1976]. Annual losses of topsoil in US agricultural areas will vary. For the Palouse region in the Pacific Northwest, the loss ranges from 50 to 100 tons per acre per year. For the Blacklands of Texas, the loss is 10–20 tons. Many cornbelt states average 10 tons. In many areas, topsoil is being lost to erosion by wind and water faster than it is being formed [Wittwer, 1982]. Soil organic matter is being reduced. Rapid subsidence of organic soils (peat, muck) is occurring. There is increasing compaction from excess and untimely tillage. Air pollution is becoming more severe. The subtle effects of acid rainfall (a product of air pollutants) on the productivity of land is now under surveillance. Additional land areas brought into cultivation may be less productive. With increasing pressure on the productive land resource base, the options for use of water, fertilizer, energy, pesticides, and mechanization become progressively fewer.

Projections for the future will see greater reliance placed on increasing yield technology, using land not presently farmed, and exploitation of potentials for more intensive cropping combinations. Projections indicate needs for yield-increasing technologies and technologies that permit additional and, perhaps, more fragile soils to be farmed and more intensive mixtures of crops to be grown on the land farmed.

Two general types of food production technologies characterize present world agriculture. One is highly mechanized, and land-, water-, and energy-intensive. The other is more biologically based and scientifically oriented and is more sparing of land, energy, and water resources. The first characterizes much of the current US agricultural production system and results in output per farmworker that is the highest in the world. Similar systems exist or are emerging in Canada, Australia, New Zealand, Brazil, and Argentina.

The second type of technology is not as productive per farmworker but yields more per unit land area, often with a higher cropping index. This system characterizes the current Japanese, Taiwanese, Western European, and Chinese systems. Because of resource constraints — cost and availability — an inevitable shift will occur in the US and worldwide agricultural systems from less of a resource- or land-based to a more scientifically and biologically based agriculture. Our world is moving from a demand-driven economy with perceived unlimited resources to a resource-limited economy. In fact, we currently see a transformation in US agriculture from a resource-based to a science-oriented industry; and from a traditional to a high-technology sector [Wittwer, 1983].

SOIL CONSERVATION AND LAND IMPROVEMENT

The land resource base can change with time and technology. Land productivity may be improved or depleted by time and by cropping. Most existing cultivated land is different from what it was in the virgin state. The original croplands of Western Europe and Japan were vastly inferior to what they are today. This is reflected by current wheat yields in Western Europe and rice yields in Japan, which are double those in the United States. Use of lime, chemical fertilizers, animal manure, green manure, and better farming practices has transformed the sandy soils of the Eastern seaboard of the United States and much of Florida into some of the most productive vegetable-growing soils in the world. The acid peat soils of Michigan and the Great Lakes area were of little agricultural value until the introduction of soil-adapted, superior strains of blueberries. These soils now support a thriving multimillion dollar industry. Bringing new land into production may be costly but not prohibitive. The challenge for the future will be to improve, optimize the use of, and preserve and protect the existing land resources.

Conservation (or reduced) tillage, usually in the absence of plowing, is an important emerging land resource conservation technology. It is a method whereby seedbed preparation and planting are completed in the same operation. It will become increasingly important in the decades ahead [Successful Farming, 1982]. Conservation tillage was used on an estimated 94 million acres of cropland in the United States in 1982. The figure represents almost a third of US cropland for 1983. This is up from 30 million acres in 1972 and from scarcely more than 2 million acres in 1962. The area in conservation tillage is expanding at the rate of 3–4 million acres a year. It is projected that 150 million acres, or half of the US cropland, will be under conservation tillage systems by the year 2000.

Conservation tillage is the most significant technology yet developed for producing crops and simultaneously controlling soil erosion [Phillip et al, 1980]. Reduced tillage can maximize the crop residue cover on the land and conserve energy, labor, water, soil, fertilizer, and organic matter in the main food-producing areas of the United States. In addition, land with steeper and longer slopes can be brought into production or planted to more profitable crops.

Successful conservation tillage requires two important inputs: first, an appropriate herbicide or mulches of plant residues that inhibit weed growth; and second, specially adapted seed drills to penetrate plant residues and operate on the more variable soil surfaces. Plunge-type planters versus the drill row are now under study.

The development and release of appropriate chemicals for killing grass and controlling weeds will continually affect the development or speed with which conservation tillage is adopted and the impact that technology will have on US land use and food production. Surface mulches associated with conservation tillage may also harbor insects, disease organisms, and rodents that can destroy the mulch and the crops. There is the potential, however, for bringing into food production tens of millions of additional acres of land heretofore not suitable for agricultural purposes and for reducing soil erosion to essentially zero on land that is now cultivated. The challenge for the future with conservation tillage will be the identification of mulches and plant residues with allelopathic properties to reduce and eventually eliminate the use of herbicides and to consider options in terms of living mulches [Putnam, 1983].

There are several types of conservation tillage. One that is receiving increasing attention is the use of a living mulch for a cover crop that is grown in the same field and at the same time as the main crop. This is in contrast to the usual procedure of leaving dead plant residues on the surface of the soil. The living mulch is designed to control soil erosion before the crop is seeded as well as after it is harvested. It functions also as a mulch in reducing weed development and in maintaining soil moisture. If a legume is used it could add substantially to the soil nitrogen level by biologic fixation. A living mulch can effectively serve in weed control if its effect on the crop is less than the combined effects of the living mulch on the weeds and on the crop. As to the availability of water, the living mulch requires water for its own growth but a reduction in tillage may lead to increased soil moisture.

Till planting on ridges is another innovative approach for conservation tillage [Robertson and Erickson, 1983]. Here the residues from the previous crop are concentrated in the valleys, and the seed is planted on the ridges, which are drier and warmer and relatively free of plant residues. This facilitates drilling of the seed and reduces the liability of soil compaction in the furrows or valleys.

With a technology such as conservation tillage, an increase in yield may be the primary objective, but an alternative perspective is that the same yields might be obtained with a reduction in inputs that are costly, both economically and ecologically. History has demonstrated that soil conservation practices must be economically attractive to be accepted by farmers.

ALTERNATIVE USES OF LAND

A crucial issue for the future is alternative agricultural uses of land. Currently there is no worldwide shortage of food. There is more food per person today on the earth than ever before. Many nations are overflowing with surplus rice, wheat, corn, and dairy products. The problems are delivery, purchasing power, and poor people [Johnson, 1982]. Here there is an obvious need to revitalize human nutrition research and review agricultural-food-human interfaces.

It has also been a tradition of many developing nations to devote extensive land areas to plantation crops (cotton, rubber, tea, coffee, sugar cane, tobacco, hemp, jute) to be grown for export and for achieving a favorable balance of trade at the expense of the production of nutritious cereal grains, legumes, and vegetables. Crops for biomass and those to be used for the extraction of alcohol as a fuel for motorized vehicles will compete with the use of land for the production of food crops. These options remain viable alternatives for nations endowed with vast land resources but no oil. Diverting agricultural lands into biomass production will become increasingly possible since projections will rely on new biotechnologies rather than more land to meet food needs.

WATER VERSUS LAND RESOURCES

The ultimate agricultural productivity of many land resources will be dependent upon water management [Jensen, 1982]. This means irrigation for arid and semiarid lands and supplemental irrigation and drainage in humid and subhumid regions. Soil moisture in the spring is the most determinant factor for agricultural productivity in the US corn and wheat belts, and July rainfall is the most important variable. Currently there is an overdraft of approximately 20–25 million acre-feet of ground water, mostly for crop irrigation in the United States. This will not only impact on future agricultural productivity but is causing land subsidence seriously affecting human habitation in many parts of the Western Hemisphere. Water resources cannot be separated from land resources in irrigated agriculture. Arid land without water is of no value for crop production. Future decisions with respect to water will have an increasingly greater impact on land use as the price of water increases [Resources for the Future, 1982]. Meanwhile, drought is the climatic hazard that farmers fear most. It greatly disrupts world food supplies and projections. Yet there are many technologies, some old and some new, for alleviation of drought and reduction of water losses from irrigation.

PHYSICAL CONSTRAINTS ON THE USE OF LAND

Soil problems (salinity, alkalinity, aluminum toxicity) constitute one of the most serious constraints on the future capabilities of land for food production. More than 3.8 million square miles of soil are too salty to grow crops in the world today. An equal land area is unproductive because of aluminum toxicity or calcium deficiency. Acid rainfall, it appears, may exacerbate the aluminum toxicity problem.

CONCLUSIONS

Many existent and emerging global and regional problems that must be resolved relate to agricultural land use and soil resources and accurate inventories of change. These include deforestation and desertification, soil erosion, loss of top soil and soil organic matter, land subsidence, overdrafts of groundwater reserves for irrigation, sedimentation and silting of rivers, lakes, and estuaries, destruction of fish and wildlife habitats, salinization and alkalinity, toxic substances in the environment and acid rainfall, and finally possible large-scale diversion from food crops to biomass production as a renewable energy resource.

The above issues will become increasingly important as to the future magnitude, stability, and safety of our food resources, more food security, and improved human nutrition [NAS, 1977]. Can we, in view of these erosions of our soil resources, increase food production at the rate of the projected necessary 4–5% per year to meet the demands of an ever increasing number of people and affluent population and at the same time establish resource-sparing technologies, create alternative production and marketing strategies, and maintain an acceptable environment? These are noble challenges for the development of new and appropriate technologies, and will in large part depend on future policy decisions relating to agricultural land use.

REFERENCES

Batie SS, Healy RG (1983): The future of American agriculture. Sci Am 248(2):45–53.

Bingham CW (1980): Forest plantations in the 21st century. Weyerhaeuser company's needs and expectations. In "Forest Plantation, the Shape of the Future." A Weyerhaeuser Science Symposium. Tacoma, WA.

Brown LR (1980): "Food or Fuel: New Competition for the World's Cropland." Worldwatch Paper 35. Washington, DC: Worldwatch Institute.

Brown LR (1981): World population growth, soil erosion, and food security. Science 214:995–1002.

CAST (1982): Soil Erosion: Its Agricultural, Environmental, and Socio-economic Implications." Report 92. Ames, IA: Council for Agricultural Science and Technology.

Eckholm EP (1976): "Losing Ground." New York: WW Norton Co.

Hodgson HJ (1980): Crops for Fuel – A Look to the Future. Paper presented in a symposium "Fuel from Crops." Detroit, MI: American Society of Agronomy Annual Meetings.

Jensen ME (1982): Water Resource Technology and Management. Paper presented at the RCA Symposium, Washington, DC.

Johnson DG (1982): The world's poor: Can they hope for a better future? In "Perspective, '83. The World Food Situation." Northbrook, IL: International Minerals and Chemical Corporation, pp 8–15.

Johnson GL, Wittwer SH (1984): Perspectives on the role of technology in determining future supplies of food, fiber, and forest products in the U.S. Michigan Agricultural Experiment Station Research Report (in press).

Larson WE, Pierce FJ, Dowdy RH (1983): The threat of soil erosion to long-term crop production. Science 219:458–465.

NAS (1977): "World Food and Nutrition Study. The Potential Contributions of Research." Washington, DC: National Academy of Sciences.

NAS (1982): "Impacts of Emerging Agricultural Trends on Fish and Wildlife Habitats." Washington, DC: National Academy of Sciences.

NASA (1983): "Land Related Global Habitability Research Program." Washington, DC: National Aeronautics and Space Administration.

Phillip RE, Blevins RL, Thomas GW, Frye WW, Phillips SH (1980): No-tillage agriculture. Science 208:1108–1113.

Putnam AR (1983): Allelopathic chemicals, nature's herbicides in action. Chem Eng News 61(14):34–45.

Resources for the Future (1982): Water for western agriculture. Resources for the Future, Washington, DC.

Robertson LS, Erickson AE (1983): "Till Planting on Ridges." Michigan Cooperative Extension Bulletin E. 1683. East Lansing, MI.

Schultz TW (1982): The Dynamics of Soil Erosion in the United States. Agricultural Economics Paper 82:8, University of Chicago. Washington, DC: Agricultural Council for America.

Successful Farming (1982): "Conservation Tillage Guide." Successful Farming, Des Moines, IA.

Wittwer SH (1981): The 20 crops that stand between man and starvation. Farm Chem 144(9): 16, 18, 23, 26, 28.

Wittwer SH (1982): New technology, agricultural productivity and conservation. In Halerow HC, Heady EO, Cortner ML (eds): Anbury, IA: Soil Science Society of America, pp 201–215.

Wittwer SH (1983): The new agriculture – A view from the twenty-first century. In Rosenblom JW (ed): Agriculture in the Twenty-first Century, Proceedings of a symposium sponsored by Philip Morris, Inc., April 11–13, pages 337–367, New York: John Wiley and Sons.

Malnutrition: Determinants and Consequences, pages 347–354
© 1984 Alan R. Liss, Inc., 150 Fifth Avenue, New York, NY 10011

Improving International Transfer of Technology

Anthony Wylie, PhD

Department of Food Technology, Fundación Chile, Santiago, Chile

Technology transfer is of great importance to both developed and developing countries. At stake is the formation of jobs, increases in productivity, production of appropriate goods and services, changes in health and nutrition, and what can in general terms be referred to as the process of improvement of living conditions.

Numerous definitions of technology can be found in the literature but perhaps the simplest of these is that it is knowledge (or know-how). In a more complete sense, especially as related to productive activities, technology is the knowledge necessary for the productive functioning of an enterprise. As such it is ever changing and complex, and according to Driscoll and Wallender [1974] it encompasses fields such as process engineering, management, marketing, and production know-how.

The transfer of technology is the process whereby the supplier of a particular technology is linked to its user. As such it occurs when technology is transmitted, received, and applied. This process is of constant occurrence in all spheres of industrial and agricultural production within a country, between research development centers and production facilities, between universities and industry, and also between countries. In this respect it is important to stress that although technology transfer is not limited to the relationship between developed and less developed countries, this chapter will focus on the process as it occurs in this context and will consider certain ways in which the efficiency of transfer mechanisms can be increased.

Perhaps one of the most complex aspects of the technology transfer process is that it necessarily involves a change in one or another aspect of the receiver's behavior. A thorough awareness and understanding of this is an essential component of any successful program in this field, especially as, in international exchanges, technological innovation usually implies changes in cultural patterns. This will be discussed in greater detail when certain means of accelerating the transfer process are considered. However, it should be remembered that changing a system is generally slow and tedious. Change will not occur overnight and the passage of long periods of time may be necessary for acceptance to take place. This indeed happens even in the most technologically advanced countries, where the period between the creation of scientific knowledge and its incorporation in technological developments has been estimated as 20 years or more on the average [Allen, 1982]. Of equal importance is the point made by Critchfield [1982] that the speed with which change can be absorbed varies substantially from one culture to another.

One aspect of the technology transfer process that has a significant impact on its success is the "appropriateness" of the technology being transferred to the real needs of the recipient, be this a country or a specific industry. Numerous programs for technology transfer with both international agency and individual country funding have been established over the last two decades as part of the increasing political pressures calling for a new international economic order. Many of these efforts have not been as successful as could have been expected because, as has been pointed out [Shaw et al, 1982; Critchfield, 1982], they have attempted to transplant technology without considering the particular cultural setting into which it's introduction is being attempted. The ideal situation in this respect would seem to be that each user should choose the technologies, bearing in mind their suitability to specific market, economic, and cultural requirements.

If the use of technology is to be increased, one of the basic requisites is to reach a thorough understanding of the various aspects of the process. These, as can be appreciated from the foregoing brief discussion, are numerous and complex, and undoubtedly the method that will be most effective in increasing the use of technology in each particular case will depend primarily on the objective that is being sought, the time in which the process is to take place, and the availability of funds and of trained personnel.

The main participants in the technology transfer process are generally considered to be the supplier and the receiver of information and know-how. It seems, however, that a third category, the transferring agent, should be included in this denomination, as the institutions or individuals that carry out this function may often serve as catalysts in the overall process. Wallender [1979] also considers the environments of both the supplier and the recipient of the technology as agents in this process, and their influence can by no means be disregarded.

In general terms, the technology transfer process involves the interlocking actions of diverse organizations, institutions, and people [Ettlie, 1983]. Traditionally all major efforts in this field can be grouped into two major categories as far as the actors are concerned, and these are the government-to-government (or institutional) programs, and the work conducted in developing countries by multinational corporations. The government-to-government projects have often involved the formation of technology centers in the developing country and have operated on the premise that direct government control over the importation and diffusion of technology is the most effective method of improving technology flows into these countries. Many of these programs have been financed and supported by international agencies and have had significant impact in certain cases, especially when the technologies being transferred have been clearly defined previously by the recipient country, so that they fit its overall socioeconomic environment. Often, however, these projects have not optimized the use of the resources assigned to them either because these considerations were not contemplated or because the link between the institution acting as the local counterpart and the actual users of the technology in the recipient country has been weak.

The role and effectiveness of the multinational corporations in the technology transfer process has been the subject of extensive reviews and debate and will not be considered at this time, except to mention that many of the constraints on and impediments to the technology transfer process that will be outlined below affect these efforts in similar ways.

It is important to keep in mind that regardless of the exact nature of any technology transfer process and of the actors involved in it, there are certain constraints that either limit its possibilities of success or unnecessarily lengthen the time required for the transfer to take place. Some of the impediments to this process are government regulations, inadequate funding, lack of trained recipients, inappropriate technology and inadequate diagnosis, lack of managerial capacity, badly defined goals, underestimation of cultural differences, and cost.

Government-to-government transfer of technology presupposes that national development goals have been established, and although this is not always the case, this tends to predetermine the nature of the technology supplier. By the same token, when a multinational corporation is involved it stands to reason that it will be the supplier of technology. In both of the above cases the needs of the actual end-users of the technology are not necessarily taken into account and the overall process may be deficient. This missing linkage can, and probably should, be filled by what has been termed a transferring agent. The agent usually is independent of both the supplier and the user of the technology required, can detect and adapt technological needs, and is equipped to search for and incorporate the most adequate technology supplier into the process. These agents are best suited for tailoring technological suppliers to users' needs by considering the resources available in consulting firms, university extension services, equipment suppliers, private volunteer organizations, and other important sources of technology.

Fundación Chile, located in Santiago, is an institution whose role is precisely that of the transferring agent indicated above. Created in 1976 as a cooperative project jointly funded by the government of Chile and the International Telephone and Telegraph Corporation (ITT), Fundacion's objective is to adapt and transfer technologies developed in Chile itself or in other countries to the needs of the local productive sector. Its main fields of action are in agriculture, marine resources, food processing, forestry, and electronics. Although it is a nonprofit organization, direct cost recovery is encouraged wherever possible in the projects undertaken. Its experience is unique, and some examples will be used to illustrate actual experience in techniques used for increasing the uses of technology.

Once a technological need has been identified, the most challenging aspect of the entire process is yet to be faced, and that is the actual introduction and implementation of a particular technology. The more general constraints on this process have been mentioned, but experience at Fundación Chile suggests that the most significant ones under conditions existing in Chile over the last 5 years are those listed in Table I. Also listed in this table are the strategies that have proven most successful in overcoming some of these impediments. It is noteworthy that of all the constraints listed in Table I, most are in areas that are not usually considered "technological." This emphasizes the need for an integrated approach, with significant roles for disciplines such as marketing and overall management, if technology transfer is to be increased. The costs involved in technology transfer are difficult to predict and the risk is high that even under proper control these may exceed the range of estimates. Awareness of this is essential at all levels, since if not considered, this factor becomes a major barrier to the process [Gartner and Naiman, 1978].

Some of the techniques used at Fundación in attempting to increase the use of technology and comments as to their usefulness are outlined below.

CONSULTANTS

One of the major tasks facing an institution whose mission is the transfer of technology is the identification of technological needs. The use of short-term consultants, preferably from industries in developed countries, for diagnostic visits has proven especially useful in meeting this requirement. When these visits have not been preceded by careful screening by local specialists of the opportunities, needs, and problem areas of the particular field being considered, their usefulness declines notoriously. The need for local counterparts to visiting specialists and their fundamental role in the process has been mentioned above and by other authors [Allen, 1982; Wallender, 1979], and experience in Fundación Chile clearly substantiates this point.

The results of various projects in which both short- and long-term consultants have been used coincide most clearly with Allen's appreciation [1982] of

TABLE I. Some of the Major Constraints on Technology Transfer Detected at Fundación Chile and the Strategies Implemented to Overcome Them

Constraints	Strategies
Lack of information	Link to technical base consultants
Financial difficulties of user	Managerial assistance
Uncertain market prospects	Product development
Scarce international marketing information	Market studies
Limited local market	Marketing and merchandising techniques
Cost of process	
User attitude	

the fact that technological problems are difficult to grasp completely without a thorough understanding of the local context. Consultants are of little value until they fully understand the local environment, and it is here where the local counterpart plays such an important role. Fundación Chile had 105 foreign consultants visit Chile and participate in its projects during 1981 and 1982. The average length of time these experts spent in Chile was one working week, and excellent results were obtained thanks to two principal factors. One is the fact that with local counterparts participating in the process, maximum use was made of the consultants' time, and their efforts were directed at key problems. The other significant factor is Fundación's capacity to locate the consultant that matches a project's or a client's needs. This is undoubtedly one of the major roles that a linking or transferring agent must play.

TECHNICAL ASSISTANCE

As used here, the term "technical assistance" means programs that try to solve industry's problems by means of supplying information, by troubleshooting problems, and by suggesting technological innovations and improvements. The comparison of two approaches to technical assistance as a vehicle for technology transfer used at Fundación Chile sheds some interesting light on this subject. In one of these instances (Case A) an industrywide (canning industry) focus was used, common services and information being offered to all parties involved in the program. The other (Case B) involved a direct approach to individual processors (cheese producers), specific work programs being designed for each of them independently. A comparison of some parameters involved in these cases is shown in Table II. As could be expected, when a program involves resource committment by the user a greater effort is needed to convince the producer to risk technological change. However, once committed to a program tailor-made for his particular industry, the technology user becomes more receptive, which makes the transfer process quicker and complete. The key elements in increasing the use of technology as suggested by

TABLE II. Comparison of Two Approaches to Technical Assistance to the
Food-Processing Industry

Activity	Case A (industrywide)	Case B (individual processor)
Time spent per user:		
Convincing industry to join	Short	Medium
Generating overall information	4 days/month	Limited
Specific problem solving	1/4 day/month	2-3 days/month
General effect on:		
Overall information level	Good	Limited
Product quality	Negligible	Significant
Industrial yield	Negligible	Excellent
Industrial sanitation	Good	Good
Product sales	Negligible	Good
Cost of project:		
Overall	High	Medium
To user	Low	High
User attitudes — willingness to:		
Implement changes	Negligible	Good
Pay for services	Poor	Acceptable-good
Trust in specialist	Medium	Good

this example are that the changes introduced have an impact on product yield, quality, and sales. Furthermore a relationship of trust was developed with the user in Case B, whereas in Case A this was more difficult.

In a more general sense what this example shows is that an approach such as the one described in Case B will have a more significant short-term effect on a productive sector than that of Case A. The long-term effect of either approach would undoubtedly be important; however, they would prove extremely costly, the prospects for recovering these costs being better in Case B. It should be pointed out that the approach used in Case A also eventually led to certain specific contracts being set up with individual industries. It would seem that this approach was less successful under present conditions in Chile than it has been elsewhere, owing probably to the fact that in a small market each industry tends toward secrecy. This difficulty is probably attributable to each participant's fear that what he disclosed would become common knowledge to others in the program.

PRODUCT DEVELOPMENT

As indicated by Stewart and James [1982], one of the most important ways in which advanced countries have changed poorer countries is through the im-

TABLE III. Product Development and Technology Transfer

Product[a]	Consumer acceptance	Investment[b] required	Implementation[c] by industry	Technology transfer
A	Good	Medium	Positive	Good
B	Good	Low	Positive	Good
C	Medium	High	Negative	Poor
D	Medium	Low	Undefined	Limited
E	Low	Low	Negative	Poor

[a]Products: A, Swiss-style yoghurt; B, beverage; C, shelf-stable fish sausage; D, processed meats; E, minced fish products.
[b]Investment required for industrial implementation.
[c]Includes payment of a royalty on sales to Fundación Chile.

pact of new products. This concept is an interesting approach to technology transfer, as product development and introduction will affect production technologies and hence unemployment and income distribution. The products developed or introduced must be adapted to local cultures, customs, and tastes and an equally important consideration is the impact their production will have on the relative usage of capital and labor.

Product development activities at Fundación Chile have concentrated on adapting and introducing products to local market and manufacturing conditions. Some of the more significant aspects (as related to technology transfer) or projects involving five different products are indicated in Table III.

As can be seen from Table III, the product development approach has been a useful means of increasing technology transfer in some but not all cases. It is interesting that, as in previous cases discussed, industry's willingness to implement change is closely linked to the consumer and market reactions to the new products. The investment required also becomes a limiting factor to the introduction of new technologies. Our experience indicates that special care must be taken in using this approach, as product development activities can be extremely costly and, unless industry's commitment is obtained early on in the process, these costs may be difficult, if not impossible, to recover.

SUMMARY AND CONCLUSIONS

Evaluation and comparison of results obtained by using different strategies in the transfer of technology are complex processes. The time frame over which this is done and results are expected is obviously an important variable, as is the measure used to quantify success.

The results of specific programs conducted by Fundación Chile stress the fact that the technology transfer process is more effective when market needs and technological opportunities are closely integrated. Applying this scheme is perhaps one of the most cost-effective and quickest ways of achieving important increases in the use of technology.

The effectiveness of technology transfer, and consequently the use of technology, is greatly enhanced by the participation of counterparts to exporting agency experts who are locally based and who have a good knowledge of the environment in which the process is occurring.

It is essential to bear in mind that there is no "good" or "bad" formula for increasing the use of technology. Perhaps the most important consideration for making technology transfer successful is the understanding of the actors involved in the process.

REFERENCES

Allen TJ (1982): Some Points Regarding Technology Transfer. Paper presented at Seminar on "The Role of Technology on a National Development Plan," held at Fundación Chile, April 1982.

Critchfield R (1982): Science and the villager: The last sleeper walks. Foreign Affairs 30:14–41, 1982.

Driscoll RE, Wallender III HW (1974): "Technology Transfer and Development: An Historical and Geographic Perspective." New York: Fund for Multinational Management Education and Council of the Americas.

Ettlie JE (1983): Organizational policy and innovation among suppliers to the food processing sector. Acad Management J 26(1):27–44.

Gertner J, Naiman CS (1978): Making technology transfer happen. Res Management 21(3): 34–38.

Shaw R, Booth RH, Rhoades R (1982): On the development of appropriate technology: A case of post harvest potatoes. Food Technol 36(2):114–118.

Stewart F, James J (eds) (1982): "The Economics of New Technology in Developing Countries." London: Francs Pinter.

Wallender III WH (1979): Technology transfer and management in the developing countries. Cambridge, Mass: Ballinger.

Malnutrition: Determinants and Consequences, pages 355–364
© 1984 Alan R. Liss, Inc., 150 Fifth Avenue, New York, NY 10011

Appropriate Technologies for Increasing Food Utilization

R.P. Bates

Food Science and Human Nutrition Department, University of Florida, Gainesville, Florida 32611

A strategy designed to overcome limitations in the quantity and quality of food and associated resources requires five distinct but highly interrelated components. These are: conservation, conversion, complementation, innovation, and implementation. Food processing and utilization entails elements of all five.

CONSERVATION

Postharvest loss prevention encompasses the major conservation strategy worldwide [Herzka, 1980]. Wasted food reflects a loss of not only critically needed nutrients but also vital, costly auxiliary inputs throughout the food chain. Furthermore, if spoiled food is consumed, serious human or animal illnesses can result.

It is estimated that 20–50% of postharvest losses are experienced in some less developed countries (LDC) [May, 1977]. When postharvest losses are combined with low production yields and preharvest losses due to environmental constraints (the vagaries of weather, poor soils, rapacious insects and pests, and persistent plant diseases), the consumable food supply that remains is often a pathetically small fraction of the total potential—a shortfall that is invariably borne by those who by nutritional and economic status can least afford it.

Postharvest food conservation occupies a high priority within the international technical assistance community [NAS, 1978]. Goals consist of 1) recovering efficiently and economically the greatest amount of edible food from a harvest, catch, or slaughter, and 2) protecting this harvest from spoilage throughout the food chain [Lindblad and Druben, 1980].

Efforts to make the most of available food resources are complicated by the perishability of foods. The tactics required to stabilize foods depend upon the type, the handling history, the intrinsic physical, chemical, and biological nature of the food, and the extrinsic interaction with the environment [Bourne, 1977; IFT, 1981; Bates, 1983]. Less developed countries can afford only the most straightforward preservation alternatives for the majority of their population, and even these techniques are severely hampered by resource limitations [Brown and Pariser, 1975]. A few of the potentially most useful methods will be presented.

Dehydration

The bulk of food staples are in the durable category. Indeed, for millenia the most practical preservation was accomplished by "letting nature take its course" in the form of sunny, dry weather at harvest time, although unseasonable rains or excessive humidity often raised havoc. The need to reduce crop moisture to about 13% (depending upon commodity) and keep the crop dry and protected from insects and pests is still a major challenge, particularly under the primitive conditions faced by the poor [LIFE, 1979].

Solar drying methods range from the simple (eg, spreading the food out during sunny days) to the elaborate (eg, mechanically ventilated drying systems) [Clark, 1976; Moody, 1980]. These involve indigenous construction materials, supplemented by industrial materials (glass, plastic sheets, screening, aluminum foil) when economically and logistically practical [Coleman et al, 1980; Doe et al, 1977; Darrow and Pam, 1981] and even indirect absorption drying [Srinivas et al, 1976].

Once the food is dry, storage facilities can be constructed from local materials such as bamboo, mud, plant fibers, ceramics, etc. Sound construction and design are necessary to protect the stored food from flooding, driving rains, and predators [Majumder, 1980; Dichter, 1980].

Since deterioration is more rapid at higher moisture contents, more extensive drying is required for semiperishables and perishables. Thus, auxiliary preservation steps, such as salting, smoking, and use of chemicals, often accompany dehydration. In these cases, the combination of salt, pH reduction, and/or smoke assist in retarding microbial growth [Labuza, 1978].

Foods of intermediate moisture content — moist enough to be eaten out of hand, yet dry enough to resist microbial growth — are a useful preservation category. Dried fruits (prunes, raisins), sugar confections, and certain cheeses are examples [Gee et al, 1977]. High concentrations of sugar, salt, or acid are the preservation agents involved. Water-activity-lowering substances such as glycerol, corn syrup, and other palatable humectants are effective, if available.

Wet Preservation

To deal with perishable foods in the moist state, methods such as thermal processing, fermentation, and chemical stabilization are applicable. The effectiveness of canning is hampered by the expense and scarcity of hermetic containers [NAS, 1974]. In the United States, home and community canning are practical operations that now rely more on reusable glass canning jars than on metal cans. Given canning jars and lids in LDCs, community canning could function as a small cottage industry or on an institutional scale [Jackson and Mehrer, 1978]. The moderate expense of a small, versatile facility is more logical in exploring and demonstrating food preservation alternatives than a "turnkey" processing plant — many of which now stand as rusting monuments to poor planning.

Fermentation is such an appropriate preservation method that there are few cultures that have not developed some type of indigenous fermentation [Beuchat, 1978; Hesseltine, 1979; Eka, 1980]. Lactic and acetic acid fermentations provide the pH-lowering effect necessary to extend shelf life [Pontecorvo and Bourne, 1978; Rao et al, 1978] or to simplify canning by reducing both process temperature and time [Worgan, 1977; Anand, 1975]. Under high-salt and anaerobic conditions the digestive enzymes of small fish reduce the flesh to a semifluid paste. While the product is salty and strongly flavored by Western standards, it is an inexpensive process that makes an important contribution to bland, high carbohydrate diets [Burkholder et al, 1968]. If cultural barriers can be overcome, similar fermentations should have potential in many LDCs. The vegetable analog of autolysis is the sprouting process, by which the enzymatic activity of viable seeds can be exploited [Fordham et al, 1975].

The preservation agent can be added to promote chemical stabilization. Wrapping cassava roots in the plant's leaves apparently decreases the rate of deterioration, presumably owing to the cyanogens present in the leaves [Aiyer et al, 1978]. The use of added acid in quick pickling; sulfur dioxide with perishables [Green, 1976]; high sugar concentration in preserves; and the many curing recipes for animal products are chemical applications. Discarded materials such as banana waste or vegetable refuse can be ready sources of acids for preservation [Adams, 1978; Bates, 1971].

There is a rather impressive inventory of preservatives available for food use in developed countries [Robach, 1980], although because of cost, availability, or safety considerations only a few are applicable to nonindustrial users in LDCs. Salt is one of the most ubiquitous chemicals and has important uses in food drying, fermentation, and curing. It is particularly valuable in the preservation of highly perishable animal products such as meat [Thomas, 1975] and fish. To overcome penetration problems, salt can be thoroughly mixed with minced fish to produce a range of stable intermediate-moisture foods [Mendelsohn, 1974].

Acid is a very useful and easily obtained preservative. When used synergistically with heat, a marked reduction in thermal-process temperature and time can be affected. Sulfur dioxide and acid can be combined to stabilize foods for reasonably long periods without the need for extensive heating [Rizvi, 1978]. Of course, chemical preservatives should be handled and applied with care and should never substitute for proper food sanitation and handling practices.

Cold preservation will receive only scant mention because of the cost and logistics associated with mechanical refrigeration in LDCs. Nevertheless, it is possible to maintain food at modest subambient temperatures by taking advantage of shade (natural or constructed), prevailing winds, and cool water or earth, and by timing harvesting and handling operations to coincide with the minimum daily temperature [Rickard and Coursey, 1979]. In arid regions with adequate water, evaporative cooling can lower the storage temperature nearly to the wet bulb [VITA, 1970]. High-temperature abuse of food is more difficult to avoid in the tropics owing to warmer heat sinks, but steps toward obtaining cool, dark, dry storage should be taken when possible.

Packaging is an essential component, since food must be protected from the environment all the way from bulk storage down to single serving containers. The cost and limited availability of hermetic containers have already been cited as serious obstacles to thermal processing. Packaging likewise limits the handling and storage associated with food preservation operations. The retort pouch is increasing in commercial importance in DCs [Mermelstein, 1978]. However, the simplicity of pouch fabrication (requiring only roll stock and an impulse sealer) is negated by the expense and sophistication of the retort system required for low-acid foods. Nevertheless, for acid foods the pouch processing system can be much simpler. Provided that the pouch stock is rugged and reasonably impermeable to oxygen, inexpensive small-scale pouch processing appears practical [Gomez et al, 1980]. The value of industrial containers — glass jars, metal cans, and plastic packaging material — to the poor in LDCs is evident by the way all sound containers are carefully salvaged and used in many household applications.

CONVERSION

The development of cooking may have been an essential response to limited food supplies that gave human access to foods hitherto toxic in the raw state [Leopold and Ardrey, 1972]. Food preparation methods stabilize foods or convert them to more valuable and convenient forms. Conversion of milk to refined dairy products, sugar cane to sugar, grains to baked products, and other staples to formulated foods, as well as most fermentations, are techniques for converting perishables to semiperishables or durables, amorphous substances to textured form, or unpalatable constituents to desirable, functional foods. The feeding of inedible crop residues, food waste, and forage to animals, thus forming meat, milk, and valuable by-products [Satterlee, 1975], exerts a significant leverage (multiplier) effect in converting low-value or even undesirable substances to important items of agriculture and commerce.

COMPLEMENTATION

Since food and resource limitations call for making the most of the least, the judicious combination of several materials in mutually complementary proportions is effective. Legumes, small quantities of animal products, leafy greens, or less conventional ingredients can significantly upgrade the nutritional value of cereal-, tuber-, and other starch-based diets [Swaminathan, 1980; Bressani and Elias, 1968]. The development of foods and feeding regimens based upon indigenous food complementation is a sound nutrition strategy in both DCs and LDCs [Rajalakshmi and Ramakrishan, 1977; Pellet and Mamarbachi, 1979].

The diverse culture-specific culinary arts attest to the importance of complementation in both nutrition and sensory appeal. Wheat flour when combined with baking ingredients, properly formulated pasta dishes, beans wrapped in a tortilla, or the typical sandwich are more nutritional and appealing meals than the separate ingredients. The use of functional foods and food ingredients to enhance the texture, flavor, appearance, storage durability, convenience, and overall commercial value is central to food technology and essential to the food industry. It is also much more applicable than appreciated in upgrading the food supply and enhancing food self-sufficiency in LDCs.

The concept of complementation promotes conservation. It implies matching raw materials, refined products, and even waste substances in order to optimize their collective usefulness.

INNOVATION

The mechanism for effectively accomplishing food and resource conservation, conversion, and complementation is innovation. Some of the best examples of innovation involve the application of well-known principles in straightforward ways. They are often deceptively simple and can consist of devices (machinery) or techniques or application of old ideas to new problems [Brown and Pariser, 1975]. As the driving force of appropriate technology (AT), innovation often consists of a blend of traditional and modern technology and takes advantage of nature.

Devices that reduce tedious, time- and raw-material-consuming, inefficient manual operations are innovative. Mechanization often makes a "quantum jump" from tedious manual operations to mechanical devices that replace many people [Ahmad and Jenkins, 1980]. Therefore, the need to make human labor more efficient without either excessive employment displacement or undue reliance upon expensive, complicated (usually imported) electric or fossil fuel-dependent machines is a delicate challenge for innovators. Hand-power devices to accomplish more efficient food refining (such as oil extraction [Donkor, 1979], staple grinding [Makanjula, 1974] and winnowing) and peddle power [Ghosh, 1978] are interesting on-farm or small-scale alternatives that are receiving attention even in the United States [Branch, 1978]. For multiple or continuous operations, animal-driven linkages can be fabricated [Scott, 1975]. A hand-held corn sheller developed by the Tropical Products Institute (TPI) [Pinson, 1977] is probably the simplest example. In fact, TPI's Rural Technology Guides (from 1977 to the present) cover a number of practical devices addressing the need for increasing the efficiency of home or small-scale industrial operations. Similarly, each issue of Appropriate Technology (from 1974 to the present) deals with innovative solutions to development problems in LDCs and provides an excellent communication forum for fieldworkers and technical experts.

Innovative energy-saving food preparation practices are minimum-water cooking, pressure cooking, and the use of soaking solutions to reduce the cooking time of refractory foods such as grain legumes. For example, chemicals [Narasunha and Desikachar, 1978; Rockland et al, 1979; Silva et al, 1981] or natural substances [Ankra and Dovlo, 1978] can significantly reduce cooking requirements for beans, thus increasing the convenience and economy of these nutritive foods. The legume storage regimen must, however, be nonabusive to take advantage of soaking solutions [Molina et al, 1976].

IMPLEMENTATION

No matter how sound the technology, urgent the need, or favorable the politics for enhancing local self-reliance in food and related resources, unless designers, practitioners, and recipients pay particular attention to the human factor, the result of their efforts is apt to be minimal or even counterproductive. It is out of many failures that AT evolved —the hopeful antonym of inappropriate technology [Harrison, 1976] by which jobs were eliminated, sociocultural linkages weakened, self-sufficiency discouraged or impeded, and the quality of life diminished. Increased access to infant foods (commercial or indigenous) could have a negative influence upon desirable breast-feeding practices, unless accompanied by an education effort. Efficient human or mechanically (wind, water, animal) powered processes appear to be desirable innovations, but only if attention is given to alternate livelihood for those replaced. The disruptive effect of such changes upon women's status has only recently been acknowledged, unfortunately, after the fact [Ahmad and Jenkins, 1980]. Wheat or other donated or subsidized imported foods can be more functional, nutritious, and acceptable than the traditional staple. However, if they are impractical to produce locally, their introduction may have potentially disastrous consequences for local agricultural incentives [Muller, 1974].

Unfortunately, the most frugal and needy — those at the poverty level — have usually already been forced to initiate the few conservation measures available to them. A major goal of technical assistance is to provide the poor with more and better alternatives. They can ill afford to initiate some promising but potentially risky endeavor. If they expend scarce resources in a failing effort, their very survival may be jeopardized. They lack "float" — the luxury of making those mistakes that are inevitable in the application and refining of new practices; they haven't the time and economic margin necessary to take chances, make errors, correct mistakes, and move confidently into unpredictable situations. Thus, the conservatism that characterizes those at the bottom economic strata has positive survival value. "If at first you don't succeed, try, try again" has little logic, if the penalty for the initial failure is starvation [Wood and Schmink, 1978].

The potential of unforeseen, undesirable side effects is inherent in any technical innovation, but much more effort must be devoted toward understanding the total consequences of change in order to eliminate or minimize serious disruptions [Dahl, 1979; Tyler, 1979; Kassapu, 1979]. It is a curious fact that those most vulnerable to food and resource limitations often survive tenaciously under very severe constraints. There is evidence of a survival strategy that works remarkably well, although subject to breakdown when the society is challenged by rapid change and diminishing resources [McDowell, 1976; Biggs, 1980]. This suggests a greater respect for traditional practices and an open dialog between AT practitioners and recipients.

There is no dearth of "how-to" literature regarding conservation, conversion, complementation, and innovation. However, the implementation steps are the most difficult and least clearly delineated. The patience, dedication, and time required by innovator, beneficiary, and administrator aren't easily quantified or described. It is uncommon in laboratory work to get a new or unfamiliar experiment to work the first time — even with the benefit of training, proper equipment, and comprehensive literature. To get the experiment functioning routinely in the field in the hands of less skilled practitioners is an even bigger hurdle. Nevertheless, experiments do eventually work, not necessarily exactly as described in the literature or as planned, but ultimately to improve our understanding of and control over natural phenomena. Thus, I am optimistic that the conservation, conversion, complementation, innovation, and even implementation strategies suggested here have positive value in overcoming global food and resource limitations. These concepts are certainly not "quick fixes" and will require far more time and attention to the human factor than to technical matters, but they must work. Indeed, what other alternatives does the world community have?

REFERENCES

Adams MR (1978): Small-scale vinegar production from bananas. Trop Sci 20:11-19.

Ahmad M, Jenkins A (1980): Traditional paddy husking – an appropriate technology under pressure. Approp Technol 7(2);28-30.

Aiyer RS, Nair PG, Prema L (1978): No-cost method for preserving fresh cassava roots. Cassava Newsletter, No. 4, pp. 8, 9. Centro Internacional de Agricultura Tropical, Cali, Colombia.

Anand JC (1975): Development of appropriate technology for a breakthrough in fruit and vegetable processing industry. Ind Food Packer 29(6):31-35.

Ankra EK, Dovlo FE (1978): The properties of trona and its effect on the cooking time of cowpeas. J Sci Food Agric 29:950-952.

Bates RP (1971): Lactic fermentation of Florida vegetables. Proc Fla State Hort Soc 84:253-257.

Bates RP (1983): Appropriate food technology. In Knorr D (ed): "Sustainable Food Systems." Westport, CT: Avi, Chap 9.

Beuchat LR (1978): Microbial alterations of grains, legumes and oilseeds. Food Technol 32(5): 193-198.

Biggs SD (1980): Informal R & D. Ceres 13(4):23-26.

Bourne MC (1977): Post harvest food losses – The neglected dimension in increasing the world food supply. Cornell International Agriculture Mimeograph 53. Geneva, NY: NY State Agric Exp Sta.

Branch D (1978): Tools for small-scale grain raising. Org Gard Farming 25(4):88-93.

Bressani R, Elias LG (1968): Processed vegetable protein mixtures for human consumption in developing countries. Adv Food Res 16:1-103.

Brown NL, Pariser ER (1975): Food science in developing countries. Science 188:589-593.

Burkholder L, Burkholder PR, Chu A, Kostyk N, Roels OA (1968): Fish fermentation. Food Technol 22:1278-1284.

Clark CS (1976): Village food technology: Solar drying of vegetables. LIFE News, April, pp 1-3.

Coleman RL, Wagner Jr CJ, Berry RE, Miller JM (1980): Building a low-cost, solar food dryer incorporating a solar reflector. USDA Citrus & Subtropical Products Lab, Box 1909, Winter Haven, FL 33880.

Dahl HA (1979): Commentary: Factors involved in the development, marketing and financing of appropriate technology in developing countries. Ecol Food Nutr 7:257-260.

Darrow K, Pam R (1981): "Appropriate Technology Source Book." Stanford, CA: Volunteers in Asia, Vols 1, 2.

Dichter D (1980): Improved mud brick silo for storing grain. Approp Technol 7(2):6-8.

Doe PE, Ahmed M, Muslemiddin M, Sachitnananthan K (1977): A polyethylene tent drier for improved sun drying of fish. Food Technol Aust 29:437-441.

Donkor P (1979): A hand-operated screw press for extracting palm oil. Approp Technol 5(4): 18-20.

Eka OU (1980): Effect of fermentation on the nutrient status of locust beans. Food Chem 5: 303–308.

Fordham JR, Wells CE, Chen LH (1975): Sprouting of seeds and nutrient composition of seeds and sprouts. J Food Sci 40:552–556.

Gee M, Farkas D, Rahman AR (1977): Some concepts for the development of intermediate moisture foods. Food Technol 31(4):58–64.

Ghosh BN (1978): A bicycle-operated PTO unit for small-scale farm jobs. World Crops 30:222–224.

Gomez JB, Bates RP, Ahmed EM (1980): Flexible pouch process development and evaluation of pasteurized-refrigerated mango slices. J Food Sci 45:1592–1594.

Green LF (1976): Sulphur dioxide and food preservation – A review. Food Chem 1:103–124.

Harrison P (1976): Inappropriate AT. New Scientist 71:236–237.

Herzka A (1980): Post-harvest food crop conservation. Prog Food Nutr Sci 4(3/4):1–138.

Hesseltine CW (1979): Some important fermented foods of Mid-Asia, the Middle-East, and Africa. J Am Oil Chem Soc 56:367–374.

IFT (1981): Open shelf-life dating of food. Food Technol 35(2):89–96.

Jackson J, Mehrer M (1978): The food preservation center: An exercise in appropriate technology. Food Technol 32(4):83–86.

Kassapu S (1979): The impact of alien technology. Ceres 12(1):29–33.

Labuza TP (1978): The properties of water in relationship to water binding in foods. A review. J Food Proc Pres 1:167–190.

Leopold CA, Ardrey R (1972): Toxic substances in plants and the food habits of early man. Science 176:512–514.

LIFE (1979): A practical method for bean storage. LIFE Newsl, May, pp 3–4.

Lindblad D, Druben L (1980): "Small Farm Grain Storage." Mt. Rainer, MD: VITA, Vols 1–3.

Majumder SK (1980): Storage and pest control strategy for preservation of foodgrains in India. J Food Sci Technol 17(1/2):55–58.

Makanjula GA (1974): A machine for preparing pounded yam and similar foods in Nigeria. Approp Technol 1(4):9–10.

May RM (1977): Food lost to pests. Nature 267:669–670.

McDowell J (1976): In defence of African food practices. Trop Doctor 6:37–42.

Mendelsohn JM (1974): Rapid techniques for salt-curing fish: A review. J Food Sci 39:125–127.

Mermelstein NH (1978): Retort pouch earns 1978 IFT Food Technology Industrial Achievement Award. Food Technol 32(6):22–32.

Molina MR, Batin MA, Gomez-Brenes RA, King KW, Bressani R (1976): Heat treatment: A process to control the development of the hard-to-cook phenomenon in black beans (*Phaseolus vulgaris*). J Food Sci 41:661–666.

Moody T (1980): Drying maize for storage in the humid tropics. Approp Technol 7(1):4–6.

Muller M (1974): Aid, corruptiion and waste. Futurist 64:398–400.

Narasunha HV, Desikachar HRS (1978): Simple procedures for reducing the cooking time of split red gram (*Cajanus cajan*). J Food Sci Technol 15:149–152.

NAS (1974): "Food Science in Developing Countries: A Selection of Unsolved Problems." Washington, DC: National Academy of Science.

NAS (1978): "Postharvest Food Losses in Developing Countries." Washington, DC: National Academy of Science.

Pellett PL, Mamarbachi D (1979): Recommended proportions of foods in home-made feeding mixtures. Ecol Food Nutr 7:219–228.

Pinson GS (1977): A wooden hand-held maize sheller. Rural Technology Guide, No. 1. London: Tropical Products Institute.

Pontecorvo AJ, Bourne MC (1978): Simple methods for extending the shelf life of soy curd (tofu) in tropical areas. J Food Sci 43:969–972.

Rajalakshmi R, Ramakrishnan CV (1977): Formulation and evaluation of meals based on locally available foods for young children. World Rev Nutr Diet 27:34–104.

Rao CS, Deyoe CW, Parrish DB (1978): Biochemical and nutritional properties of organic acid-treated high-moisture sorghum grain. J Stored Prod Res 14:95–102.

Rickard JE, Coursey DG (1979): The value of shading perishable produce after harvest. Approp Technol 6(2):18–19.

Rizvi SRH (1978): Appropriate technology for preservation of food in unsealed covered containers. Pakistan J Sci Ind Res 21(3/4):147–149.

Robach MC (1980): Use of preservatives to control microorganisms in food. Food Technol 34(10):81–84.

Rockland LB, Zaragosa EM, Oracca-Tetteh R (1979): Quick-cooking winged beans (*Psophocarpus tetragonolobus*). J Food Sci 44:1004–1007.

Satterlee LP (1975): Improving utilization of animal by-products for human foods — A review. J Anim Sci 41:687–697.

Scott D (1975): Animal power boosts new crop production. Approp Technol 2(1):7–9.

Silva CAB, Bates RP, Dene JC (1981): Influence of presoaking on black bean cooking kinetics. J Food Sci 46:1721–1725.

Srinivas T, Raghavendra Rao SN, Bhashyam MK, Desikachar HSR (1976): Studies on the use of dry earth as a contact medium for absorbing moisture from paddy. J Food Sci Technol 13:142–145.

Swaminathan M (1980): Development of supplementary foods and their usefulness in applied nutrition programs. J Food Sci Technol 17(1/2):78–81.

Thomas PL (1975): Dried meat products. Food Res Q 35:73–78.

Tyler PS (1979): New crop varieties store up problems. Third World Agric 1(2):18–20.

VITA (1970): "Village Technology Handbook." Mt. Rainer, MD: Volunteers in Technical Assistance.

Wood CW, Schmink M (1978): Blaming the victim: Small farmer production in an Amazon colonization project. Studies in Third World Societies, Publ. No. 7, "Changing Agriculture Systems in Latin America," pp 77–93.

Worgan JT (1977): Canning and bottling as methods of food preservation in developing countries. Approp Technol 4(3):15–16.

MALNUTRITION: DETERMINANTS AND CONSEQUENCES; CARIBBEAN CASE STUDIES

Moderators

Norge W. Jerome, PhD
Kansas City, Kansas

Noel W. Solomons, MD
Cambridge, Massachusetts

Malnutrition: Determinants and Consequences, pages 367–368
© 1984 Alan R. Liss, Inc., 150 Fifth Avenue, New York, NY 10011

Introduction: Caribbean Case Studies

Norge W. Jerome, PhD
Department of Community Health, Community Nutrition Division, University of Kansas College of Health Sciences, Kansas City, Kansas 66103

The Caribbean islands have been described in an earlier section (Picou). They are a string of tropical isles encircling the Caribbean sea (Fig. 1). Some are tiny dots, others are relatively large. Regardless of size, each has its unique culture and historical background; some are Spanish-speaking, others are French- or Dutch-speaking, but the majority are English-speaking. Most are independent countries. Most are now poor. In 1980, the total population was reported as 5.3 million.

The balance of trade between Caribbean island countries and the metropolitan capitals of the West is uneven, and it follows patterns established during the colonial era. Raw agricultural products are exported—sugar, cocoa, coffee, bananas, pineapples, limes, rum, spices, arrowroot, and tobacco. Processed foods are imported—sugar, cocoa, coffee, salted codfish, smoked herring, flour, rice, butter, milk, salt, etc. Essentially, staple foods are imported and garnishes are produced locally. Other consumer goods are also imported. These include textiles, footwear, and clothing; household equipment such as stoves and refrigerators; farm and office equipment of all types; and bicycles and automobiles. Children's toys are also imported.

Caribbean island peoples participate in the international cosmopolitan culture (clothing, fashion, hairstyles, food and eating styles, music) purely as consumers, not as decision makers or power brokers. They have not been allowed to participate as equals in such activities as market pricing, international trade, and the developing bilateral international agreements. This mode of functioning is a direct result of geographic insularity, language differences, and old colonial trading patterns. The newly independent countries continued the economic strategies of a past era while the world economies were undergoing major transformations.

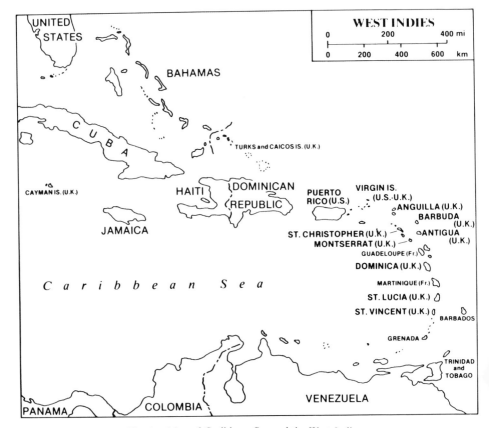

Fig. 1. Map of Caribbean Sea and the West Indies.

Economic systems in the Caribbean become more "underdeveloped" as economic relations between Caribbean countries and rich metropolitan countries increase. The economic relations often follow the patterns outlined during the colonial era. The features of underdevelopment in a stagnant economy are present everywhere — rural migration to local cities and metropolitan capitals, poverty, idleness, underemployment, high infant mortality rates, and malnutrition.

Thus, the determinants of malnutrition in the Caribbean stem from the economic system and sociocultural structures of the colonial past, from the economic and social constraints of the neocolonial present, and from contemporary patterns of living. These determinants will be elucidated in four mini-case-studies from large and small island nations: English-speaking Jamaica and St. Lucia; and the Spanish-speaking Dominican Republic and French-speaking Haiti, both on the island of Hispaniola.

Malnutrition: Determinants and Consequences, pages 369–372
© 1984 Alan R. Liss, Inc., 150 Fifth Avenue, New York, NY 10011

Comfort Castle, Jamaica

Dorothy Blake, MD, MPH

Project for Development of Health Services, Bureau Sanitaire Panamericain, Port-au-Prince, Haiti

Comfort Castle is a small, rural community (population 2,000) situated in a high, land-locked valley in the parish of Portland in the northeast section of Jamaica. Jamaica is the largest of the English-speaking territories in the Caribbean with a population of 2.2 million and a land surface of 11,000 sq. km. The population density is 195 per sq. km. The main economic activities are bauxite mining, tourism, and agriculture. The GNP per capita in 1980 was $1,200.00. See Table I for selected health statistics.

Approximately 32% of Jamaican households are headed by women, many of whom have the sole responsibility for the support of their children and many of whom are either unemployed or underemployed. There is a high rate of unemployment among 15- to 19-year-olds. Teenage pregnancy has increased considerably in the last 5 years.

A series of financial measures has been taken recently that has effectively devaluated the Jamaica dollar, even while subsidies on many basic food items have been lifted.

Undernourishment continues to be a problem. In 1981, 3% of the population 0–4 years old were moderately to severely undernourished, according to the Gomez weight-for-age classification, and 15% were mildly undernourished. Seventy-two percent of the children in this age group were adequately nourished. However, the general picture of the island should not mask the realities of many rural areas. Comfort Castle, a rural community in the Rio Grande Valley, exemplifies some of the nutritional problems in rural pockets in Jamaica.

As depicted in Table II, the nutritional status of the population 0–4 years old in Comfort Castle has been consistently lower than that of the island and parish.

TABLE I. Health and Social Indicators: Jamaica

Life expectancy	
Male	69 years
Female	73 years
Infant mortality	20/1,000 live births
Safe water	
Rural	74% of the population
Urban	87% of the population
Adequate exreta disposal	95% of the population
Access to health service (7-km radius)	100% (approx.) of the population

TABLE II. Percentage of the Population (0–4 years of age) at Three Levels Showing Normal Nutritional Status From 1979 to 1982 Based on the Gomez Weight-for-Age Classifications

Location	1979	1980	1981	1982
Jamaica		78.1	72.5	74.2
Portland Parish	70.3	75.1	70.8	72.2
Comfort Castle community	45.0	51.6	47.0	52.6

FINDINGS

In 1979, in light of the high malnutrition figures registered in Comfort Castle, a community diagnosis of the area was carried out. The findings were as follows:

Geography

Comfort Castle is situated in a high, land-locked valley.

Population, 2,000.

Rainfall ranges between 200 and 300 inches a year and is the highest in the island.

The area is subject frequently to landslides and high winds, and less frequently to hurricanes.

Economy

Agriculture-based.

The average size of agricultural holdings is one-quarter to one-half acre. No cultivated holding is greater than 5 acres.

Average income per capita is $450 per annum (compared to $1,200 overall for Jamaica).

Bananas for export and domestic use are the chief cash crop and basic staple.

Dasheen and yam, both tubers, are grown for sale but are mostly consumed by local households. Green and yellow vegetables grown in smaller quantities are mostly sold in the towns on the coast.

Bananas are transported on the backs of donkeys. This results in 50% rejection at buying stations.

Dasheen has an unstable market.

Fruits are abundant; however, they are not marketed unless buyers go to the field and collect them. Otherwise they are left to rot.

Small livestock (goats, pigs) are raised; cattle are rare.

Marketing of goods is wasteful and uneconomical. Often goods are not marketed because the cost of picking, packaging, and transport is not recovered after sales.

Male community members migrate to towns in search of jobs; this results in decreased agricultural production and broken families, women being left to bring up the children as single parents.

Sociocultural Findings

The people are of African origin and are geographically isolated. More specifically, they are Maroons whose runaway slave forebears wrested autonomous enclaves from the British. Recently, however, there has been intermarriage and migration, as well as inflow of outsiders.

The community is very religious, Seventh Day Adventist being the dominant religion. Members of this denomination do not eat the abundantly available river shrimp, busu (a small river snail), and wild pigs.

Bush teas (ie, leaves such as cerasee, mint, aralia) are used extensively during the weaning process and for illnesses.

Family sizes are large: six children on an average, with a range of 3 to 12.

Women are usually the sole providers in these large families. The young female teenager becomes a mother (often having left school because of pregnancy). The infant's father leaves very soon after, usually to find a job further down the valley or in town. The young mother enters union with another man mainly for economic reasons and has one or two other children before she is abandoned again. At age 26 she will have had 4–5 children from two or three different men. The current consort usually gives her only enough money for herself and his child if there is one. The mother tries to stretch this to support all other children; alternatively, she leaves the children with her mother to support and raise.

Biological

High incidence of gastroenteritis and intestinal parasites linked to poor sanitation.

High incidence of anemia, linked to both gastroenteritis and intestinal parasites.

Profile of Families With Malnourished Children

A study conducted by medical students on rural clerkships [Case Study by University of West Indies Medical Students on Rural Clerkship, 1980] showed that four features distinguished families with malnourished children from those with well-nourished children. The former usually had younger mothers, more often teenagers. The mothers often had more than five children before the age of 26. Such families typically had a single parent, or absentee parents, often with a grandparent bringing up the child(ren). And these families are affected by a greater poverty, with average income below US$25 per month.

Furthermore, it was noted that proportionately more undernourished children were female.

CONCLUSIONS

Comfort Castle can be seen as a concentrate of some of the key determinants of undernutrition in Jamaica. To summarize, these are:

1. Populations sequestered in hilly or mountainous enclaves.

2. Limited land availability.

3. Major agricultural efforts expended in the production of cash export crops, which implies a decline in production and cash as export markets decline.

4. Low income levels limiting the purchase of staple foods such as rice and flour, both imported, and protein foods.

5. Male urban drift.

6. Single, very young, undereducated, underemployed or unemployed women having the sole responsibility of child rearing, or coparenting with grandparents from a distance.

7. Low levels of sanitation.

8. Dietary practices apparently incompatible with proper nutrition both qualitatively and quantitatively.

Malnutrition: Determinants and Consequences, pages 373–377
© 1984 Alan R. Liss, Inc., 150 Fifth Avenue, New York, NY 10011

La Romana, Dominican Republic

Haydée Rondón, MD

University Autonoma of Santo Domingo, and Nutrition Department, Public
Health Ministry, Santo Domingo, Dominican Republic

La Romana is a province located in the eastern part of the Dominican Republic in Regional Health Zone 5. In 1981, there were 103,946 individuals over 5 years of age living in the urban and rural sections of La Romana. Rural-urban distribution is shown in Table I.

At the present time, the city of La Romana is the best-known tourist resort in the country and includes the well-known Casa de Campo Hotel and the artists' city, Altos de Chavon. A large number of jobs have been created in the urban areas with the installation of industrial free zones. By contrast, 50% of the land in the rural areas is devoted to sugar cane production and is owned by the Gulf and Western Company. La Romana, the focus of our case study, is but one small area of the country known as the Dominican Republic.

THE DOMINICAN REPUBLIC: GENERAL STATISTICS

Hispaniola is the second-largest island (after Cuba) in the Caribbean. It consists of 48,440 km². The island is shared by two countries, Haiti and the Dominican Republic, which speak different languages but have very good commercial and political relations. The countries are both small, with dependent economies and high rates of illiteracy, poverty and malnutrition.

According to the 1981 census, the total population of the Dominican Republic numbers 5,647,977. Children under 5 years of age make up 43.1% of the total and the 5–14 years age group make up 27.1% of the total population. The population is almost evenly divided between urban and rural residents; 51% live in urban areas and 49% in rural communities. The monthly income of 72% of the rural population and 50% of the urban dwellers is below RD$200.00. Urban unemployment rates are very high; the national unemployment rate in 1981 was 35%.

TABLE I. Rural-Urban Distribution of La Romana Residents Over 5 Years of Age (1981 data)

	Urban	Rural
Adults	60,529	28,238
Children	10,350	4,829
Total	70,879	33,067

The general death rate is 4.7 per 1,000; infant mortality is 30.5 per 1,000, and preschool mortality is 3 per 1,000. However, these statistics should be taken with reservations, since there is a 50% rate of underregistration of deaths. Life expectancy at birth is 62.5 years for both sexes.

HEALTH ORGANIZATION AND SERVICES IN 1983

The Secretariat of Public Health is responsible for health and medical services throughout the country. However, the armed forces provide health care to their members and their immediate family members.

Health services are offered free of charge to the low-income population; people who are employed obtain health care at the social security clinics or at private clinics. There are 13 hospitals in Santo Domingo, the capital city; the majority are specialized units. Also, there are 27 rural and 8 regional hospitals, 55 health centers, and 337 rural clinics.

The country is divided into seven health zones; each provides prophylactic and medical treatment. Staffing includes supervisors in maternal and infant health and in human nutrition, 2,518 medical doctors (ie, 0.5 per 1,000 inhabitants), 413 registered nurses (ie, 0.08 per 1,000 inhabitants), and 3,922 practical nurses (ie, 0.84 per 1,000 inhabitants). Primary health care workers now number 5,259 (2.3 per 1,000 inhabitants).

THE NUTRITIONAL PICTURE

Recent data from the Children's Hospital in Santo Domingo show that 50% of the population admitted to the hospital for other illness also suffer from malnutrition. Currently, the Secretariat of Public Health has, through its Nutritional Vigilance Project, diagnosed several variable degrees of malnutrition, depending on the socioeconomic and environmental conditions present in each zone. The situation is worse in the frontier zone and in the country's southwest, where 65% of the children are undernourished. This is also true of the slum areas located near the capital city. In the agricultural zone (Cibao) and in the eastern portion of the country, 40% of preschool children are undernourished.

On the basis of these statistics, we involved primary health workers in making a nutritional diagnosis of La Romana district in 1981.

THE LA ROMANA STUDY

A Nutrition Division team spent three days in the rural zone training the primary health worker in basic nutrition. They were taught to identify clinical signs of malnutrition, to weigh and measure children, and to classify and chart their nutritional status. In addition, workers were taught how to conduct a small nutrition survey in their communities and to summarize the information obtained. These summaries were collected by a supervisor and processed first at the appropriate regional office and then at the national level by the Nutrition Division. At the end of 3 months all data were collected, summarized and processed, and a nutritional diagnosis was established. A special day was set aside for a luncheon meeting with the community, primary health workers, local Public Health officers, and representatives from other institutions such as ODC (Community Development Office), the Secretariat of State for Agriculture, Gulf and Western Industries, etc.

Results of the La Romana Study

Some demographic data obtained in La Romana are presented in Table I. In addition, the rural population consisted of 1,019 children under 5 years of age.

Social and economic conditions are bleak. The sugar industry provides work for most of the rural population. The monthly income of 70% of the population is less than $200.00. The majority (92.7%) of the rural population is landless; 3.5% own less than 10 hectares of land. The schooling level of adults is extremely low; 33% are illiterate and 55% are marginally literate. Only 12% had received secondary education. Most of the houses in which the people live are owned by the Gulf and Western sugar mill; 33% of the houses have no water except that trucked in from a distance. Sewage disposal is inadequate in 35% of the homes.

The illnesses most often reported for children under 5 during the survey were respiratory infections (38%), diarrhea (30%), and intestinal parasites (60%). Skin and other diseases were also reported. The general mortality was 60 per 1,000. Infant mortality was 40.5 per 1,000 and preschool mortality was 5.1 per 1,000. The data obtained in the rural community were higher than those for the country as a whole.

The Nutritional Situation

Data on the nutritional status of 83% of the rural population less than 5 years old (849 children) from 260 homes were analyzed by the district and province. The provinces were Guaymate and Romana. The districts were Guaymate, Higueral, Sabana de Chavon and Aleton. The results are presented in Table II.

TABLE II. Diagnosis of Malnutrition in the Region of La Romana (rural preschool population), 1981

Province	Section	No. of children studied	Normal	%	Malnutrition[a]						Total (I-III)		Population according to 1980 census	
					I	%	II	%	III	%	No.	%	5 year	Total
Guaymate	Guaymate	196	113	57.6	59	30.1	19	9.7	5	2.6	83	42.3	206	1,808
	Higueral	273	148	54.2	96	35.2	26	9.5	3	1.1	125	45.8	338	2,099
	Sabana de Chavon	85	52	61.2	28	32.9	5	5.9	–	–	33	38.9	96	1,036
Romana	Aleton	295	188	63.7	87	29.5	19	6.4	1	0.3	107	36.7	379	2,609
	Total	849	501	59.0	270	31.8	69	8.1	9	1.1	348	41.0	1,019	7,552

[a]Diagnosis of mild (I), moderate (II), and severe (III) malnutrition.

Of the 849 children, 501 (59%) were adequately nourished and 348 (41%) were undernourished. Of that 41% the majority showed signs of mild undernutrition and a very low percentage showed signs of severe undernutrition.

The nutritional diagnosis was discussed with members of the community and local authorities. As a result, a series of local intervention projects designed to improve the nutritional situation in the sugar mill was developed. These included vegetable gardens for selling vegetables at a low price and to eliminate wholesalers; sale of low-priced meat; donation of a cow to produce milk for sale in the rural communities, etc.

We believe that this was a good experience that motivated the authorities to develop food availability projects and improve sanitary conditions.

Public health services have been supplementing the undernourished children with CARE foodstuffs which are stored in the rural clinics and distributed to children either in their homes or, in severe cases, at the rural clinic or hospital.

SUMMARY

A study of the nutritional situation of the La Romana area was carried out with the primary health workers of the area. Eighty-three percent of the preschool children were evaluated in a small survey of 260 rural homes in a 3-month period.

The results show that 59% of the preschool children living in the rural area of La Romana are adequately nourished and 41% are undernourished in several degrees. There is a 1.1% rate of chronic malnutrition, an 8.2% rate of moderate malnutrition, and a 31% rate of mild malnutrition on the basis of weight-for-age classification.

The rural population is made up of sugar cane cutters with low incomes. Thirty-three percent of the homes visited lack adequate sanitary installations, and 33% of the parents are illiterate. Infant mortality was reported at 40.5%, higher than the national rate, and preschool mortality, at 5.1%, was also higher than the national rate.

The results of this study were shown to the local authorities including those of the sugar mill. Several projects were planned to improve the nutritional condition of the rural population living in La Romana.

Malnutrition: Determinants and Consequences, pages 379–381
© *1984 Alan R. Liss, Inc., 150 Fifth Avenue, New York, NY 10011*

Haiti

William Fougère, MD
Ministry of Health, Port-au-Prince, Haiti

Malnutrition in Haiti stems from three broad areas—the environmental, host, and food determinants.

ENVIRONMENTAL DETERMINANTS

In tropical regions such as the Caribbean in general and Haiti in particular, poor agricultural and biological conditions, or lack of food and inadequate hygiene and sanitation, are major determinants of malnutrition.

Periodic droughts and hurricanes are very often registered in those areas, causing acute malnutrition and death to human beings and animals. Haiti has experienced several periodic droughts and hurricanes during the last 20 years, causing a great damage to its agriculture and economy.

Potable water is scarce and water from polluted springs and streams causes diarrhea and other waterborne diseases. Infectious diseases exacerbate malnutrition. In 1980, only 12.6% of the Haitian population had access to potable water. This included 0.67% for the rural population and 46.9% for urban areas other than Port-au-Prince, the capital city, and 45.0% for Port-au-Prince.

Lack of transportation and lack of roads impair food distribution. Traditional food conservation systems and lack of silos expose food to insects and other contaminants.

HOST DETERMINANTS

Host determinants are viewed largely as population characteristics, and the ratio of population to food and other resources. In Haiti, the population was estimated as 500,000 in 1804, the year of independence of the nation. In 1844, the Haitian population was 833,000. By 1960, 4,155,597 Haitians were living in the country. According to the Haitian Institute of Statistics, the Haitian population in 1980 was estimated at 5,008,500 with 72.5% living in rural areas. Crude reproduction rate was 2.46%, true reproduction rate 1.84%. The crude birth rate was estimated at 36.78% and the crude death rate at 14.48%. The natural rate of increase was found to be 22.30% with a true increase rate at 1.8%.

Population density is 181 inhabitants per square kilometer. Haiti consists of 27,000 square kilometers of land area of which 21,000 are mountainous, mostly unproductive land, and 6,700 square kilometers are plains and highlands. Only 33.0% of the country is cultivated; 39.0% is not. Forest occupies only 9.0% and grazing land 18.0% of the total area. As a result, the population density for cultivable land is 431 inhabitants per square kilometer.

The vulnerable age group, 0–4 years, represents 15.4% of the population. Vulnerabilities are also seen in the high illiteracy rate (about 80% of the population) and low level of income per capita ($186.00). Lack of education and nutrition information are responsible for limited and improper choices of food. In this regard, shifts in world market prices, causing inflation, raise food expenditures and widen the gap in family budget.

In Haiti, iron deficiency anemia is one of the most important nutritional problems, requiring serious intervention measures. It is particularly serious among vulnerable groups, including young children and pregnant women.

FOOD DETERMINANTS

Poor nutrient intake is very often due to lack of diversity of food. Lack of animal protein imposes a limited choice of starchy foods in the family diet. Absence of modern food technology or other practical means of food preservation is responsible for food spoilage. Toxic foods, sometimes high in cyanate or other toxic ingredients, are very often consumed in rural areas during droughts. Finally, lack of suitable weaning foods exposes young children to malnutrition due to the introduction of inappropriate food components into their diets. Shortening the breast-feeding period or suppression of breast feeding is also responsible for infant deaths.

CONSEQUENCES

In Haiti, as in many other countries of the Caribbean, undernutrition causes death and physical and psychological deterioration chiefly among vulnerable groups.

Calorie intake is around 1,700 kcal per day, with a deficit of 500 kcal. Protein intake is 41 gm per person per day with a deficit of 14 gm per person. Several mineral and vitamin deficiencies have been discovered by nutritional surveys. An official organization of the Haitian government has estimated the annual food deficit at 650,000 metric tons.

The last national nutrition survey carried out by the Haitian Bureau of Nutrition and the US Centers for Disease Control showed that 70% of the pre-school children were malnourished, 27% sustaining moderate and severe (grades II and III malnutrition). Infant mortality is high, 149 per 1,000; and mortality for children 1–4 years of age is 45 per 1,000.

CONCLUSIONS

Undernutrition is a public health problem in the Caribbean in general and in Haiti in particular. Since there are several determinants, it is imperative that approaches to solving nutritional problems take into consideration all factors or determinants involved in its causation. Nevertheless, it is important to emphasize the role of education, economic improvement, food availability, environmental betterment, and adaptation of family size to family income for a more comprehensive planning method in nutrition strategy.

Malnutrition: Determinants and Consequences, pages 383–384
© 1984 Alan R. Liss, Inc., 150 Fifth Avenue, New York, NY 10011

St. Lucia

A.J. D'Souza, MBBS, DPH, DIH
Ministry of Health and Local Government, Castries, St. Lucia, West Indies

IMPACT OF COMMUNITY NUTRITION PROGRAMS ON NUTRITIONAL STATUS OF INSULAR POPULATIONS IN THE CARIBBEAN

To most people, the Caribbean islands are beautiful beaches, coconut palms, and spectacular scenery. But they also are characterized by the health and nutrition problems associated with developing countries. Historically the determinants of undernutrition have been poverty, lack of proper nutrition information, and disease. In recent years, community nutrition programs have had a considerable impact on the nutritional status of the people living in the islands of the Caribbean. However, community nutritional status is dependent on four main factors: 1) economics; 2) education; 3) food availability, accessibility, and utilization; and 4) public health measures.

In the Caribbean, it is the mother and the child who have suffered most from malnutrition. Until recently, two-thirds of all deaths in the age group 0–4 were due to gastroenteritis/malnutrition or related causes resulting in the deadly sequence of poverty → malnutrition → infection → death.

The characteristics of the malnourished child are related to 1) age (age 6–36 months), 2) distance from clinic, 3) sex (more common among females), and 4) duration of breast feeding. Factors that may be associated but have not been proven statistically are mother's age (< 20 years), birth weight (< 6 lb.) and left arm circumference.

Initially, some community nutrition programs were established primarily as health service programs for the purpose of reducing high childhood malnutrition and mortality by nutritional interventions.

In the Hanover Health Surveillance and Nutrition Education Program in Jamaica, community health workers surveyed preschool children, carried out home visits, and provided nutrition education and nutritional supplements on a selective basis to those identified as malnourished. This program did reduce the prevalence of malnutrition and reduced excess child mortality over a period of four years, 1972–1975. However, there was also an associated improvement in the socioeconomic status of the population during this period. The largely curative nature of the program did produce a short-term decrease in the prevalence of undernutrition, but it did not significantly influence the incidence of malnutrition.

The need for continuing nutrition education was, therefore, obvious. Most Caribbean islands now have community-based nutrition education programs where mothers are educated in the following: 1) various food groups and how to use locally grown foods; 2) the importance of breast feeding; 3) how to feed the child from the family pot; 4) the importance of regular monitoring of the child's weight at the clinic; 5) good environmental sanitation practices; and 6) backyard or kitchen gardens to grow fruits and vegetables.

The child's progress is charted in a child Health Passport, a patient-held record that was adapted in St. Lucia by Dr. Ed Cooper from the original used in Africa by David Morley.

Voluntary community-based organizations and international agencies have helped (eg, CANSAVE has established a day nursery and a child-feeding program in St. Lucia; and the Seventh-Day Adventists World Services are actively supporting the Ministry of Health in St. Lucia in their nutrition programs). Continuing education programs for health workers have also been established.

Perhaps the most significant impact in reducing mortality in the young child in recent times has been the introduction of oral rehydration. Although it has not directly attacked undernutrition, its impact in minimizing the debilitating effects of gastroenteritis and the consequent nutritional loss cannot be underestimated.

The Caribbean Islands have come a long way since the 1950s and 1960s. Our infant mortality ranges between 20 and 30 per 1,000 and the malnourished child nowadays presents mainly with mild to moderate malnutrition. To be successful, nutrition programs have to be preventive, promote good health and nutrition, and be carried out in a primary health care program. The future would be brighter if local food production in the islands were geared to producing more local foods, reducing the need for imported goods, and if the arable land at our disposal were more efficiently utilized and not used largely for export crops. There is also need for better intersectional coordination between the Ministries of Health, Education, and Agriculture.

The Caribbean is at present in a transitional phase — as we conquer the problems of undernutrition, diseases like diabetes and hypertension also demand our attention.

Malnutrition: Determinants and Consequences, pages 385–386
© 1984 Alan R. Liss, Inc., 150 Fifth Avenue, New York, NY 10011

Summary of the Open Discussion

Norge W. Jerome, PhD
Department of Community Health, Community Nutrition Division, University of Kansas College of Health Sciences, Kansas City, Kansas 66103

The four Caribbean case studies and papers were discussed by panel members and the approximately 60 Congress participants attending the session. The following points were emphasized.

1. Malnutrition assumes two major forms in the Caribbean: 1) overnutrition, as indicated by the large numbers of obese adults, particularly women, and the high prevalence of the "diseases of affluence"—obesity, coronary heart disease, hypertension, and diabetes; and 2) undernutrition, particularly mild and moderate undernutrition in the children under 5 years of age.

2. Both forms of malnutrition can be traced to the trading and marketing policies and practices of the colonial past. These include a) the peculiar agricultural production-for-export system that forced each island to specialize in a specific cash crop for export rather than diversify the economic systems to meet regional and local economic and nutritional needs; b) the peculiar food import system that forced each island to sell raw materials (cash crops) abroad and import processed foodstuffs such as coffee, cocoa powder, and sweetened condensed milk, which are available locally and at less cost when left unprocessed (at present, the Caribbean area imports 62% of its protein and 46% of its energy from abroad); and c) the traditional dietary pattern consisting of imported starchy, salted, and fatty staples (wheat flour, rice, dried and salted cod and herring, pickled beef, pigs' tail and snout, and lard and butter) and garnishes from local foods.

3. Undernutrition appears to be limited to young mothers and children and is closely associated with social and economic conditions such as unemployment, underemployment, low wages; migration of young men to local, regional, and metropolitan cities; mating patterns; and family size, structure,

and dependency ratio. Obviously, the role and status of women are linked to undernutrition.

4. Poor hygiene and sanitary conditions, and insufficient potable water are important determinants of malnutrition in some island nations.

5. Inadequate transportation and undeveloped infrastructures are significant factors in malnutrition.

6. Community nutrition services including nutritional assessments, nutrition education, food cooperatives, food production, and food subsidy programs play a role in alleviating problems of malnutrition. However, these programs are supplementary and self-limiting. Program participants will not continue to derive nutritional benefits from such programs once a certain delivery point has been reached. Specific actions must also be taken to drive the economy for sustained, long-term growth and its concomitant economic, social, and nutritional benefits.

7. Economists, nutritionists, nutrition planners, and policy makers from outside the Caribbean area have very limited roles in modifying the nutritional picture locally. However, they can be extremely valuable in their home settings by careful consideration of the points raised in items 1–6 above. For example, the Caribbean Basin initiatives of the Reagan administration should be reassessed to determine disparities in country participation and in the potential benefits to specific countries in the region. These experts could initiate a North-South dialogue on the real issues that directly counter nutritional well-being in the region, including the inability of well-trained Caribbean-born nutritionists to secure good positions in the region, and the absence of Caribbean leaders in decision-making positions concerning the economic well-being of the region.

8. The complex nutritional problems of the Caribbean can be solved if addressed as a problem of the Caribbean region within the context of the Western Hemisphere, but with due consideration of the unique characteristics and special needs of each island nation.

(A) IATROGENIC MALNUTRITION AND (B) FOLK MEDICINE AND SELF-TREATMENT

Malnutrition: Determinants and Consequences, pages 389–401
© 1984 Alan R. Liss, Inc., 150 Fifth Avenue, New York, NY 10011

Iatrogenic Contributions to Cancer Cachexia

Rajender K. Chawla, PhD, David H. Lawson, MD, and Daniel Rudman, MD

Department of Medicine, Emory University School of Medicine, Clinical Research Center (R.K.C., D.R.), and VA Medical Center (D.H.L.), Atlanta, Georgia 30322

OVERVIEW OF CANCER CACHEXIA

Introduction

Progressive wasting, weakness, anorexia, and anemia are frequent complications of neoplastic disease. As the tumor enlarges, the host's muscle mass and adipose mass are depleted; contrastingly the liver, kidney, adrenal glands, and spleen may actually enlarge. In the early stages, total body protein may be unchanged, although nitrogen is redistributed from muscle to tumor. Later, when anorexia is pronounced, total body protein declines.

This syndrome has been extensively studied and reviewed in both man and rodent [1]. While some features of cancer cachexia are seen in both species, there are several differences. The transplanted rodent tumors are antigenically foreign, more rapidly growing than most human cancers, and larger (20–40% of body weight) at the time of death than most malignancies seen in people. One reason the rodent tumors achieve a larger size than human tumors is their subcutaneous location and lack of metastatic potential; they can enlarge substantially without lethal mechanical, hemorrhagic, or infectious complications. Most human tumors lead to fatal mechanical or hemorrhagic complications at a comparatively earlier stage. Finally, the tumorous rat is studied in the untreated state, whereas most humans have been or are being treated with surgery, radiation therapy, or chemotherapy, all of which tend to impair nutrition.

Prevalence of Clinical Cancer Cachexia

Cachectic cancer patients frequently have not only protein-calorie undernutrition (PCU) but also depletion of vitamins and minerals. Nevertheless, it is the protein-calorie depletion that has engaged the interest of most investigators. Most surveys have concentrated on weight loss, contraction of lean body mass, depletion of fat mass, and hypoproteinemia as indicators of cancer cachexia [2].

DeWys and co-workers studied the history of weight loss among patients who were subjects of the Eastern Cooperative Oncology group [3]. None of these patients had received chemotherapy, and all had disseminated disease. In the preceding 6 months, 54% of these patients had lost some weight and 32% had lost greater than 5% of their usual weight.

Nixon and co-workers studied anthropometric parameters, creatinine: height index, and serum albumin and vitamin levels in a series of hospitalized patients with various types of cancer and at various stages in the natural history of their disease [4]. Forty-two percent of these patients had less than 80% of standard adipose stores, as determined by triceps skinfold measurements, and 53% had less than 60% of standard. The serum albumin concentration was subnormal in 31% of these patients. Furthermore, among patients who had lost at least 60% of their premorbid weight, 45% had subnormal serum concentrations of vitamins A and C, and 20% had decreased levels of serum folate.

These studies demonstrate a high frequency of nutritional abnormalities in cancer patients, confirming the widely held clinical impression. However, it must be emphasized that PCU is not unique to cancer [5]. On the contrary, 30–50% of hospitalized patients presently have some degree of PCU, and most chronic, fatal, nonneoplastic diseases terminate in a cachectic state (eg, chronic disseminated infections, or prolonged insufficiency of heart, lungs, liver, kidneys, or the small intestines).

Relationship of PCU to Survival in Cancer Patients

Recent studies have documented the association between undernutrition, usually as measured by weight loss, and decreased survival. DeWys and co-workers found that median survival time was significantly shorter in patients who had lost weight, and this was true in all the tumor types examined except acute nonlymphocytic leukemia, pancreatic carcinoma, and gastric carcinoma [3]. The relationship of more specific nutritional indicators to survival has also been examined. In a study involving patients with a variety of tumor types, visceral protein and lean body mass depletion (as measured by serum albumin concentration and creatinine:height index) had a worse prognostic import than adipose depletion (as measured by triceps skinfold thickness) [4]. Twelve of 27 patients (44%) with triceps skinfold measurements less than 60% of standard died within 70 days of nutritional evaluation compared to 7 of 31 (23%) with greater adipose stores; this difference was not significant ($P > 0.05$). On the other hand, 53% (16/30) of patients with serum albumin concentrations less than 3.5 gm/dl died within this time period, compared to only 18% (7/39) of patients with higher serum albumin concentrations ($P < 0.05$). Similarly, 56% (18/32) of patients with a creatinine:height index less than 60% of standard died within 70 days of study, compared to only 4% (1/26) of patients with higher values ($P < 0.05$).

In an often quoted study Warren, in 1932, attempted to determine the cause of death in 500 autopsied cancer patients [6]. In 114 cases, the charts documented progressive weakness, wasting, and anemia, and at autopsy no clear cause of death could be discerned. Warren concluded that these 22% of his patients died of cancer cachexia. He commented that cachexia was also present in many, but certainly not all, of the other patients, and thus could have contributed to death from other causes, such as infection. Nevertheless, it is recognized that many cancer patients die in a well-nourished state from mechanical effects of the tumor on specific organ sites or from infection or bleeding.

Although these studies demonstate a general association between PCU and survival in cancer patients, they do not establish a cause-and-effect relation [7,8]. Primary PCU is known to have an adverse effect on resistance to some infections, on wound healing, and on cardiorespiratory, hepatic, and renal functions; these factors must contribute to cancer mortality. However, the precise mechanisms by which the cancer cachexia syndrome may cause death in some patients and perhaps contribute to it in others are not completely understood.

ENDOGENOUS MECHANISMS OF CANCER CACHEXIA

The following factors contribute to loss of weight: reduced food intake, gastrointestinal malabsorption, and endogenous metabolic abnormalities leading to various combinations of impaired protein synthesis, accelerated protein breakdown, or hypermetabolism. An additional mechanism, unique to cancer, is the redistribution of protoplasmic elements from host to tumor [1], which erodes lean body mass and adipose tissue even in the absence of weight loss.

Advanced cancer in rodents and in patients is associated with hypophagia. In patients, mechanical factors (dysphagia, GI obstruction, ascites) and anorexigenic chemotherapeutic drugs are major contributors. Many cancer patients and laboratory animals, however, show pronounced food aversion in the absence of such factors. In the rat, the degree of hypophagia is not regularly correlated with tumor size [9]. For some tumor types, food intake declines when tumor/body weight ratio is 5%; for others intake does not decline until this ratio exceeds 30%. If, however, the food's nutrient density is reduced by unabsorbable bulk, the hypophagia often becomes demonstrable at an earlier stage, for example, when tumor/body weight ratio is still < 1%. Animal studies suggest that the hypophagia could result in part from a potent biochemical property of the tumor.

About 30% of the locomotor activity of the rat is feeding activity. Feeding motor activity is reduced in parallel with food intake. In some cases, feeding activity commences at normal intervals, but is terminated abnormally rapidly, as though responsiveness to preabsorptive signals is intact but satiety signals are hyperactive [10].

Abnormalities of taste are often demonstrable in both rats and patients with cancer [2]. In both, the threshold for sucrose rises. In humans, additionally, the threshold for urea falls, but the thresholds for HCl and NaCl remain unchanged. Hypersensitivity to the bitter taste of urea correlates with aversion to meat. The altered taste thresholds tend to parallel the degree of hypophagia among different patients and in the same patients over time. There may also be a correlation with tumor burden.

The metabolic mechanisms by which tumors depress appetite have been the subject of much discussion [2,9]. Leading possibilities are the following: Since appetite is related to amino acid composition of diet and plasma, the frequently altered aminogram in cancer suggests that a disorder of amino acid metabolism could depress appetite; since glucoreceptors in the liver are believed to influence food intake, the known abnormalities in hepatic carbohydrate metabolism, especially increased glucose synthesis, could depress appetite; lactic acid, often elevated in cancer patients' blood, is anorexigenic; bioactive factors released from tumors, including products of necrosis, inflammation, and infection, could depress appetite.

Gastrointestinal malabsorption occurs frequently in clinical cancer and contributes significantly to the wasting [11]. However, the malabsorption is not tumor-directed, but instead is caused either by treatment (resection of a portion of the GI tract, or enteropathic effects of chemotherapeutic drugs or irradiation), or by the neoplastic infiltration of mesenteric lymphatics, or by the nonspecific intestinal atrophy caused by semistarvation.

In both rat and man, erosion of muscle and adipose tissue frequently precedes a detectable fall in food intake. In undernourished cancer patients, moreover, measured food intake fails to correlate with degree of PCU [12,13]. Finally, when control rats are pair-fed with tumorous rats, the atrophy of muscle and adipose mass in the latter exceeds that in the former. These observations show that anorexia is only a partial cause of the wasting process [1]. Evidently there are metabolic disturbances within the tumor or within the host tissues, or both, that also contribute. Two general types of mechanism are suspected: a) increased uptake of carbohydrate and amino acid nutrients by the tumor cells, and b) release of bioactive materials that cause anorexia and catabolism in the host lean body mass. See extensive recent reviews for discussions of these topics [1,9,14].

Other manifestations of a catabolic state in many cancer patients are decreased protein synthesis in muscle, insulin resistance, and increased lipolysis [15–19]. Opinions vary as to whether these characteristics are intrinsic properties of the neoplastic state, or merely secondary consequences of semistarvation, since all of these changes do occur under conditions of negative caloric balance.

Growth of the tumor is often contrasted with that of the fetus. Both tumor and fetus are highly anabolic systems that trap nitrogen and other protoplasmic elements. In the latter situation, hyperphagia allows the host to maintain normal nutrition of the lean body mass. In the former state, food intake is relatively depressed; consequently, adipose and muscle masses atrophy. These events have been extensively documented by implanting tumors in rats and thus eliminating mechanical interference with nutrition or therapeutic factors. They show the potency of nonmechanical, endogenous mechanisms in the pathogenesis of cancer cachexia.

Endogenous mechanical factors also can contribute to malnutrition in cancer patients. These include mechanical obstruction, infiltration of the small intestine or its lymphatics by tumor cells causing gastrointestinal malabsorption, or metastasis to the central nervous system [20,21].

EXOGENOUS MECHANISMS

The patient with cancer is bombarded with therapy that often propels him towards PCU [22].

Surgery

Surgery leads to PCU by the catabolic response to injury, by surgical alterations of the pharynx that cause hypophagia, or by resection of the GI tract leading to malabsorption and diarrhea [23].

Radiation

Radiation causes PCU by various mechanisms depending on the target. Head and neck radiation leads to xerostomia, loss of taste, and dysphagia. Radiation of the thorax causes esophagitis, esophageal stenosis, and dysphagia. Radiation of the abdomen and pelvis causes radiation enteropathy [23].

Antineoplastic Agents

Antineoplastic agents may cause malabsorption, anorexia, stomatitis, and dysgeusia [23–25]. These compounds are capable of inhibiting a number of metabolic processes involved in the synthesis of such nutrients as choline, carnitine, tyrosine, cysteine, and polyamines. These nutrients are physiologically essential although nutritionally nonessential because in normal individuals they are readily synthesized endogenously. Increasing numbers of cancer patients are being maintained on liquid elemental diets (enteral or parenteral) that contain the 40 essential nutrients, including vitamins, minerals, energy source, and essential amino acids. All nonessential nutrients are expected to be synthesized in optimal quantities by endogenous biosynthetic pathways. Some of these pathways, however, are compromised by chemotherapy. Special nutritional problems, therefore, may arise for cancer patients on elemental nutrition as well as those with limited intake. Representative examples of metabolic blocks caused by eight different types of chemotherapeutic drugs are listed below.

Metabolic effects of methotrexate. Methotrexate, an antifolate, inhibits dihydrofolate reductase and blocks the formation of tetrahydrofolate, which is required as a cofactor in the biosynthesis of thymine nucleotides and purines [26,27]. As a result, this drug prevents the synthesis of RNA and DNA and thereby prevents the rapid proliferation of tumor cells.

One well-documented side effect of this drug is the systemic depletion of tetrahydrofolate. However, a not so well recognized metabolic property of methotrexate is its capacity to competitively inhibit dihydrobiopterin reductase, an enzyme required for regeneration of tetrahydrobiopterin [26]. The latter is a cofactor for a group of enzymes – aromatic amino acid hydroxylases – that are involved in conversion of phenylalanine to tyrosine, tyrosine to dihydroxyphenylalanine (Fig. 1), and tryptophan to serotonin. Therefore, a

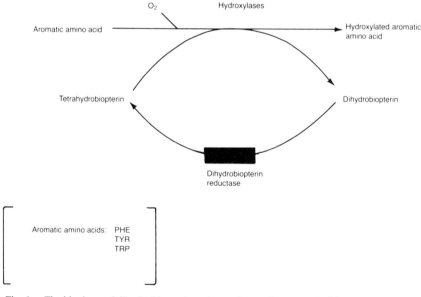

Fig. 1. The blockage of dihydrobiopterin reductase by methotrexate (solid square) in the conversion of phenylalanine to tyrosine, tyrosine to DOPA, and tryptophan to hydroxytryptophan and serotonin.

patient undergoing methotrexate therapy is at nutritional risk owing to the following: a) acute deficiency of tetrahydrofolate; b) elevated plasma levels of phenylalanine analogous to those observed in type II phenylketonuria, which is described by Kaufman (cited in Hilton et al [26]); c) depressed plasma levels of tyrosine, if the patient is being maintained on a tyrosine-free synthetic amino acid diet; and d) impaired synthesis of serotonin and dopa.

Metabolic effects of adenine arabinoside. This drug—also known as ara-A or 9-β-D-arabinofuranosyladenine—is used alone or with an adenosine deaminase inhibitor as an oncostatic and an antiviral agent. Its therapeutic effect is attributed to its capacity to inhibit virus-specific DNA-polymerase [28].

Recent work by Sacks et al [29] and Helland and Ueland [30] has conclusively shown that ara-A also irreversibly inhibits S-adenosylhomocysteine hydrolase, the enzyme that converts S-adenosylhomocysteine to homocysteine in the transsulfuration pathway (Fig. 2). This property may also contribute to the therapeutic effects of the drug. However, it also leads to an intracellular and extracellular accumulation of S-adenosylhomocysteine and a depletion of homocysteine in the host. S-Adenosylhomocysteine is a competitive inhibitor

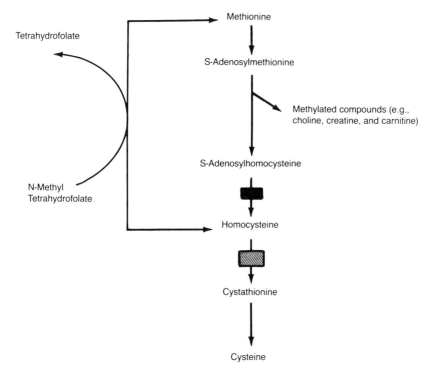

Fig. 2. The blockage of 1) S-adenosylhomocysteine hydrolase by ara-A (solid square) in the conversion of S-adenosylhomocysteine to homocysteine and 2) cystathionine synthetase by methylglyoxal bis-(guanylhydrozone) (hatched square) in the formation of cystathionine from homocysteine.

for most transmethylation reactions, which are of vital importance to the organism. These may be effectively blocked during ara-A therapy.

The nutrition-related side effects of blockage of transmethylation processes are as follows: a) deficiency of carnitine, choline, and creatine due to lack of an effective transmethylation process (this deficiency will be especially pronounced in patients maintained on commercially available synthetic amino acid diets that do not contain any of these micronutrients); b) low plasma levels of methionine due to its depressed de novo synthesis from homocysteine (consequently, the patient may go into negative nitrogen balance); c) acute folate deficiency (in the absence of adequate levels of homocysteine, methyltetrahydrofolate will accumulate in the so-called tetrahydrofolate trap); d) hypocysteinemia due to depressed biosynthesis of cysteine (the patient kept on cysteine-free nutritional solutions will be at greater risk).

Metabolic effects of 6-azauridine triacetate. This drug blocks the de novo synthesis of pyrimidine by inhibiting the activity of orotidinic acid-5'-phosphate decarboxylase. In the late 1960s, it was observed that 6-azauridine triacetate also produced homocystinuria and hyper-β-alaninemia [31]. The drug inhibits cystathionine synthetase (Fig. 2), thus causing accumulation of homocysteine. The activity of β-alanyl-α-ketoglutaric amino transferase is also suppressed by this agent (Fig. 3), with the resultant accumulation of β-alanine [31,32].

The metabolic consequences of the drug-induced block of cystathionine synthetase are as follows: a) hypermethioninemia due to increased enzymatic recycling of homocysteine (Fig. 2) (elevated plasma methionine levels may have toxic effects on the patient); and b) hypocysteinemia (this will be especially true in patients maintained on cysteine-free parenteral or enteral formula).

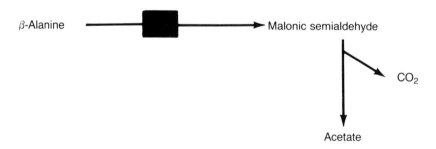

Fig. 3. The blockage of β-alanyl-α-ketoglutaric amino transferase by ara-A (solid square) in the conversion of β-alanine to malonic semialdehyde.

Metabolic effects of cyclophosphamide. This widely used antitumor drug is activated by hepatic mixed-function oxidases; in this process, phosphoramide mustard and acrolein are generated. Phosphoramide mustard is the effective chemotherapeutic moiety, whereas acrolein is a toxic by-product that can cause hemorrhagic cystitis [33]. Both cysteine and hepatic glutathione protect the organism from these toxic effects by forming a complex with acrolein. In this process, there is an overall depletion of cysteine and glutathione. It is apparent that the host's requirements for these sulfhydryl-containing compounds will be elevated during cyclophosphamide therapy. If these requirements are not completely fulfilled, the patient may go into negative N balance, especially if he is receiving cysteine-free total parenteral or enteral formula.

Metabolic effects of enzyme therapy. Many tumor cells lack enzymes required for the synthesis of one or more nonessential amino acids or have an increased requirement for these amino acids and depend on a high concentration of these amino acids in body fluids for optimal growth. In recent years, specific enzymes (eg, asparaginase-glutaminase, histidase, and cystinase) capable of degrading these amino acids in the circulation have been employed to deplete their systemic levels and thus to kill tumor cells [34,35]. It is likely that a prolonged enzyme therapy would lower the host's overall capacity to synthesize the nonessential amino acids for normal tissues, and put him at risk of a negative nitrogen balance.

Another use of enzyme therapy may be the potentiation of chemotherapeutic agents. In this regard, it is of interest that specific nutrients may have effects on the action of the drugs, just as the drugs affect nutritional status. For example, the cellular uptake of melphalan (L-phenylalanine mustard) is an active, carrier-mediated process. In the L1210 murine leukemia model this apparently occurs by an amino acid transport system of the leucine-preferring (L) type. Physiologic concentrations of the L-isomers of leucine and glutamine reduced the uptake of melphalan by these cells in vitro to one-sixth that of control cells incubated without these amino acids, whereas L-valine had only a minimal effect [36]. Similar results have been obtained in primary cultures of human ovarian carcinoma cells, and it has been shown that glutamine and leucine are present in the ascites fluid of these patients at concentrations sufficient to exhibit this protective effect [37]. These findings suggested that a reduction of leucine or glutamine concentrations in vivo might enhance the therapeutic effectiveness of this drug, and this was found to be true. Mice bearing L1210 tumors were "cured" more often by the concomitant systemic administration of the enzyme acinetobacter glutaminase-asparaginase and melphalan than by the administration of either agent alone [38]. In humans this concept has been applied to patients with advanced carcinoma of the ovary. These patients often have disease confined to the peritoneal cavity, making them ideal candidates for treatments localized to this region. Furthermore, the enzyme acinetobacter glutaminase-asparaginase is cleared slowly from the peritoneal space, in contrast to its more rapid clearance from plasma [38]. Three patients with advanced ovarian carcinoma were treated with peritoneal lavage followed by intraperitoneal glutaminase-asparaginase and, 1 hr later, melphalan. One of these patients had a complete response despite previous resistance to oral melphalan. Depletion of glutamine in the ascitic fluid was demonstrated [39]. This strategy of enhancement of the cellular uptake of melphalan by the depletion of a competing nutrient is promising.

Metabolic effects of methylglyoxal bis-(guanylhydrazone). The therapeutic effect of this drug is based on its capacity to inhibit irreversibly and competitively the activity of S-adenosylmethionine decarboxylase and thus prevent the formation of polyamines, which are required for cellular proliferation [40]. The deleterious metabolic effects of this drug on the host are largely unknown. The polyamines are vital for cellular multiplication and protein biosynthesis. These molecules bind with and stabilize double-stranded polynucleotides. Increased polyamine synthesis precedes DNA replication in the cell. If intracellular polyamine contents are depleted, cellular morphology is altered and growth slows. The consequences of polyamine depletion on DNA and RNA functions in the host's tissues are not known.

Metabolic effects of cis-platinum. Treatment with cis-platinum (cis-dichlorodiamine platinum (II)) causes hypomagnesemia in the majority of patients treated [41–43]. In some cases this may be associated with hypocalcemia and/or hypokalemia. Tetany has been reported, but apparently occurs primarily when both hypomagnesemia and hypocalcemia are present [43]. The mechanism for the hypomagnesemia is renal wasting, presumably due to renal tubular damage caused by this agent. Although serum magnesium concentrations eventually return to normal in most patients, the mean duration of hypomagnesemia was 118 days in one study (range: 2–622 days) [41,42], and not infrequently the defect lasted until the patient's death. Thus, in these patients, the nutritional complications of chronic hypomagnesemia will be superimposed on the other cancer-associated nutritional problems.

Cardiac toxicity of adriamycin. In some instances chemotherapeutic agents can cause effects resembling those seen with specific nutritional defects without in fact depleting the host of that nutrient. An example is the cardiomyopathy associated with the anthracycline antibiotic adriamycin [44]. The cytoplasmic vacuolization, loss of myofilaments, and cellular necrosis in adriamycin cardiotoxicity resemble the changes seen with vitamin E deficiency. The muscle changes of α-tocopherol deficiency are thought to be due to peroxidation of membrane lipids as a result of free-radical reactions. Similar reactions have been noted in association with drugs that contain quinone and hydroxyquinone groups. Since adriamycin contains both groups, it was felt that a similar mechanism might be operative, and that administration of large doses of vitamin E might be protective against myocardial damage [44]. Although this was proved to be true in cases of acute toxicity in animals [45], no protective effect in humans on chronic adriamycin therapy could be seen [46,47]. Nevertheless, the possibility that α-tocopherol in conjunction with other agents might be efficacious remains open.

CONCLUSIONS

The untreated cancer patient has a host of nutritional and metabolic defects that appear to have a deleterious, though poorly defined, effect on the prognosis. Treatment often adds other abnormalities, some obvious and others more subtle. The effect of these superimposed metabolic and nuritional aberrations on morbidity and mortality remains to be determined.

ACKNOWLEDGMENTS

This work was supported in part by RR00039 and by the R and D Career Development Program of the Veterans Administration.

REFERENCES

1. Lawson DH, Richmond A, Nixon DW, Rudman D (1982): Metabolic approaches to cancer cachexia. Annu Rev Nutr 2:277–301.
2. DeWys WD (1979): Anorexia as a general effect of cancer. Cancer 43:2013–2019.
3. DeWys WD, Begg C, Lavin PT, Band PR, Bennett JM, Bertino JR, Cohen MH, Douglas MD, Engstrom PE, Ezdinli EZ, Morton J, Johnson GJ, Moertel CG, Oken MM, Perlia C, Rosenbaum C, Silverstein MN, Skeel RT, Sponzo RW, Tormey DC (1980): Prognostic effect of weight loss prior to chemotherapy in cancer patients. Am J Med 69:491–497.
4. Nixon DW, Heymsfield SB, Cohen AE, Kutner MH, Ansley J, Lawson DH, Rudman D (1980): Protein calorie undernutrition in hospitalized cancer patients. Am J Med 68:683–690.
5. Heymsfield SB, Horowitz J, Lawson DH (1981): Enteral hyperalimentation. In Berk JE (ed): "Developments in Digestive Diseases." Philadelphia: Lea and Febiger, Vol 3, pp 59–83.
6. Warren S (1932): The immediate causes of death in cancer. Am J Med Sci 184:610–615.
7. Houten L, Reilley AA (1980): An investigation of the causes of death from cancer. J Surg Oncol 13:111–116.
8. Harnett WL (1952): "British Empire Cancer Campaign: A Survey of Cancer in London." London: British Empire Cancer Campaign.
9. Garattini S, Bizzi A, Donelli MG, Guaitani A, Samanira R, Spreafico F (1980): Anorexia and cancer in animals and man. Cancer Treat Rev 7:115–140.
10. Morrison SD (1982): Control of food intake in the experimental cancerous host. In "Proceedings of the 34th Annual M.D. Anderson Hospital Tumor Institute Symposium on Fundamental Cancer Research." Houston: The Institute, pp 1323–1326.
11. Lawrence W (1979): Effects of cancer on nutrition: Impaired organ system effects. Cancer 43:2020–2029.

12. Burke M, Bryson EI, Kark AE (1980): Dietary intakes, resting metabolic rates and body composition in benign and malignant gastrointestinal disease. Br Med J 280:211–215.
13. Costa G, Lane WW, Vincent RG, Siebold JA, Aragon M, Bewley PT (1980): Weight loss and cachexia in lung cancer. Nutr Cancer 2:98–103.
14. Holrode CP, Gabuzda TG, Putnam RC, Paul P, Reichard GA (1975): Altered glucose metabolism in metastatic carcinoma. Cancer Res 35:3710–3714.
15. Lundholm K, Bylund AC, Schersten T (1977): Glucose tolerance in relation to skeletal muscle enzyme activities in cancer patients. Scand. J Clin Lab Invest 37:267–272.
16. Fenninger LD, Mider GB (1954): Energy and nitrogen metabolism in cancer. Adv Cancer Res 2:229–253.
17. Ramaswamy K, Lyon I, Baker N (1980): Dietary control of lipogenesis in vivo in host tissues and tumors of mice bearing Ehrlich ascites carcinoma. Cancer Res 40:4606–4611.
18. Schein PS, Kisner D, Maller D, Blecher M, Hamosh M (1979): Cachexia of malignancy: Potential role of insulin in nutritional management. Cancer 43:2070–2076.
19. Lundholm K, Holm G, Schersten T (1978): Insulin resistance in patients with cancer. Cancer Res 38:4665–4669.
20. Donaldson SS, Lenon RA (1979): Alterations of nutritional status. Impact of chemotherapy and radiation therapy. Cancer 43:2036–2052.
21. Copeland EM, Daly JM, Dudrick SJ (1981): Nutrition and Cancer. Intern Adv Surg Oncol 4:1–13.
22. Ohnuma T, Holland JF (1977): Nutritional consequences of cancer chemotherapy and immunotherapy. Cancer Res 37:2395–2406.
23. Dionigi R, Campani M (1981): Nutritional and immunological abnormalities in malignant disease. Acta Chir Scand (Suppl) 507:435–474.
24. Donaldson SS, (1982): Effects of therapy on nutritional status of the pediatric cancer patient. Cancer Res 42:7295–7365.
25. Dudrick SJ (1977): Nutrition as an adjunct to cancer treatment in the adult. Cancer Res 37: 2451–2455.
26. Hilton MA, Kmetz DR, Patel CC (1975): Plasma amino acids during high-dose methotrexate-citrovorum rescue. Biochem Med 16:9–15.
27. Moran RG, Werkheiser WC, Zakrzewski SF (1976): Folate metabolism in mammalian cells in culture. J Biol Chem 251:3569–3575.
28. Benet LL, Shanon WM, Allan PW, Arnett G (1975): Studies on the biochemical basis for the antiviral activities of some nucleoside analogs. Ann NY Acad Sci 255:342–358.
29. Sacks SL, Merigan TC, Kaminska MJ, Fox IH (1982): Inactivation of S-adenosylhomocysteine hydrolase during adenine arabinoside therapy. J Clin Invest 69:226–230.
30. Helland S, Ueland PM (1982): Inactivation of S-adenosylhomocysteine hydrolase by 9-β-D-arabinofuranoxyladenine in intact cells. Cancer Res 42:1130–1136.
31. Hyanek J, Bremer HJ, Slavik M (1969): "Homocystinuria" and urinary excretion of β-amino acid in patients treated with 6-azauridine. Clin Chim Acta 25:288–290.
32. Slavik M, Lovenberg W, Keiser MR (1973): Changes in serum and urine amino acids in patients with progressive systemic sclerosis treated with 6-azauridine triacetate. Biochem Pharmacol 22:1295–1300.
33. Gurto HL, Hipkens JH, Sharma SD (1981): Role of glutathione in the metabolism-dependent toxicity and chemotherapy of cyclophosphamide. Cancer Res 41:3584–3591.
34. Holcenberg JS, Roberts J (1977): Enzymes as drugs. Annu Rev Pharmacol Toxicol 17:97–116.
35. Roberts J, Schmid FA, Rosenfeld HJ (1979): Biologic and antineoplastic effects of enzyme-mediated in vivo depletion of L-glutamine, L-tryptophan, and L-histidine. Cancer Treat Rep 63:1045–1054.

36. Vistica DT, Toal JN, Rabinovitz M (1978): Amino acid-conferred protection against Melphalan: Characterization of melphalan transport and correlation of uptake with cytotoxicity in cultured L1210 murine leukemia cells. Biochem Pharmacol 27:2865–2870.

37. Vistica DT, von Hoff DD, Torain B (1981): Uptake of melphalan by human ovarian carcinoma cells and its relationship to the amino acid content of ascitic fluid. Cancer Treat Rep 65:157–161.

38. Vistica DT, Rabon A, Rabinovitz M (1978): Enhancement of melphalan therapy with glutaminase:asparaginase. Res Commun Chem Pathol Pharmacol 22:83–91.

39. Holcenberg J, Anderson T, Ritch P, Skibba J, Howser D, Ring B, Adams S, Helmsworth M (1983): Intraperitoneal chemotherapy with melphalan plus glutaminase. Cancer Res 43: 1381–1388.

40. Warrell RP, Burchenal JH (1983): Methylglyoxal-bis-(guanylhydrazone)(methyl-GAG): Current status and future prospects. J Clin Oncol 1:52–65.

41. Schilsky RL, Anderson T (1979): Hypomagnesemia and renal magnesium wasting in patients receiving cis-platin. Ann Intern Med 90:929–931.

42. Davis S, Kessler W, Haddad BM, Maesaka JK (1980): Acute renal tubular dysfunction following cis-dichlorodiamineplatinum therapy. J Med 11:133–141.

43. Hayes FA, Green AA, Senger N, Pratt CB (1979): Tetany: A complication of cis-dichlorodiamineplatinum (II) therapy. Cancer Treat Rep 63:547–548.

44. Myers CE, McGuire W, Young R (1976): Adriamycin: amelioration of toxicity by α-tocopherol. Cancer Treat Rep 60:961–962.

45. Wang Y-M, Madanat FF, Kimball JC, Gleiser CA, Ali MK, Kaufman MW, Van Eys J (1980): Effect of Vitamin E against Adriamycin-induced toxicity in rabbits. Cancer Res 40: 1022–1027.

46. Legha SS, Wang Y-M, MacKay B, Ewer M, Hortobagyi GN, Benjamin RS, Ali MK (1982): Clinical and pharmacologic investigation of the effects of α-tocopherol on Adriamycin cardiotoxicity. Ann NY Acad Sci 393:411–418.

47. Weitzman SA, Lorell B, Carey RW, Kaufman S, Stossel TP (1980): Prospective study of tocopherol prophylaxis for anthracycline cardiac toxicity. Curr Ther Res 28:682–686.

Malnutrition: Determinants and Consequences, pages 403–404
© 1984 Alan R. Liss, Inc., 150 Fifth Avenue, New York, NY 10011

Hospital Malnutrition: What Does It Mean? (Abstract)

Douglas W. Wilmore, MD
Department of Surgery, Harvard Medical School and Brigham and Women's
Hospital, Boston, Massachusetts 02115

It has been suggested that malnutrition is widespread among patients hospitalized longer than 2 weeks. It has also been said that many of these changes are avoidable or that they are related to the disease process or its treatment. With the advent of specialized tube feedings and a variety of parenteral formulas for intravenous infusion, nutrient requirements can be met in almost all hospital patients. With the issue of cost-effective medical care central to the planning of much of our medical and surgical therapy, the decision as to how to feed hospitalized patients is an extremely important one. Do patients in US hospitals really become malnourished? If so, can this malnutrition be prevented with newly devised techniques of enteral and parenteral nutrition? Is this cost-effective therapy? Finally, will nutritional intervention improve patient outcome?

Malnutrition is usually defined as a state of nutrient(s) excess or deficiency, the normal nutritional state being measured in a precise manner. For example, the components of the body have been determined and for any given age and sex a norm with 95% confidence limits has been established. For any individual patient, lean body mass, total body fat, muscle mass, organ size, and concentrations of nutrients in biologic fluids and tissues can be determined and these measurements compared with norms to determine if nutrient excess or deficiency exists. However, such quantitations are done at a single point in time and contribute very little to our appreciation of the nutritional state as it relates to the past medical history of the patient or to the future therapy.

Another approach has been to use indicators that are utilized to define nutritional status of large populations. By using such tests, it has been reported that 79% of the patients remaining 2 weeks or longer in a large university hospital demonstrated a decline in average arm muscle circumference, that 75% lost weight during their hospitalization, that 64% had a fall in hematocrits (average hematocrit decrease of 8%), and that serum albumin declined in 47% of the subjects (average of 0.4 gm/dl). From a purely nutritional point of view, such changes are appalling, but when integrated into the hospital course of a patient, it may not be surprising that individuals who are bedridden with an arm strapped to an IV board will show some change in arm muscle circumference, that people who cannot eat because of treatment or disease will show some loss of body weight (weight loss would be viewed as an asset in over 25% of the adult population), that a hematocrit fall associated with operative procedures or blood drawing may not reflect iron deficiency, and that a decline in serum albumin concentration following a major operative procedure or illness may reflect redistribution of the albumin in an enlarged compartment, rather than nutritional inadequacy. Therefore, such criteria serve to alert the medical professionals that an individual is not normal (and that is usually why the person is hospitalized), but they rarely quantitate nutritional inadequacies that have occurred.

A final approach is more integrated and provides a functional definition of malnutrition for the hospitalized patient. That is to say, hospital malnutrition occurs when nutritional deficiencies interact with the disease process to prolong illness, to increase hospitalization, or to increase the degree of disability. By such a definition, normal body composition or nutrient concentration would not need to be rigidly maintained. Rather, safe limits would be set and nutritional intervention would be required when these limits were approached. Most, if not all, hospitalized patients, after 5-7 days, would receive some form of nutritional support containing protein or amino acid equivalents, although some degree of weight loss would be acceptable. Necessary changes in body composition that occur with sophisticated medical and surgical therapy associated with bed rest would be appreciated and minimized by physical therapy. More vigorous nutritional support would subsequently be instituted if indicated.

In the well-nourished patient with a severe catabolic disease, a weight loss of more than 10% body weight would not be allowed. In the malnourished patient vigorous nutritional support would be carried out to achieve weight maintenance; more aggressive nutritional care would be given with resolution of a catabolic disease when the neurohormonal environment favored tissue anabolism. Long-term rebuilding of body mass under such situations would be integrated with the home care, and this could be done by the patient, the family, and/or the visiting nurse with modified dietary care tube feedings or home intravenous nutrition.

If objective evidence of the benefits of nutritional support were not present, then nutritional support would be offered in a manner that would limit risks and minimize costs. If objective evidence demonstrated that nutrition integrated with medical and surgical therapy improved outcome, then vigorous nutritional therapy would be pursued. In such a manner, valuable hospital resources would be judiciously administered to patients where benefits and gains are clear-cut and nutritional therapy would be modified where gains are minimal and risks and costs unacceptable.

Malnutrition: Determinants and Consequences, pages 405–413
© 1984 Alan R. Liss, Inc., 150 Fifth Avenue, New York, NY 10011

Effects of Fad Diets for Weight Reduction

Richard L. Atkinson, MD
Department of Internal Medicine, School of Medicine and Clinical Nutrition
Center, University of California at Davis, Davis, California 95616

INTRODUCTION

During the last century Americans have become the most overweight people on earth. This epidemic of excess adipose tissue has several origins, including an abundance of relatively inexpensive food, changes in the types of food eaten, increasing availability of food, and a progressive decrease in the activity associated with daily living. As obesity has become more prevalent it has lost its status as a symbol of affluence and has become a social liability. This fact, coupled with the known medical complications of obesity, has stimulated a mania for thinness that itself has reached epidemic proportions. The ideal body weight as perceived socially has steadily decreased and now is below the levels thought to be desirable by life insurance company statistics (Metropolitan Life Insurance Company). This preoccupation with thinness has resulted in a steady stream of new diets and commercial and university-based weight reduction programs. Some of these diets and programs are sensible, but others are nonsensical, having no basis in scientific observations, and may even be dangerous [White and Selvey, 1982]. Most of these diets and weight reduction programs are unsuccessful because they do not alter the person's long-term eating habits and lifestyle and they are not developed with recognition of the physiologic factors that regulate body weight at a given level [Keesey, 1980]. This chapter will briefly survey some of the current fad diets for weight reduction and will discuss in detail the most popular, very-low-calorie formula diets. Most new diets can be classified as one of the following: balanced low-calorie diets, one-food diets, "magic" diets, diets based on elimination of one or more nutrients, and what may constitute a new fad, high-fiber diets.

BALANCED LOW-CALORIE DIETS

These diets contain a mix of protein, carbohydrate, and fat in a general ratio of about 20%, 40%, and 40% of calories, respectively. By cutting back on portion sizes, total calorie intake is reduced and weight loss theoretically ensues. This type of diet is usually prescribed by physicians and nutritionists as being a safe, nutritionally sound method of losing weight. Unfortunately the long-term success rate with such diets in treating obesity is less than 5% [Stunkard and McLaren-Hume, 1959]. Psychologically it is difficult to restrict oneself continuously to small amounts of food when food is so generally available. In addition, it appears that there may be physiologic factors that stimulate hunger and increase energy efficiency when body weight deviates significantly below a "setpoint" [Keesey, 1980].

ONE-FOOD DIETS

The most widely known diet of this category is the "rice diet" originated by Kempner at Duke University [Kempner, 1949]. Other examples of this genre are the "banana diet," the "ice cream diet," and the "steak diet." The success of these diets depends upon monotony. Although unlimited quantities of the food may be allowed, after a few meals the subject no longer wishes to eat much. As a result, calorie intake declines and weight is lost. These diets are not suitable for long periods because of the risk of deficiencies of vitamins or other nutrients. They do not incorporate any mechanism for changing the lifestyle, and in general are useful only for modest weight loss over a short period of time. Large weight loss requires almost constant supervision on an inpatient status.

"MAGIC" DIETS

Many diets foisted upon the public require suspension of rationality. Netter [1975] nicely summarized the appeal of diets that promise easy weight loss with minimal effort. The common factors of such diets are that they are promoted by unqualified or self-proclaimed "nutritionists," they promise easy weight loss, and they have little or no basis in scientific observation. An older example is the "grapefruit diet." Supposedly, grapefruit has a factor that allows the dieter to "burn off" excess calories. Thus, the dieter may eat as much as is desired as long as grapefruit is included. Another recent diet is the "Beverly Hills Diet." The author [Mazel, 1981] devised a complicated scheme of food intake based predominantly on fruit. Fruit assumes the magical property of enhancing metabolism and ridding the body of fat. Certain foods cannot be eaten together, as the combination causes loss of the beneficial effects. No documentation of these claims was provided. The hazards of this diet and of eating fruit to the exclusion of other foods were pointed out by Mirkin and Shore [1981].

The Zen macrobiotic diet is heavily endowed with mysticism and in its purest form consists only of brown rice and tea [Berland, 1974]. This diet, which was a fad more than a decade ago, has been severely criticized and may be dangerous if followed for long periods, as protein malnutrition may occur [Berland, 1974].

REDUCTION OR ELIMINATION OF ONE OR MORE NUTRIENTS

This category comprises most of the popular diets in the lay press. The diet with by far the most variations is the low-carbohydrate diet. This diet consists of predominantly protein and fat foods (mainly meat) and contains little or no carbohydrate. This diet has resurfaced many times since 1863 [Banting, 1863] with the name of a person or place attached. Recently it has been promoted as "Dr. Atkins' Diet Revolution" [Atkins, 1972], "The Complete Scarsdale Medical Diet" [Tarnower and Baker, 1978], "The Last Chance Diet" [Linn, 1977], and as a variety of formula diets such as Optifast, Modifast, and The Cambridge Diet.

There are several reasons for the popularity and effectiveness of this diet. The low level of carbohydrate results in diuresis, with losses of sodium and water that accelerate initial weight loss [Sigler, 1975; DeHaven et al, 1980]. Persons staying on this diet only briefly may lose fairly large amounts of weight. This provides immediate reinforcement, and for those remaining longer on the diet the low calorie intake of most of these diets causes sustained weight loss of relatively large amounts each week. The mechanism of the sodium and water loss is thought to be the combination of decreased insulin secretion, increased glucagon secretion, and production of ketone bodies [Saudek et al, 1973; DeHaven et al, 1980]. Insulin has a sodium-retaining effect on the kidney, whereas glucagon causes a natriuresis [Saudek et al, 1973]. In the absence of carbohydrate and insulin, fatty acids are broken down into ketones, which may be used for energy. Keto acids are negative ions excreted in the urine that must carry a positive ion to maintain chemical equilibrium. The most commonly excreted positive ions are sodium, potassium, and ammonium, thus furthering the natriuresis and diuresis and helping to maintain a lower body weight as a result of decreased total body water.

A second reason low-carbohydrate diets are popular is that hunger decreases on such diets. The increased production of ketones has been said to diminish hunger [Howard, 1981]. However, this has been challenged, and in a controlled setting, subjects on normal versus low-carbohydrate diets had a similar loss of hunger sensation. Regardless of changes in hunger sensation, our anecdotal observations of patients on very-low-calorie formula diets containing low carbohydrate levels show that such diets are better tolerated for longer periods than are balanced low-calorie diets. The explantion for this difference may be that formula diets are easier to follow than diets containing small amounts of food. Psychologically, it is easier to eat no food than to eat small amounts.

Blackburn et al [1973] and Genuth et al [1974] described the use of a low-calorie, low-carbohydrate, moderate-protein diet that could be followed for long periods of time with minimal nitrogen loss. These basic observations were presented to the lay public as "The Last Chance Diet" [Linn, 1977]. This diet consisted of about 1–1.5 gm of protein per kilogram of body weight per day and minimal to no carbohydrate intake. The protein source recommended was hydrolyzed collagen. Surveys after the fact estimated that several hundred thousand people used this diet, and 58 deaths were attributed to cardiac arrhythmias secondary to the diet [Sours et al, 1981]. Sours et al evaluated 17 of the 58 patients for whom no other predisposing factors for arrhythmias were apparent. The etiology of the arrhythmias remained unclear, but the US Food and Drug Administration acted to require a warning label on hydrolyzed collagen diets, and their use has almost ceased. Other investigators have described problems in patients on hydrolyzed collagen diets including anecdotal reports of death or serious arrhythmias [Michiel et al, 1978; Siegel et al, 1981]. Lantigua et al [1980] studied six patients for 40 days on a hydrolyzed collagen diet and found arrhythmias on Holter monitors in three. However, when this study was repeated with high-quality protein, no excess arrhythmias, compared to control, were noted (Lockwood, personal communication). This suggests that there may be some toxin in the hydrolyzed collagen that causes arrhythmias. Alternately, the hydrolyzed collagen may lack enough of the essential amino acids that this deficiency in some way predisposes to arrhythmias.

Other explanations have been advanced for the etiology of cardiac arrhythmias in patients on very-low-calorie diets. Since ketogenic diets are associated with potassium loss, hypokalemia is a possible cause. Several of the subjects who died had hypokalemia, but many did not [Frank et al, 1981]. Factors other than hypokalemia must play a role, but few patients had measurement of other ions, such as magnesium and only one had measurements of the trace elements copper and zinc.

In addition to the deaths and arrhythmias reported on very-low-calorie ketogenic diets (VLCKD), a number of lesser side effects have been noted [Bistrian et al, 1976; Atkinson and Kaiser, 1981]. Many patients complain of headache, nausea, diarrhea, constipation, lethargy, and lack of stamina [Atkinson and Kaiser, 1981]. We noted gout in several patients who had a prior history of gout [Atkinson and Kaiser, 1981], but we have never seen the new onset of gout in a patient on a VLCKD. Serum uric acid rises initially in virtually all patients whose carbohydrate intake is less than 40 gm per day. In the majority of these patients uric acid decreases towards baseline and may even fall below baseline after a few weeks on the diet.

The importance of the negative nitrogen balance in subjects on a VLCKD is a matter of great controversy. The initial reports demonstrated that, on the average, subjects achieve nitrogen balance after a few days or weeks on a

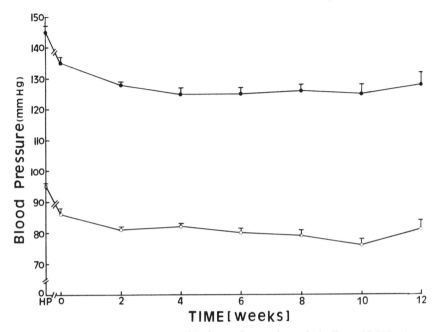

Fig. 1. Blood pressure response to weight loss and a very-low-calorie diet. Initial blood pressure was taken during the initial physical exam. Week 0 is at the end of phase I of the weight reduction program. Weeks 2–12 are on VLCKD. From Atkinson and Kaiser [1981], with permission.

VLCKD [Howard, 1981]. However, more recent studies have pointed out that it may take up to 6 weeks to achieve nitrogen balance, and some patients never achieve equilibrium, but remain in negative balance. For those who do achieve nitrogen equilibrium, this early loss of nitrogen may not be important, as several studies have shown that significantly obese subjects have a greater lean body mass. However, the long-term consequences for those patients who do not go into nitrogen balance are unknown, and further research is needed to prove the long-term safety of a VLCKD.

Despite these obvious disadvantages of a VLCKD, we have found these diets to be clinically useful in the controlled setting of our university-based outpatient weight reduction program. A VLCKD allows rapid weight loss in the severely obese with a minimal degree of hunger. Problems such as hypertension and sleep apnea may resolve very quickly with rapid weight loss on a VLCKD. We found that approximately 40% of our obese outpatients had hypertension [Atkinson and Kaiser, 1981]. Mean blood pressure fell by 19 mm Hg shortly after the start of a VLCKD and remained lower for the duration of the diet (Fig. 1). However, many patients became hypertensive again when they went off the VLCKD if they began to overeat and regain some of their lost weight.

Sleep apnea occurs fairly frequently in massively obese subjects, but in many cases it responds to small amounts of weight loss. We recently treated a patient with severe sleep apnea and concomitant congestive heart failure and hypersomnolence (Pickwickian syndrome). She was admitted to the hospital for weight loss. Using a low-calorie diet (Cambridge Diet mixed with milk, supplying about 800 kcal per day), she lost about 50 pounds in 6 weeks. Repeat sleep studies showed a marked improvement with virtual resolution of the sleep apnea.

Type II diabetes mellitus also responds rapidly to a VLCKD [Bistrian et al, 1976]. We did preliminary studies on 20 obese diabetic patients and found that 80% were able to achieve blood sugars below 150 mg% after 1–28 days on a VLCKD [Atkinson et al, in press].

A number of low-calorie formulas are available commercially. Optifast is the original product developed by Genuth and co-workers [1974], although the protein content has been increased from 45 gm to 70 gm per day. It is sold only through physicians who have received training in the use of the VLCKD by the manufacturer. The Cambridge Diet is currently the most popular fad diet. It was developed by Howard in Cambridge, England and contains 33 gm of good-quality protein and 45 gm of carbohydrate [Baird et al, 1974]. The distribution system is through lay "counselors" who receive a percentage of the profit for each can sold. This counselor system has advantages and disadvantages. The counselors are required by the company to hold frequent small-group meetings to provide support and encouragement, and to answer questions. This support system may be helpful in maintaining weight loss and is similar to other organizations such as TOPS or Overeaters Anonymous. The disadvantage of the counselor system is that the counselors are not trained in nutrition and may overstep their competency in advising their customers. Although all customers are encouraged to see their private physician before going on the diet, this is not required for purchase of the formula.

Despite the controversy surrounding the use of the VLCKD, we have used such diets in our outpatient weight reduction program, keeping the patients under close medical supervision. We believe a VLCKD can be useful when combined with a long-term, comprehensive program for weight maintenance once target weight is achieved. The use of a VLCKD for rapid weight loss in the absence of such a long-term plan for weight maintenance cannot be condoned.

HIGH-FIBER DIETS

High-fiber diets are developing into a fad in this country. The diet by Pritikin and McGrady [1979] and "The F-Plan Diet" [Eyton, 1982] are examples of this type of diet. Unlike many of the other fad diets, high-fiber diets do have support in the medical literature. Several investigators demonstrated improvement in glucose tolerance [Kiehm et al, 1976; Simpson et al, 1981] and in serum lipid levels [Anderson and Chen, 1979] with the use of high-fiber diets. Other claims that a high-fiber intake may decrease the incidence of cancer of the colon, diverticulitis, heart disease, and various other diseases have not been scientifically proven. The evidence that high-fiber diets are useful for weight reduction is scanty. A few studies have shown weight loss with a high-fiber diet [Bosello et al, 1980; Mickelsen et al, 1979], and Weinsier et al [1982] have proposed a theoretical mechanism by which fiber might promote decreased calorie intake and weight reduction. Weinsier's belief is that the time required to chew high-fiber foods, coupled with their relatively low calorie content, results in a time-calorie displacement and reduced energy intake. Numerous investigators have reported that vegetarians, who consume a high-fiber diet, weigh less and have a lower incidence of hypertension, heart disease, and diabetes than do nonvegetarians [Ophir et al, 1983]. In our laboratory we tend to believe that high-fiber diets will prove beneficial. Further research is necessary to confirm the initial findings of beneficial effects and the mechanisms of action of high-fiber diets.

SUMMARY

Obesity is a chronic disorder that requires lifelong alterations in lifestyle and eating habits. Fad diets generally address only short-term weight loss and not long-term maintenance of body weight. Diets may be classified according to the amount and proportions of fat, carbohydrate, and protein. The currently popular very-low-calorie formula diets have the potential to be abused, but may be useful in a controlled setting as part of a comprehensive program for the long-term treatment of obesity. High-fiber diets are becoming more popular and may be the fad of the future. Long-term use of a high-fiber, low-fat diet is theoretically optimal for weight reduction, but further studies are necessary to demonstrate the clinical usefulness of this diet.

ACKNOWLEDGMENTS

I thank Carolyn Russ for editorial assistance and Tamra Barker for typing the manuscript.

REFERENCES

Anderson J, Chen W (1979): Plant fiber, carbohydrate and lipid metabolism. Am J Clin Nutr 32:346–363.
Atkins RC (1972): "Dr. Atkins' Diet Revolution: The High Calorie Way to Stay Thin Forever." New York: David McKay, Inc.

Atkinson RL, Kaiser DL (1981): Nonphysician supervision of a very low calorie diet; results in over 200 cases. Int J Obesity 5:237-241.

Atkinson RL, Berke LK, Kaiser DL, Pohl SL (in press): Effects of very low calorie diets on glucose tolerance and diabetes mellitus in obese humans. In Blackburn GL (ed): "Proceedings of a Symposium on Very Low Calorie Diets." New York: Alan R. Liss.

Baird IMcL, Parsons RL, Howard AN (1974): Chemical and metabolic studies of chemically defined diets in the management of obesity. Metabolism 23:645-657.

Banting W (1863): "Letter on Corpulence, Addressed to the Public." 2nd Ed. London: Harrison, p 22.

Berland T (1974): "Rating the Diets." Chicago: Rand McNally, pp 266-278.

Bistrian BR, Blackburn GL, Flatt JP, Sizer I, Scrimshaw NS, Sherman M (1976): Nitrogen metabolism and insulin requirements in obese diabetic adults on a protein-sparing modified fast. Diabetes 25:494-504.

Blackburn GL, Flatt JP, Clowes GHA Jr, O'Donnell TF, Hensle TE (1973): Protein sparing therapy during periods of starvation with sepsis or trauma. Ann Surg 177:588-594.

Bosello O, Ostuzzi R, Armellini F, Miccido R, Scuro L (1980): Glucose tolerance and blood lipids in bran-fed patients with impaired glucose tolerance. Diabetes Care 3:46-49.

DeHaven I, Sherwin R, Hendler R, Felig P (1980): Nitrogen and sodium balance and sympathetic-nervous-system activity in obese subjects treated with a low-calorie protein or mixed diet. N Engl J Med 302:477-482.

Eyton A (1982): "The F-Plan Diet." New York: Crown.

Frank A, Graham C, Frank S (1981): Fatalities on the liquid-protein diet: An analysis of possible causes. Int J Obesity 5:243-248.

Genuth SM, Castro JH, Vertes V (1974): Weight reduction in obesity by outpatient semistarvation. JAMA 230:987-208.

Howard AN (1981): The historical development, efficacy and safety of very-low-calorie diets. Int J Obesity 5:185-208.

Keesey RE (1980): A set point analysis of the regulation of body weight. In Stunkard AJ (ed): "Obesity." Philadelphia: WB Saunders, pp 144-165.

Kempner W (1949): Treatment of heart and kidney disease and of hypertensive and arteriosclerotic vascular disease with rice diet. Ann Intern Med 31:821-856.

Kiehm T, Anderson J, Ward K (1976): Beneficial effects of a high carbohydrate, high fiber diet on hyperglycemic diabetic men. Am J Clin Nutr 29:895-899.

Lantigua RA, Amatruda IM, Biddle TL, Forbes GB, Lockwood DH (1980): Cardiac arrhythmias associated with a liquid protein diet for the treatment of obesity. N Engl J Med 303:735-738.

Linn R (1977): "The Last Chance Diet Book." New York: Bantam.

Mazel J (1981): "The Beverly Hills Diet." New York: Macmillan.

Michiel RR, Sneider JS, Dickstein RA, Hayman H, Eich RH (1978): Sudden death in a patient on a liquid protein diet. N Engl J Med 298:1005-1007.

Mickelsen O, Makdani DD, Cotton RH, Titcomb ST, Colmay IC, Gatty R (1979): Effects of a high fiber bread diet on weight loss in college-age males. Am J Clin Nutr 32:1703-1709.

Mirkin GB, Shore RN (1981): The Beverly Hills Diet. Dangers of the newest weight loss fad. JAMA 246:2235-2237.

Netter F (1975): "Fad Diets Can Be Deadly." Hicksville: Exposition Press, pp 3-18.

Ophir P, Peer G, Gilad J, Blum M, Aviram A (1983): Low blood pressure in vegetarians: The possible role of potassium. Am J Clin Nutr 37:755-762.

Pritikin N, McGrady PM Jr (1979): "The Pritikin Program for Diet and Exercise." New York: Grosset and Dunlap.

Saudek CD, Boulter PR, Arky RA (1973): The natriuretic effect of glucagon and its role in starvation. J Clin Endocrinol Metab 36:761–765.

Siegel RJ, Cabeen WR Jr, Roberts WC (1981): Prolonged QT interval-ventricular tachycardia syndrome from massive rapid weight loss utilizing the liquid-protein-modified-fast diet: Sudden death with sinus node ganglionitis and neuritis. Am Heart J 102:121–123.

Sigler MH (1975): The mechanism of the natriuresis of fasting. J Clin Invest 55:377–387.

Simpson H, Lousley S, Geekie M, Simpson RW, Carter RD, Hockaday T, Mann J (1981): A high carbohydrate leguminous fibre diet improves all aspects of diabetic control. Lancet 1: 1–5.

Sours HE, Frattali VP, Brand CD, Feldman RA, Forbes AL, Swanson RC, Paris AL (1981): Sudden death associated with very low calorie weight reduction regimes. Am J Clin Nutr 34: 453–461.

Stunkard AJ, McLaren-Hume M (1959): The results of treatment for obesity. A review of the literature and report of a series. Arch Intern Med 103:79–85.

Tarnower H, Baker SS (1978): "The Complete Scarsdale Medical Diet." New York: Rawson, Wade.

Weinsier R, Johnston M, Doleys D, Bacon J (1982): Dietary management of obesity: Evaluation of the time-energy displacement diet in terms of its efficacy and nutritional adequacy for long-term weight control. Br J Nutr 47:367–378.

White PL, Selvey N (1982): Nutrition and the new health awareness. JAMA 247:2914–2916.

Malnutrition: Determinants and Consequences, pages 415–421
© 1984 Alan R. Liss, Inc., 150 Fifth Avenue, New York, NY 10011

Food and Nutrition Mythology

William T. Jarvis, PhD
Department of Public Health Science, Loma Linda University, School of Allied Health Professions and California Council Against Health Fraud, Loma Linda, California 92354

Dictionaries vary in their definitions of "myth." One definition is "an unfounded belief held uncritically..." [Gove, 1972]. Some examples of food myths are the following.

According to a fourth century B.C. poet, a taboo against eating pork arose among the Galatians because Attis the Phrygian was killed by a wild boar [Pyke, 1970]. Beet juice is believed to be beneficial for the blood because it resembles blood. This notion is based upon the Doctrine of Signatures advanced by Paracelsus, the sixteenth century alchemist. Paracelsus developed the Doctrine of Signatures from the Unity of All Nature concept and its principle that "like cures like."

The Chinese, and others, classify diseases and foods as "hot" or "cold." When a person gets a chill and feels unwell, the common treatment is to cut a few chips of raw ginger and brew it with water and red sugar. The patient drinks it while it is still hot. The idea is to counter the "cold" disease with "hot" foods. In this case, it is not the hot temperature, but the symbolic hotness of these foods that is important [Whang, 1981]. The principle of treating symptoms with "opposites" is completely contrary to the "like cures like" belief. It is compatible with the humoral theory and allopathic medicine established by Hippocrates.

These food myths are easily dismissed by sophisticated Westerners as primitive folklore. However, modern Western man also has developed some food myths. Modern food myths are diverse enough to include all of the major food groups. Furthermore, both positive and negative attributes are assigned to foods in each grouping. For instance, in the milk group, yogurt enjoys a positive image for aiding longevity, while cow's milk is sometimes condemned as being designed for calves, not humans. Meat group myths include the notion that eating raw meat makes a person fierce, leading some boxers to eat a bloody, raw steak before combat. Conversely, vegetarians have argued that the great beasts of burden of the world are herbivores and have extolled a non-meat diet for endurance (Eskimo sled dogs notwithstanding). In the cereal and bread group, negative myths center around "devitalized" white bread; whole wheat is viewed as the "staff of life." Bread myths are among the most romantic in our culture. In times past a woman's worth was judged by the quality of her homemade bread [Fishbein, 1932]. Foods in the fruit and vegetable group suffer from a stigma placed upon them by medical doctors promoting low-carbohydrate diets. On the other hand, they also are often praised beyond reason by vegetarians and fruitarians.

While the four food groups can provide a means for cataloging food myths, modern food mythology is more apt to divide foods into just two groups, "good" and "bad." The term "junk food," although scientifically undefinable [Benarde, 1981; Guthrie, 1977] has nevertheless come into wide use. "Natural," "organic," and "health" foods have become synonymous with "good" foods even though they are also undefinable according to the Federal Trade Commission [Donegan et al, 1978]. Whether a food is mythologized as "good" or "bad" is most likely to be based upon its emotional symbolism. Honey is extolled but sucrose is condemned even though they differ insignificantly in their composition or physiologic effects.

A highly negative mythology has grown up around food additives. Over half of the public view food additives negatively [General Mills, 1980]. This is unfortunate because there is reason to believe that food additives actually aid health and longevity. The food industry apparently has decided not to fight the negative image of food additives despite their knowledge of their safety and health-protecting qualities. By extolling the absence of additives and preservatives in their products they are reinforcing this negative myth.

A recent incident in California illustrates how various nutrients have come to symbolize good or evil. A woman contacted the fraud unit of the Food and Drug Section of the state Department of Health, presenting a pill for analysis that was being touted as a "nonsurgical intestinal bypass pill." Supposedly, the pill would enable "your body to absorb the vitamins and minerals from food while the calories went on through!" The public apparently views "calories" as demons to be exorcised from foods, whereas vitamins and minerals are like the foods of the gods.

Sucrose is often condemned as having only "empty calories." It is unimaginable to a nutrition scientist how a calorie can be considered empty. While sucrose may be devoid of vitamins and minerals, so are vitamins and minerals devoid of caloric value. The body needs both calories and vitamins and minerals for proper functioning, but somehow "empty nutrients" are considered all right by the public while "empty calories" are abhorred.

No aspect of modern food mythology is more interesting than the faith the public places in vitamins. Vitamins are so idolized that politicians have sought to remove them from the rational control of government regulators who must oversee the safety and effectiveness of a wide variety of foods, drugs, and cosmetics. It is enigmatic that an agency like the United States Food and Drug Administration, which must regulate the most potent pharmaceutical chemicals, is prevented from exercising reasonable control over vitamins. Paradoxically, Senator Proxmire, who is famous for his "golden fleece award," is the author of the bill that has caused millions of Americans to be fleeced by the vitamin promoters. The Proxmire Bill was described by the FDA Commissioner Alexander M. Schmidt as "a charlatan's dream" [Consumer's Union, 1980], because it permitted the marketing of supplements like bioflavonoids, para-amino benzoic acid, lecithin, etc. that are unnecessary in the human diet. In 1981, Senator Orrin Hatch introduced S.1277 with the pompous title of "The Voluntary Vitamins Act of 1981." It would have removed FDA's option to regulate vitamins or minerals as drugs or food additives. Such legislation can only be seen as bizarre by anyone with a modicum of understanding about the functioning of biologically active chemicals. The dose, not the substance, determines whether a substance should be regarded as a food, drug or poison [Oace, 1982].

The emotional significance of vitamins may be understood best when viewed historically. Working backward in time we find that historic misconceptions were compounded resulting in today's vitamin mythology. The word "vitamin" is a conjugation of "vital amine" done by Funk [Williams, 1969] when he thought he had discovered the essential element in food that was "vital" to life. The "amine" portion of the word is based upon Funk's belief that the vital substance was a protein. The idea that the vital element in food was a protein stemmed from the work of Magendie, who in 1816 had determined that animals needed nitrogen-containing foods to survive. Twenty-two years later (1838), utilizing the Greek word meaning "first," Mulder gave the name "protein" (ie, "first foods") to nitrogen-containing (termed "albuminous foods") foods because they were thought to contain *the essential element necessary for life* [Lowenberg et al, 1968]. The belief that food contained a basic vital element can be traced back through the alchemists, who searched for the Elixir Vitae [MacKay, 1977], to Galen, who espoused the doctrine of Vitalism [Garrison, 1929]; Hippocrates, who thought foods contained a single principle [Young, 1978]; and the magical thinking of antiquity [Mahdihassan, 1979], which espoused the Unity of All Nature principle. While nutrition science uses the term to classify organic substances needed exogenously in the diet, the work "vitamin" seems to conjure up in the public's mind a great deal of the mystification inherent in the ancient search for the life-sustaining essence in food [Bitensky, 1973].

The ultimate nutrition myth in Western society is set forth in the homely expression "You are what you eat." This statement fits Pyke's description of a food myth. He says, "A food myth, although basically fictitious, may yet contain some element of truth" [Pyke, 1970]. The concept of "you are what you eat" contains an element of truth, but is misleading. It is often employed to advance the exaggerations that characterize food faddism. Part of the falsity of the phrase "you are what you eat" may be seen in a joke told by comedienne Phyllis Diller, who says that when she heard people are what they eat she "followed Raquel Welch around for months eating everything Raquel ate, but it didn't help a bit!" Diller's bit of humor illustrates the importance of genetics in nutrition, a factor that extends beyond external beauty and includes metabolism, as is clear in familial hypercholesterolemia. As important as genetics is, the role of physical activity is also dominant. This can be illustrated by an experiment that will produce results so certain that one need not conduct it. Take a pair of healthy, identical-twin, college athletes. Feed both the same 3,000-calorie-a-day diet. Have one do high-resistance exercises and run several miles a day while the other is restricted to bed rest. In a few weeks, noticeable differences in their body compositions will surely emerge in these genetically and nutritionally identical subjects.

The notion of "you are what you eat" can be traced to antiquity. It is revealed in the Unity of All Nature concept. This was expressed in the animistic beliefs of primitives who saw nature as all one piece. They didn't make a distinction between human beings and animals or between animate and inanimate existence. Animals could be ancestors of men and people could change into animals. Trees and stones could possess souls that were transferrable to a man [Nida, 1959]. This Unity of All Nature idea is what leads to the belief that the body parts of certain animals have medicinal value. The rhinoceros and the tiger are threatened with extinction because so many of their body parts are exploited by folk medicine [McNeely et al, 1981]: The tiger's heart may be eaten to acquire strength, courage and cunning. Its penis can be used as an aphrodisiac as can the rhino's horn. All of this is based upon the "like makes like" principle that emerges from the Unity of All Nature concept.

The "you are what you eat" belief was predominant in the health reform movement of the nineteenth century. The American Vegetarian Society, founded in 1850, declared that "comparative anatomy, human physiology, and...chemical analysis...unitedly proclaim that...the human race should subsist upon the productions of the vegetable kingdom." Meat-eating was blamed for all manner of evil. English poet Percy Shelley charged that it was responsible for the bloody excesses of the French Revolution. The vegetarians believed that diet made a difference in the basic physiology and body composition of the eater. They were sure that diet also affected moral behavior [Whorton, 1977]. Today, food faddists are again claiming that diet is the primary cause of juvenile delinquency and criminal behavior.

In California, the man who murdered the mayor of San Francisco invoked the now famous "Twinkie defense" in which he claimed that his having eaten "junk foods" was responsible for his bizarre behavior. Exaggerated notions about "you are what you eat" are also key elements in cancer quackery today. A "holistic health" clinic in California states that "if you are what you eat, then you aren't what you don't," and "it doesn't really matter what it is, whether it's arthritis or migraines or cancer. If you get the system working properly, the body will cure itself." Such thinking combines the "you are what you eat" notion with a faulty naturopathic principle that underlies beliefs in "diet cures." The faulty principle is that "health is *natural* and disease is *unnatural*"; therefore, if you *eat* right and *do* right, you will *be* all right. This false principle is so nearly alike Hippocrates' basic principle that "nature cures" that some fail to distinguish between them. Hippocrates meant to differentiate between natural and supernatural forces. However, the naturopathic notion erroneously applies the concept to its nostrums, which purport to be "natural" and, therefore, superior, although most are no more natural (eg, coffee enemas, dimethyl sulfoxide, laetrile) than conventional modalities. To discover the error in the naturopathic premise one must consider basic natural laws. The first law of thermodynamics states that you cannot make something out of nothing. This law is compatible with the "you are what you eat" statement. At least one death has resulted from an attempt to become a "breatharian," that is, a holy man who could live on air alone. A young Philadelphia college teacher starved to death in his extreme attempt to be "holistic"! It is the second law of thermodynamics, entropy, that makes the "health is natural, disease is unnatural" idea false. According to the law of entropy, orderly systems eventually become random. Therefore, even if one lives an idealized, healthful life the steady-state mechanisms will eventually fail and disorder will occur within the cells. Disease, death, and decomposition —the natural processes of entropy —will follow. By applying these most fundamental natural laws it can be understood that disease is as natural as health. It is only correct to state that disease is abnormal and health is normal [Tabor, 1965].

Interestingly, the same faulty thinking described above is represented in so-called "orthomolecular" therapy. "Ortho" represents "right" and "molecular" stands for molecules, ergo "the right molecules." The concept is that if the right molecules are put into the cells (meaning megadoses of vitamins) they will be healthy. Like the unsound naturopathic theory it ignores the limitations imposed by the intracellular steady-state mechanisms.

In his discussion of the development of food myths, Pyke observed that not only do food myths sometimes contain some truth, but some "articles of doctrine which appear to us to be based upon nutrition science may...include some degree of error which itself may develop into a new myth which modern nutritionists may...come to believe and propagate" [Pyke, 1970]. One doesn't have to search far for examples in which this error may be operative. The dietary recommendations for reducing cancer and heart disease advanced by various "scientific authorities" that are based upon uncertain epidemiologic evidence can be cited. I don't wish to be too hard on the well-meaning people in preventive medicine. Unfortunately, having to make recommendations for lifestyle based upon shaky scientific data is one of the frustrating tasks of practitioners in preventive medicine.

Although we must willingly admit that both "nutrition myths" and some "nutrition truths" are apt to contain a mixture of truth and error, we must hasten to emphasize that they are nevertheless by no means equal in credibility. Traditional myths have little mechanism for change. They are perpetuated by the faulty self-validation of personal experience (ie, it works for me!), selective self-affirmation (ie, recalling the times it worked, while forgetting the failures), and situational application in the manner of common-sense cliches (eg, "haste makes waste" and "he who hesitates is lost" are contradictory common-sense expressions that make sense when applied post hoc in an appropriate situation). On the other hand, beliefs based upon science have a built-in mechanism for correction because one of the unique features of the scientific process is its continual self-criticism [Nagel, 1961].

Perhaps, the reason nutrition myths often triumph over nutrition science is that educational efforts focus too much upon nutrition and not enough upon science — particularly science as a process of testing beliefs. Focusing upon the importance of specific nutrients, overemphasizing the function of each nutrient on specific organs (eg, vitamin A is good for the eyes, B vitamins for the nerves, etc), and creating unnecessary anxiety about nutrient losses in food preparation may be counterproductive. Levine [1973] warns nutritionists of "the human failing whereby the very act of examining a subject in great detail tends to exaggerate its importance." I suspect that almost every nutrition educator has probably told a class, "You are what you eat," without adequately pointing out the basic fallacies inherent in that statement.

One of the great failings of education at all levels has been the failure to develop an appreciation for the scientific process. Science is more than simply a body of knowledge, or logical thinking. It is a process whereby people arrive at beliefs. Nutrition myths are fictions, resulting from faulty processes for arriving at beliefs. Mythology will disappear only when people come to know how to evaluate propositions, understand how easily they can fool themselves with faulty self-validation, and learn to apply the basic rules of scientific thinking. There is no reason why scientific thinking cannot become commonplace. Einstein said that scientific thinking is nothing more than a refinement of everyday thinking [Einstein, 1954]. Experiences with food and nutrition are also everyday occurrences. Only when people begin to think scientifically about foods will nutrition mythology join the now defunct myths of the past such as geocentrism, a flat-earth, sea serpents and mermaids in the sea, and fairies in the woodlands.

REFERENCES

Benarde MA (1981): What's the junk in junk foods. In "The Food Additives Dictionary." New York: Simon and Schuster, Chap 5, pp 31-36.

Bitensky R (1973): The road to Shangri-La is paved with vitamins. Am J Psychiatry 130:1253-1256.

Consumer's Union (1980): "Nutrition as Therapy." Consumer Rep, January, pp 21-24.

Donegan TJ et al (1978): "Proposed Trade Regulation Rule on Food Advertising, Staff Report and Recommendations." Washington, DC: Federal Trade Commission.

Einstein A (1954): "Ideas and Opinions." New York: Dell.

Fishbein M (1932): "Fads and Quackery in Healing." New York: Covici, Friede, pp 255-256.

Garrison FH (1929): "History of Medicine." Philadelphia: W.B. Saunders.

General Mills (1980): "A Summary Report on U.S. Consumers' Knowledge, Attitudes and Practices About Nutrition – 1980." Minneapolis: General Mills, pp 34-36.

Gove P (1972): "Webster's Seventh New Collegiate Dictionary." Springfield, Mass: G. & C. Merriam Co.

Guthrie HA (1977): Concept of a nutritious food. J Am Diet Assoc 71:14-19.

Levine R (1973): Carbohydrates. In Goodhart RS, Shils ME (eds): "Modern Nutrition in Health and Disease." Philadelphia: Lea & Febiger, Chap 3, p 114.

Lowenberg ME, Todhunter EN, Witson ED, Feeney MC, Savage JR (1968): "Food and Man." New York: Wiley, pp 10-11.

MacKay CL (1977): "Extraordinary Popular Delusions and the Madness of Crowds." New York: Noonday Press, pp 98-256.

Mahdihassan S (1979): A comparative study of Greek and Chinese alchemy. Am J Chin Med 7:171-181.

McNeely JA, Wachtel PS (1981): They use everything but the cat's meow. Int Wildlife, May-June, pp 14-19.

Nagel E (1961): "The Structure of Science." New York: Harcourt, Brace & World, pp 1-14.

Nida EA, Smalley WA (1959): "Introducing Animism." New York: Friendship Press.

Oace S (1982): Reader's forum. J Nutr Educ 14:46-47.

Pyke M (1970): The development of food myths. In Blix G (ed): "Symposia of the Swedish Nutrition Foundation, VIII: Food Cultism and Nutrition Quackery." Uppsala: Almqvist and Wiksells, pp 22-29.

Tabor CW (1965): "Cyclopedic Medical Dictionary." 10th Ed. Philadelphia: FA Davis.

Whang J (1981): Chinese traditional food therapy. J Diet Assoc 78:55-57.

Whorton JC (1977): 'Tempest in a fleshpot': The formulation of a physiological rationale for vegetarianism. J Hist Med, April, pp 115-139.

Williams SR (1969): "Nutrition and Diet Therapy." St. Louis: CV Moseby, p 72.

Young JH (1978): The agile hole of food: Some historical reflections. In Hathcock J (ed): "Nutrition and Drug Interrelations." New York: Academic Press, p 5.

Malnutrition: Determinants and Consequences, pages 423–429
© 1984 Alan R. Liss, Inc., 150 Fifth Avenue, New York, NY 10011

Food Ideology and Medicine in Mexico

Luis Alberto Vargas, MD, PhD

Instituto de Investigaciones Antropológicas, National University of Mexico,
04510 México DF, Mexico

INTRODUCTION

This chapter attempts to summarize the way the Mexican traditional culture perceives the relations between food and health care. Most of the information is drawn from the author's field work and from recent papers in Spanish that may be little known to English-speaking scholars.

A title suggested by the organizers of the VII Western Hemisphere Nutrition Congress was "Food Myths and Folk Medicine in Mexico." I considered this title inadequate, for it would convey the idea of an ancient mythology that has survived unchanged in Mexico, a relic of a mysterious past. This is partly true, since Mexico has a popular culture, deeply rooted in its Indian past. This culture, however, changes constantly, incorporating new ideas and concepts and influencing other cultures, among others our own so-called Western culture. A second problem with the original title is the word "myth," which has a precise meaning in anthropological literature, a meaning different from the common use of "myth" to mean something which has no basis in truth or fact. As we shall see, most of the popular ideas on food in Mexico are not necessarily based on the scientific method, but some of them have proven to be effective. Still others are based on a logical "cause-effect" relationship, although their principles may not prove to be true. Finally, I think that the most important aspects to be included in a volume on "Malnutrition: Determinants and Consequences" are the ideas that move people to adopt a certain diet and foodways. For these reasons I have renamed this article "Food Ideology and Medicine in Mexico."

MEDICAL SYSTEMS IN MEXICO

Readers from developed countries find that in their own environment, where they have grown and worked, scientific medicine is the only valid and visible form for the provision of medical care. People often obtain their ideas on health, disease, and medicine from both an educational system and a socializing process, and as a result almost everybody in a society has a similar set of concepts about these issues. For instance, Europeans living in urban areas, as well as most people in the United States, have been taught through their lifetimes that germs exist and that antibiotics kill germs. They also know about mental illness, for instance. The individual confirms his ideas through mass media, and can easily visit a physician to deal with his problems, either in a hospital or in private practice.

In countries such as Mexico, the situation is very different. Scientific medicine may be accessible for only a small part of the population. For instance, the Mexican Minister of Health has acknowledged that at least 15 million Mexicans lack the means to use the resources of scientific medicine [Soberón, 1983]. In large cities such as Mexico City, Guadalajara, Monterrey, or Morelia, a patient can find a type of medical care that is similar in quality to that of industrialized countries. In smaller communities, the *pasante de medicina*, a medical student who has completed all his degree requirements, is the only source of scientific medical care. These *pasantes* have to practice in small and isolated places as a way of repaying the Mexican people and the government for their education.

According to the 1970 census estimates [Collado, 1976], Mexico had only one physician for every 1,414 inhabitants. Although this figure seems adequate, in reality it is deceiving. Most physicians in the Mexican Republic practice in large cities and several states have very diverse ratios of physicians to inhabitants. They vary from 1 per 474 in Mexico City to 1 per 5,601 inhabitants in Chiapas [López Acuña, 1980]. Forty-seven percent of Mexico's municipalities (the smallest political division of the country, roughly equivalent to a county), lack a physician [Collado and García-Torres, 1975]. This means that health care must be sought elsewhere, and the usual resource is a host of local healers known as *curanderos*. This is a catch-all term, since these people can be as highly specialized as their scientific counterparts. For instance, some deal only with childbirth and others practice bone setting; some will treat only specific diseases like *susto* or *mal de ojo* or they handle a special type of therapy based on herbs or certain curing ceremonies.

Countries like Mexico do not have a single unified medical system, but rely on what has been called a series of parallel medical systems [Vargas, 1979], that is, systems that coexist in the same area, interacting with each other. Thus, a Mexican patient decides what type of healer to consult according to diverse factors. For instance, it has been found that an important issue in this process is the diagnosis that the patient or his family has made of the disease [Casillas, 1979]. Among administrative personnel of the National University of Mexico, 32.35% stated that they used only the free scientific medical services of their social security system. The rest usually shopped around among several types of healers, including physicians, depending on what illness they thought they had. A similar study was conducted in a rural area of the state of Morelos [Rodríguez Domínguez et al, 1979]. This study ascertained the type of health care received before patients went to the government-sponsored medical center. Self-care, self-medication, and home remedies were the resources most used, and folk medical practitioners came next. Unfortunately, there is little information on the decision-making process and the choices for medical care in most areas of Mexico.

This situation is certainly full of contradictions. How can a person with pain and tenderness in his throat decide whether to seek a physician for advice, or to take a home remedy such as an herbal infusion, or to go to a *curandero* to have a healing ceremony, or to buy a pack of antibiotic lozenges over the counter in the local drugstore? Apparently there exists a set of very important concepts that involve what this person believes is afflicting him, what his symptoms mean and what type of treatment he should choose. In one situation the patient may adopt the germ theory; in another he may believe in a magical or supernatural cause; or he can see his troubles as part of life's daily afflictions, for which nature has provided handy remedies.

From what I have mentioned, one can conclude that the popular ideology in relation to medicine is very diverse. It is difficult to characterize an individual's concept of health and disease, since it is likely to be a mixture of ideas from the varied systems to which he has access. This is also the case with traditional medical practitioners. Some *curanderos* may refer a patient to the hospital, if he has a disease that the *curandero* considers beyond his resources to heal. We have found that students in a nursing school in Mexico City were very familiar with concepts and practices of popular or traditional medical systems. Some of them are daughters of *curanderas* and they use their scientific resources together with what they learned from their mothers. A perception of magical healing may also be found among medical students, and it is not uncommon to find that Mexican physicians prescribe, or at least accept, the use of folk remedies by their patients.

FOOD AND MEDICINE

Food in Mexico is considered a powerful therapeutic resource. It is important not only as the fuel and building material for the human body, but also as a drug having therapeutic effects *on* the body. This idea certainly has a pre-Hispanic origin. Using the work of López Austin [1975, 1980], a distinguished Mexican historian, I will briefly introduce some of these ancient beliefs.

One of the basic aspects of the Nahuatl concept of the universe relates to its geometry. The universe was perceived as a confrontation of opposites: It was divided horizontally by a plane on which stood the earth, a flat surface surrounded by the sea. Seawater rose at the four edges of this surface to support the heavens and it descended forming the walls of the underworlds. The central part of the square or rectangle of the earth was its navel, the center of everything. There the four directions or regions of the world met. A tree stood at each corner of this world and communicated between the underworlds, the world, and the heavens. The feature to be emphasized is that in this vision the heavens had a set of characteristics that were opposite and complementary to those of the underworld. The heavens were considered as the dwelling of the Father god: They were masculine, hot, dry, and full of light and were related to the day and to fire. They were represented by the eagle. The underworlds were naturally the home of the Mother goddess, being feminine, cold, humid, and dark and related to night and to the wind. They were represented by the jaguar.

Man was a microcosm. He was sensible to changes in his environment, and his own body could change his equilibrium with the environment. And this was indeed a very easily disturbed equilibrium, for many factors could affect it. The most important ones were sex, age, personality, physiological changes such as menstruation or pregnancy, fatigue, sexual activity, and a series of external agents, such as temperature, the evil eye, supernatural forces and, of course, food. Several diseases had their origin in a disturbed equilibrium. I will discuss the disturbances in equilibrium that have been studied the most: The interaction between hot and cold.

HOT AND COLD QUALITIES IN FOOD, DISEASE, AND HEALING

Hot and cold qualities seem to be an important part of the Nahuatl world view. They had and still have an important impact on food choices. Although this is not the only quality involved in beliefs about disease and health, the opposition between hot and cold has attracted the most attention.

Hot and cold are not to be understood in terms of temperature. In this context they are qualities, and they can behave in ways that may seem bizarre. For instance, in some cases, cold may push heat into another part of the body without mixing with it and becoming tepid.

Although the concepts of hot and cold seem similar to the yin-yang of the Orient or the humoral ideas of ancient Greece or other parts of the world, we cannot establish the origin of the hot-cold dichotomy for the Nahuatl people. It would seem logical that it is based on common experiences and observations such as the different temperatures of certain parts of the body (cold feet, hot abdomen), the effect of temperature on the organism (heatstroke, frostbite), the effect of behavior on the body (blushing or getting red with anger and becoming pale with fear) and changes present in disease (fever, hot abscess).

What has become clear is that the Nahuatl believed that these qualities could change as a result of external influences and could cause disease.

Among today's Indian groups and in many Mestizo towns or even in large cities, the use of the hot-cold system can be found, not as a relic of the past, but as a very *dynamic* way of thinking about nature. The amount of information that we have from ethnographic sources is larger and better documented than that from pre-Hispanic sources. It has been a matter of controversy whether the present situation is simply derived from ancient ways of life or whether it was influenced by such European concepts as the humoral theory of disease. Foster [1953, 1978] and López Austin have contributed to this debate. The important fact is that the hot-cold dichotomy exists today and influences people's habits.

This can be seen in many places, from very isolated Indian towns to the big cities. It is very difficult to find anyone who can explain the logic behind the system, since it is applied in daily life in an unconscious manner. Nevertheless, in most places it is relatively easy to ask people to classify foods and diseases according to their hot or cold qualities. In some circumstances people state a third quality: *cordial* or *templado*, meaning something in between the polar extremes. The basic criterion for calling some food *cordial* or *templado* is that it will not harm babies or small children. One can easily make up a similar list showing the qualities of common diseases and medicines. Several authors have published lists of this type [Alvarez Heydenreich, 1981; Foster, 1967; Madsen, 1960; Ryesky 1976; Villa Rojas, 1978].

One finds, in conversation with the people who use the classification, that several criteria operate simultaneously in classifying food, disease, and medicine. For instance, a food may be classified as hot if it comes from the hotlands or if it is brightly colored, or if it lives exposed to the sun, as in the case of fruits that grow high on trees; or, again, by its effect on the body as in the case of chile peppers. Cold foods usually grow near or in the water; they may come from the highlands, have darker colors or be protected from the effects of the sun, by having a thick shell or peel. This classification can have striking consequences. In the Western culture, probably the coldest edible item a person could think of would be ice; but in some places in Mexico ice is considered hot. People will say that if the frost can "burn" plants, it must be hot, or that pork is cold but lard is hot.

Diseases or changes in the body have similar classifications. Pregnant women are hot, since they have an extra body inside producing heat. Frightened people are cold whether their fright is natural, or supernatural as in the case of the disease called *susto*. Sunstroke is of course hot, but with other diseases the relation is less obvious. Diseases that involve some kind of irritation of the body or that cause redness are hot. Diarrhea can be hot if the stools are dark or red, but it is cold if they are whiteish. Women after childbirth are cold, and if they continue to get colder they may become sterile. Ailments that have to do with air, that result in water retention or edema, or that involve skin eruptions that do not itch or are not red are considered cold.

The connection between food and disease in this system is apparent. Basic therapeutic measures counteract the quality of the disease by means of the appropriate food or medicine, in order to regain an equilibrium. Thus the food that was acceptable for a hot, pregnant woman may be inadequate once childbirth has left her cold.

Cooking and other forms of preparing foods can alter their basic quality. Boiling can turn cold foods hot or *templado*. Adding chile or other condiments can also change them. *Curanderos* and, indeed, almost everyone in a rural area can very easily choose a good diet for a patient based on the disease that he or she has.

The dichotomy between hot and cold is certainly one of the most interesting aspects of Mexican food classification. New studies are published every year. Its potential uses in dietary guidance have become apparent. If a nutritionist or a physician recommends to a pregnant woman foods that she may consider too hot for her condition, she may reject not only the dietary counseling, but also the entire complex of Western medical care.

OTHER FOOD CATEGORIES

Mexicans have many adjectives for foods, depending on their characteristics. *Pesado* and *ligero*, *aguada* y *seca*, *indigesta*, *ácida* and many other terms are used in relation to the effect of food on health. Menstruating or lactating women are not supposed to eat acid fruits lest their milk or their menstrual fluids be retained, with deleterious effects on their well-being. These categories are being studied, and they certainly influence food choice. Some products may be eaten in the morning and others only at night. Others must start or end a meal. Mixtures of particular foods or dishes are considered dangerous.

The task before Mexican anthropologists dealing with nutrition and medicine is large. There may be conceptual dichotomies as important as that between hot and cold. What is most important, however, is that these traditional ideas become part of the knowledge of all of those interested in Mexico's health problem [Aguirre Beltrán, 1980].

REFERENCES

Aguirre Beltran G (1980): "Programas de salud en la situación intercultural." México City: Instituto Mexicano del Seguro Social (Colección salud y seguridad social).

Alvarez Heydenreich L (1981): "La enfermedad y la cosmovisión en Hueyapan, Morelos." Dissertation, Mexico: Escuela Nacional de Antropología e Historia.

Casillas LE (1979): El uso de recursos médicos en el hogar: estudio de familias urbanas y suburbanas de la Ciudad de México. Ests Etnobot y Antro Med 3:95-114.

Collado R (1976): "Médicos y Estructura Social." Mexico City: Fondo de Cultura Económica (Archivo del Fondo 70).

Collado R, García Torres JE (1975): Los médicos en México en 1970. Sal Pub Mex 17(3):309-324.

Foster G (1953): Relationships between Spanish and Spanish American folk medicine. J Am Folklore 66:201-217.

Foster G (1967): "Tzintzuntzan. Mexican Peasants in a Changing World." Boston: Little Brown and Company.

Foster G (1978): Hippocrates' Latin American legacy: "Hot" and "cold" in contemporary folk medicine. In RK Wetherington (ed): "Colloquia in Anthropology." Dallas: Southern Methodist University, pp 3-19.

López Acuña D (1980): "La Salud Desigual en México." Mexico City: Siglo XXI Editores.

López Austin A (1975): "Textos de Medicina Náhuatl." Mexico City: Universidad Nacional Autónoma de México.

López Austin A (1980): "Cuerpo Humano e Ideología. Las Concepciones de los Antiguos Nahuas." Mexico City: Universidad Nacional Autónoma de México.

Madsen W (1960): "The Virgin's Children." New York: Greenwood Press.

Rodríguez Domínguez J, Vandale S, López Acuña D, Yáñez BL, Meljem Moctezuma J (1979): Tratamientos no médicos de la enfermedad en el medio rural mexicano. Estudio de los usuarios de un centro de salud C en el estado de Morelos. Sal Pub Mex 21(1):13-30.

Ryesky D (1976): "Conceptos tradicionales de la Medicina en un Pueblo Mexicano. Un Análisis Antropológico." Mexico City: Secretaría de Educación Pública (Sep Setentas 309).

Soberón G (1983): Carecen de servicios de salud 15 millones de personas. Uno Más Uno, June 11, p 7.

Vargas LA (1979): Definición y características de la relación médico-paciente. Estud Etnobot Antrop Med 3:19-36.

Villa Rojas A (1978): "Los Elegidos de Dios. Etnografía de los Mayas de Quintana Roo." Mexico City: Instituto Nacional Indigenista (Serie antropología social 56).

THE SEARCH FOR SOLUTIONS

Moderator

José María Bengoa, MD
Former Chief, Nutrition Unit
World Health Organization
Geneva, Switzerland

Malnutrition: Determinants and Consequences, pages 433–445
© 1984 Alan R. Liss, Inc., 150 Fifth Avenue, New York, NY 10011

Nutritional Anthropology in the Search for Solutions to Problems of Malnutrition

John R.K. Robson, MD

Department of Family Medicine, Medical University of South Carolina, Charleston, South Carolina 29425

INTRODUCTION

Traditional nutritional deficiency diseases have declined in recent years, but the Third World is being increasingly affected by protein-energy malnutrition especially in the urban slums [Pellett, 1983]. By contrast, the affluent Western World is afflicted by diet-related degenerative diseases, such as atherosclerosis, cancer, diabetes, and obesity [Trowell and Burkitt, 1981]. In studying these diet-related problems, nutritionists and others have tended to focus on the immediate or etiologic causes of malnutrition.

Thirty years ago kwashiorkor and marasmus were considered to be confined to the tropical and subtropical areas of the world. Both diseases were recognized as being the result of protein and energy deficits; kwashiorkor was attributed to poor weaning practices and marasmus was blamed on failure of breast feeding and the introduction of artificial feeding with cow's milk. This analysis was found to be too simplistic and it was subsequently shown that malnutrition was not due simply to an interruption in energy or nutrient supply but a variety of other remote causes. These included marketing systems, agricultural systems imposed by Western scientists, international monetary systems, tribal land tenure systems, and traditional tribal law and customs [Cox, 1981; Robson, 1974].

An increasing interest in the more remote (ecologic) causes of diet-related disease has led to the involvement of students of human behavior in nutrition research. This involvement by anthropologists has led to the recognition of even wider vistas of untapped nutritional information that may have a very great influence on the health of all peoples.

To explore these new areas of nutritional information, it is first necessary to review changes in the dietary habits of man during his evolution. These changes may have been responsible for some of the food-related diseases of Western Civilization. (It seems likely that it may lead to the demise of millions in the Third World if the inhabitants in those areas continue to mimic the development of the West.) The eras concerned may be conveniently divided into three. The first is the time of the emergence of man, covering perhaps a million or more years when he was omnivorous. Because of his limited tools and hunting skills it is probable that his main food resources were plant materials supplemented by easily caught insects, reptiles, fish, and small animals [Brothwell and Brothwell, 1969; Tannahill, 1973]. The eating pattern would be characterized by continuous gleaning, although after fire was discovered, an evening-cooked meal eaten in a more leisurely fashion would become an established habit. After grasses were domesticated, about 10,000 years ago, a more steady supply of food became available but the need to cultivate and care for the primitive wheat, corn, and other cereals reduced the time available for hunting and gathering, thereby leading to dietary specialization. As the Agricultural Evolution continued, so did meal patterns become more important in the lifestyle, and in times of plenty, the practice of eating large amounts at one time became a prevalent habit.

In the last 200 years food resources and eating habits were completely changed by the Industrial Revolution. Food processing, marketing pressures, the need to work long hours away from home, convenience in packaging foods, all resulted in the exploitation of fewer basic food resources, the wider spacing of meals, the consumption of highly refined carbohydrates, and a reduction in plant protein foods. Table I summarizes these events and identifies contemporary populations that provide an insight into the diets of earlier times. The work of Schlegel and Guthrie [1973] with the Tiruray demonstrates the changes in the utilization of food resources that occurred during transition from an aboriginal to a peasant mode of life (Table II). It can be seen, for example, that there is a drastic reduction in the number of food resources exploited. McArthur [1960] provides similar details of the complexity of the diet of the Australian Aborigines, which contrasts strongly with the relatively few cereal, fruit, meat, and vegetable resources used by expatriate settlers.

There is an increasing interest in the significance of these changes, and it is here that the work of the physical and cultural anthropologist has to be recognized. Highly skilled research is needed to produce sound and accurate data relating to the food habits and dietary resources of tribes such as the Tasaday in the Philippines. We should also be prepared for moving promptly should new Stone Age tribes be discovered, for it is recognized that social events outside reservations have affected the lifestyle of isolated groups very quickly. Furthermore, the process of acculturation will also affect the natural habitant and

TABLE I. Changes in Food Habits During Human Evolution

Time scale	Events	Mode of food behavior	Contemporary examples
? ↓ 10,000 BC		Hunting and gathering	Tasaday Australian Aborigines
↓ AD 0	Agricultural evolution	Swidden and peasant agricultural	Philippine Tiruray
↓ 1800			Peasant farming in Africa, Asia, and the Americas
↓ 1983	Industrial revolutions	Intensive farming Food processing	Cities in developing countries
			Industrialized nations

TABLE II. Numbers of Sources of Food in Tiruray Aborigines and Peasants

	Source		Starchy staples	Viands	Others	Total
Aboriginal	Swidden		6	19	17	42
	Hunting and gathering		1	52	9	62
		Totals	7	71	26	104
Peasant	Cultivated		3	13	6	22
	Purchased		4	13	16	33
	Gathered		0	4	0	4
		Totals	7	30	22	59

Adapted from Schlegel and Guthrie [1973].

hence the diet of the indigenous population. The fact that the dietary changes of the past have undoubtedly led to increased morbidity and mortality in Western man implies that similar mimicking by the Third World should be avoided and brings a sense of urgency to data collection.

Data already available provide a framework for some hypotheses that need to be explored, and as the type of research and new needs for research are described, it is clear that anthropologists have a vital role in future studies. It is also apparent that traditional research strategies may require considerable modification if the information needed is to be devoid of Western biases.

TABLE III. Gain in Weight (kg) With Age in Rural and Urban Black Males

Age (years)	Zulu		Venda		UK
	Rural	Urban	Rural	Urban	
20–29	57.4	59.9	56.8	60.1	70.0
30–39	58.5	63.3	58.9	63.5	75.5
40–49	60.4	64.5	56.7	64.6	80.0
50–59	60.0	66.0	54.9	65.8	73.2

Data from Walker [1974], with permission.

A HYPOTHESIS

The general hypothesis that needs to be tested is "Dietary changes under-gone by man during his evolution have resulted in metabolic adaptation." The corollary that metabolic adaptation can be genetically transmitted is an ad-junct to this hypothesis.

The first step is to demonstrate evidence of metabolic changes during evolu-tion. Contemporary populations can be used for this, and they provide limited data, suggesting that changes in diet have led to changes in carbohydrate and fat metabolism. Tables III–V show the trends that are characterized by in-creases in weight, blood sugar, triglycerides, cholesterol, and growth hormone levels during social and economic development. Obviously, much more data are required, and, as will be discussed later, much of the burden for research will have to be borne by anthropologists. In the meantime, these findings need to be related to the Western diseases that plague civilization and the increasing prevalence of these diseases in developing populations [Trowell and Burkitt, 1981].

The Western diseases of obesity, diabetes, heart disease, and cancer are all diet-related. It is possible that these diseases have origins in metabolic changes needed to cope with the dietary alterations that have taken place. The stresses imposed on metabolism mainly appear to affect carbohydrate metabolism, which in turn affects fat metabolism.

Metabolism and metabolic control mechanisms vary according to the state of feeding of the individual [Cahill, 1981]. In the individual exposed to long-term food deficits, the ability to withstand starvation is dependent on fat stores. It can be argued, therefore, that the facility with which an individual can deposit fat may be fundamental to survival. In the normal fed state, the metabolism responds to the influx of carbohydrate by secreting insulin. This facilitates the conversion of glucose into glycogen in the liver and muscles and also helps the entry of amino acids into cells, where they can be incorporated into proteins during the process of anabolism. Glucose not converted into gly-

TABLE IV. Fasting Blood Sugar (ranked by increasing values) and Insulin Levels and Insulin/Glucose Ratios in Selected African Groups

Group	Fasting blood sugar (mg/dl)	Fasting insulin (mU/ml)	Insulin/ glucose	Source of data
!Kung Bushmen	60	nd[a]	nd	Jenkins et al [1974]
Saharan Nomads	64	18	0.23	deHertogh et al [1975]
!Kung Bushmen	95[b]	10[b]	0.10	Joffe et al [1971]
Uganda prisoners	65	nd	nd	Tulloch and Patel [1969]
S. African urban laborers	73	6	0.08	Rubenstein et al [1969]
Nonobese urban S. African laborers	76	14	0.18	Seftel et al [1973]
Rhodesian students	76	19	0.25	Wapnick et al [1972]
S. African urban workers	78	15	0.19	Joffe et al [1975]
Rhodesian urban cleaners	79	16	0.20	Wapnick et al [1972]
Obese urban S. Africans	81	20	0.26	Joffe et al [1975]
Obese urban S. Africans	83	21	0.25	Seftel et al [1973]
S. African urban diabetics	205	12	0.25	Asmal and Leary [1975]

[a]nd = no data.
[b]Nonfasting levels.

cogen undergoes glycolysis and the substrates formed by the breakdown of glucose become available for entry into the Krebs cycle, where they are broken down further with the production of energy. However, when the supply of cal-orifers exceeds the demands of the Krebs cycle, the redundant substrates are synthesized into fatty acids, which combine with glycerol to form fat. It may seem logical to expect that in the nonfed state there will be no synthesis of fat (which is true) and that fat in adipose tissue will be broken down to provide the necessary energy. The latter phenomenon does not occur in any significant amount, however, during food deprivation that lasts only a few days. Perhaps the body recognizes that the fat stores are life-saving and protects the utilization of fat until the food deprivation is serious. Although some 150–200 gm of fat may be lost during the first few days of starvation, the fat stores are largely untouched while other mechanisms come into play. First, glucagon, a hormone antagonistic to insulin, mobilizes the glycogen stores. Glucagon also has the ability to break down protein, and the amino acids produced become available for conversion to carbohydrate in the process called gluconeogenesis. This results in the destruction of tissue protein, and in the first few days of starvation, losses of 500 gm of flesh can be expected daily. This metabolic system ensures that if the interruption in food supplies is of short duration then fat stores will be left intact for a more serious threat. Any muscle protein lost can be quickly replaced as physical activity and a more normal diet resume.

TABLE V. Human Growth Hormone, Triglyceride, and Cholesterol Levels in Selected African Populations

Group	Human growth hormone (ng/ml)	Triglycerides (mg/100 ml)	Cholesterol (mg/100 ml)	Source of data
Kalahari Bushmen	2.0	89–105	111–120	Joffe et al [1971] Wilmsen [1978] Truswell and Hansen [1968]
Pygmies	2.9	nd	nd	Rimoin et al [1968]
Tarahumara Indians Mexico	nd[a]	120	125	Connor et al [1978]
Botswana Bushmen	nd	95	130	Truswell and Mann [1971]
Masai pastoralists	nd	nd	135	Biss et al [1971]
Rural Bantu	nd	92	143	Truswell and Mann [1971]
Bantu laborers	nd	75	166	Bronte-Stewart et al [1955] Antonis and Bersohn [1960]
Bantu medical students	nd	95	197	Truswell and Mann [1971]
Bantu hospital workers	nd	132	197	Truswell and Mann [1971]
S. African diabetics	2.7	126	215	Asmal and Leary [1975]
Nonobese urban Bantu		127	169	Joffe et al [1975]
Obese Bantu laborers	3.2	146	203	Seftel et al [1973]
Obese urban Bantu		143	208	Joffe et al [1975]
Nonobese Bantu laborers	4.2	74	153	Rubenstein et al [1969]
Nonobese Bantu laborers	8.0	130	168	Seftel et al [1973]

[a]nd = no data.

DIETARY AND METABOLIC INTERRELATIONSHIPS

The dietary changes during development have resulted in increases in insulin and growth hormone secretion. This increased hormone activity, associated with the social and economic development of man, appears to have resulted in hyperglycemia, hyperlipidemia, obesity, and diabetes. The question now arises whether these morbid conditions are a maladaptation of the metabolic systems that were present in emerging man and designed for his mode of life.

TABLE VI. Theoretical Glycolytic Activity in Different Individuals

	Subject A	Subject B
Resource substrates	100 units	100 units
Delivery rate of substrate	50 units/hr	20 units/hr
Rate of utilization of substrates in Krebs cycle	40 units/hr	40 units/hr
Rate of accumulation of substrates	10 units/hr	0 units/hr

Early man ate almost continually as he gathered food. Although some sucrose was undoubtedly a dietary component, it would not be the readily assimilable sucrose of the modern world. Food grains, seeds, nuts, roots, and berries would be subject to a continual relatively slow digestive process and only after a meal would the products of digestion enter the metabolic system in large amounts. This would explain the low blood glucose levels observed during the day in hunters and gatherers. In these circumstances, glucagon is mobilizing glycogen to serve as a substrate for energy metabolism; at the same time there is a slow, continual turnover of protein. This would ensure a supply of glucose for energy metabolism. Also, the mixture of high-quality amino acids derived from body tissues would facilitate the protein synthesis that continues even in the nonfed state. After a meal there would be an influx of monosaccharides (mainly glucose and fructose from the maltose and other complex carbohydrates consumed). Blood sugar levels would then rise and insulin secretion would be stimulated.

In the Bushmen, however, the insulin response to carbohydrate loads appears to be poor. In the studies by Joffe et al [1971] and Jenkins et al [1974], blood sugar levels remained high 2 hr after a 50-gm glucose load. This suggests that hunter-gatherers (and therefore early man) had an intolerance of carbohydrate even at very small loads; handling of high blood glucose levels probably was not a serious problem, however, because growth hormone levels were also low. In such circumstances, the tissues tend to be more sensitive to insulin, representing an economy of insulin needs.

With increasing carbohydrate challenges, demands for insulin would nevertheless increase in order to avoid a diabetic state. This would increase adiposity and eventually lead to exhaustion of the β-cells of the pancreas.

Traditionally it has been assumed that caloric equilibrium is measured over a minimum of one day and that if an individual's daily caloric requirements are exceeded, fatness will result. It can be postulated, however, that the phenomenon of lipogenesis is not time-related but is determined by the rate at which calorifers are presented to the Krebs cycle. In Table VI, it is assumed that two subjects with identical caloric needs are provided with the same number of calories, and that their Krebs cycles are both accepting substrates at the same rate. In subject A, however, the calories are provided in a few large boluses during the day; hence the delivery rate of substrates to the Krebs cycle is far higher than the delivery rate in subject B. As a consequence, subject A has an excess of substrates that then form fatty acids. A similar situation can arise when one subject eats readily assimilable carbohydrates such as are found in the refined-sugar diets of the Western World and the other eats the more slowly digested and absorbed starchy diets of early man. Therefore, it is possible that despite identical caloric intakes, the type of eating as well as the type of carbohydrate can lead to adiposity.

There is evidence also that the enzymes in the glycolytic cycle can be induced by high substrate concentrations as well as by insulin. Individuals with readily inducible enzymes would have facilitated fat deposition, which would also encourage adaptations in peripheral fat. For example, it has been shown that Pima Indians have an increased adipose tissue lipoprotein lipase activity, which facilitates deposition of fat [Reitmen et al, 1982]. Over thousands of years, whole populations may have survived because of their ability to induce their glycolytic pathways and deposit fat. While they would come to little or no harm with limited food supplies, they would be destined to become morbidly obese with the newly acquired food affluence associated with acculturation.

One other explanation for differences in obesity in modern and acculturated man relates to the phenomenon of thermogenesis. Nonshivering thermogenesis (NST) [Himms-Hagen, 1981] is a physiologic response to cold and is brought about by the activity of brown adipose tissue (BAT). Originally noted in hibernating animals and in the newborn, NST was assumed to be a mechanism whereby the body could be protected from cold by the generation of heat by BAT. In the early days of man, cold stress would be considerable in the unclothed or partially unclothed state. This would be true even in the desert areas of the tropics and subtropics, where the night can be very cold. While BAT would provide more comfort, it would also be wasteful of energy and it would not be so important in the humid areas of the world, where nocturnal temperatures are high. During evolution, as housing and clothing developed, cold stress would be diminished, and the need for BAT would be less. It is possible, however, that there are genetic differences in the amounts of BAT provided at birth, and therefore, considerable differences in the capacity of individuals to generate (waste) heat.

Table VII shows a hypothetical situation in which there is a difference in thermogenesis in two persons of identical body size, body composition, physical activity, and basal energy metabolism who are fed the same amount of food energy. Subject D is more heat-efficient than subject C, and as a consequence the former has additional energy for disposal. In these circumstances, this energy will be stored as fat. Because thermogenically efficient persons will deposit fat at lower caloric intakes than their thermogenically less efficient counterparts, the heat-efficient individual would be more likely to survive dur-

TABLE VII. **Adiposity Risks in Two Individuals With Different Thermogenic Efficiency**

	Subject C	Subject D
Intake	2,000 kcal	2,000 kcal
BMR	400 kcal	400 kcal
Physical activity	1,000 kcal	1,000 kcal
Heat	600 kcal	500 kcal
Total	2,000 kcal	1,900 kcal
		100 kcal excess for fat

ing food shortages. Because of genetic selection, no doubt certain ethnic groups or even populations themselves have survived because of thermogenic efficiency, but they are now faced with problems of disposing of the extra energy as modern life increases their caloric intake or decreases their physical activity.

The hypothesis that dietary changes during human evolution have produced metabolic adaptation has at least two components. The first relates to the patterns of food behavior. It appears that "gorging" and the consumption of refined carbohydrates may have led to changes in hormonal control and enzyme activity that encourage adiposity. A second component likely to be associated with survival is the presence of BAT, which may be one of several mechanisms determining whether a person is heat-efficient or heat-inefficient. If these postulates are true, then individuals, groups, or even populations may have varying risks for obesity and diabetes. At greatest risk are those who have Western dietary habits and who have never had a need in the past for BAT to counter cold stress and who have also developed readily inducible glycolytic pathways, or increased lipoprotein lipase activity.

Contemporary populations who, through recently developed acculturation, are passing through the dietary evolution of Western man in the space of a few years may not have had time to adapt to the changes or develop genetic resistance to diet-related diseases through natural selection. This may explain the very high morbidity and mortality of certain groups recently exposed to Western life.

Since cancer and heart disease are serious health problems for modern man that may have resulted from the change in diet, this response may represent a maladaptation. The origin of these diseases can also be explained by glycolytic overload brought about by gorging, the consumption of refined carbohydrates, high fat intake, and possible enzyme induction. Figure 1 shows the interrelationships between glycolysis, cholesterol synthesis, and the synthesis of sex hormones. It is postulated that the control of cholesterol synthesis can be overwhelmed by overloading glycolytic pathways; consequently abnormally

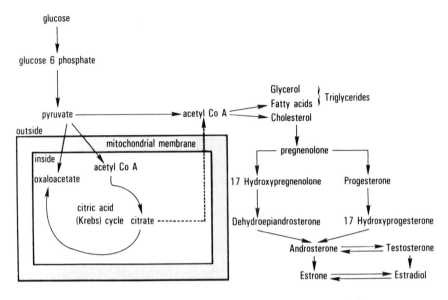

Fig. 1.   Glycolysis, fat, cholesterol, and sex hormone synthesis.

high cholesterol levels can occur even in the absence of dietary cholesterol [Robson et al, 1983].

Because hypercholesterolemia is an index of risk of heart disease, glycolytic overload may be an important etiologic factor in atherosclerosis. In addition, glucose overload may also induce the production of pregnenolone, a steroid precursor of progesterone, androgens, and estrogens. These hormones are produced not only in the gonads, but also in peripheral fat where interconversions can take place. As a consequence, powerful estrogens such as β-estradiol may be produced in excessive amounts while gonadal production of inhibitors of β-estradiol remain constant. There would thus be a relative excess of β-estradiol. A third possibility, that abnormal sex hormones may be produced, also has to be considered. In conditions where there is glycolytic overload, adiposity increases and allows greater hormonal transformations and an increased risk of generation of abnormal sex hormones.

A very important ethical point is therefore raised that relates to the role of the Western World in bringing about (by accident or design) changes in traditional food habits. At the worst, if the West imposes its agricultural marketing and food consumption practices on the Third World, it may be that these countries are inevitably being exposed to risks of diabetes, obesity, heart disease, and cancer. Certainly the evidence from studies of acculturation confirm the high risks of obesity and diabetes. It is also significant that coronary artery disease and cancer appear to be increasing in the Third World and it may not all be due to better reporting and diagnosis.

THE ROLE OF THE ANTHROPOLOGIST IN SOLVING NUTRITIONAL PROBLEMS

Research into the physiology and biochemistry of peoples at varying stages of social and cultural development is a vital component of the understanding of the significance of change. Yet the acquisition of the data cannot be effectively carried out by scientists trained in medicine, phsyiology, or biochemistry alone. It is important to relate the observations to human behavior, but even more fundamental is the need for persons knowledgeable in human behavior to have proper input into the research projects. Individuals and groups living in remote areas present special problems for nutrition research. In all cases careful preparation is needed to ensure that the target population will be willing to participate in the research. Anthropologists have a primary role in this phase, but first they themselves need to know what kind of data are required.

Studies of metabolic adaptation will require the acquisition of data ranging from the very mundane, such as assessment of longevity and collection of anthropometric data, to the measurement of metabolic parameters. The latter present a major problem in that collection of blood (and possibly urine) samples will be necessary, a procedure that may not be acceptable to the isolated populations. The protocol will also call for measurements of heat production and energy expenditure. This presents problems relating not only to the logistics of providing power supplies but also the cultural impact of these technical innovations on persons living at the lower levels of social organization.

Another major problem relates to the duration of the project, which may have to cover several seasons. In some areas, collection of body fluids has been successful, and very informative data on carbohydrate and fat metabolism and hormones have been collected. Therefore, an examination of the future needs and how the problems can be overcome is already justified.

It is obvious that a team is required. Clinical observations require a physician, and the highly technical procedures involved in measuring metabolism will require the services of a physiologist/biochemist. The anthropologist must be seen as a key member of the team who may have several functions. The first entails a long preparatory phase in which the anthropologist makes contact with the group alone and determines what investigations are acceptable. For those procedures that are not immediately acceptable, the anthropologist is needed to find ways of overcoming the difficulties.

While the traditional training of anthropologists is essential for this task, further training in nutritional studies would be required. An understanding of the procedures planned, their technical difficulties, and the essentials of quality control would be a necessary part of the education of the field anthropologist. This has implications for the basic educational program in anthropology.

If studies are initiated then consideration has to be given to the role of the nonanthropologists on the team. It is vital that the sensitivities of the participants in the study be respected. This would imply that one of the first steps is to persuade physicians, biochemists, and other scientists that they require special training if they wish to be successful and innovative in field research. Anthropologists, therefore, need to be involved increasingly in the training of field researchers.

It seems unlikely that clinicians and other scientists will be able to spend their time profitably in remote areas for prolonged periods. The possibility that anthropologists may be able to take over the role of data collection needs to be examined. At the present time, it seems improbable that a comprehensive study of metabolic adaptation can be undertaken on any one group. If this topic is to be given a high priority, one of the immediate steps to be taken should be an interdisciplinary discussion of problems of field work in isolated areas. The interdisciplinary nature of this discussion is obvious and seems sufficiently important to justify support from national sponsors.

REFERENCES

1. Antonis A, Bersohn I (1960): Serum-triglyceride levels in South African Europeans and Bantu and in ishaemic heart-disease. Lancet 2:998–1002.
2. Asmal AC, Leary WP (1975): Carbohydrate tolerance, plasma insulin, growth hormone and lipid levels in Indian and Black diabetics. S Afr Med J 49:810–812.
3. Biss K, Ho KJ, Mikkelson B, Lewis L, Taylor CB (1971): Some unique biologic characteristics of the Masai of East Africa. N Engl J Med 284:694–699.
4. Bronte-Stewart B, Keys A, Brock JF, Moodie AD, Keys MH, Antonis A (1955): Serum cholesterol, diet and coronary heart-disease. Lancet 2:1103–1107.
5. Brothwell D, Brothwell P (1969): "Food in Antiquity." New York: Frederick A. Praeger.
6. Cahill GF (1981): Physiology of acute starvation in man. In Robson JRK (ed): "Famine: Its Causes, Effects and Management." New York: Gordon and Breach, pp 51–60.
7. Connor WE, Cerqueira MT, Connor RW, Wallace RB, Malinow RM, Casdorph RH (1978): The plasma lipids, lipoproteins, and diet of the Tarahumara Indians of Mexico. Am J Clin Nutr 31:1131–1142.
8. Cox GW (1981): The ecology of famine: An overview. In Robson JRK (ed): "Famine: Its Causes, Effects and Management." New York: Gordon and Breach, p 5–18.
9. DeHertogh R, Vanderheyden I, de Gasparo M (1975): Glucose tolerance in a Saharan nomad population — The Broayas, from the Toubou ethnic group. Diabetes 24:983–987.
10. Himms-Hagen J (1981): Non-shivering thermogenesis, brown adipose tissue and obesity. In Beers RF, Bassett EG (eds): "Nutritional Factors: Modulating Effects on Metabolic Processes." New York: Raven, pp 85–95.
11. Jenkins T, Lehmann H, Nurse GT (1974): Public health and genetic constitution of the San ("Bushmen"): Carbohydrate metabolism and acetylator status of the !Kung of Tsumkwe in the north-western Kalahari. Br Med J 2:23–26.
12. Joffe BI, Jackson WPU, Thomas ME, Toyer MG, Keller P, Pimstone BL, Zamit R (1971): Metabolic responses to oral glucose in the Kalahari Bushmen. Br Med J 4:206–208.
13. Joffe BI, Goldberg RB, Seftel HC, Distiller LA (1975): Insulin, glucose and triglyceride relationships in obese African subjects. Am J Clin Nutr 28:616–620.
14. McArthur M (1960): In Mountford CP (ed): "Records of the American-Australian Scientific Exhibition to Arnhem Land. 2. Anthropology and Nutrition." Melbourne: Melbourne University Press, pp 1–26, 139–143.

15. Pellett PL (1983): Changing concepts in world malnutrition. Ecol Food Nutr 13:115–125.
16. Reitman JS, Kosmakos FC, Howard BV, Taskinen M-R, Kuusi T, Nikkila EO (1982): Characteristics of lipase activities in obese Pima Indians. J Clin Inv 70:791–797.
17. Rimoin DL, Merimee TJ, Rabinowitz D, Cavalli-Sforza LL, McKusick VA (1968): Peripheral subresponsiveness to human growth hormone in the African Pygmies. N Engl J Med 281:1383–1388.
18. Robson JRK (1974): The ecology of malnutrition in a rural community in Tanzania. Ecol Food Nutr 3:61–72.
19. Robson JRK, Campbell CT, Dias JK (1983): Plasma cholesterol and glucose metabolism (letter). Am J Clin Nutr 38:489–491.
20. Rubenstein AH, Seftel HC, Miller K, Bersohn I, Wright AD (1969): Metabolic response to oral glucose in healthy South African White, Indian, and African subjects. Br Med J 1: 748–751.
21. Schlegel AS, Guthrie HA (1973): Diet and the Tiruray shift from swidden to plow farming. Ecol Food Nutr 2:181.
22. Seftel HC, Spitz IMG, Bersohn I, Goldin AR, Joffe BI, Rubenstein AH, Metzger BE (1973): Metabolic features of Johannesburg Bantu with myocardial infarction. S Afr Med J 47:1571–1575.
23. Tannahill R (1973): "Food in History." New York: Stein and Day.
24. Trowell HC, Burkitt DP (1981): "Western Diseases: Their Emergence and Prevention." London: Edward Arnold, pp 427–435.
25. Truswell AS, Hansen JDL (1968): Serum-lipids in Bushmen. Lancet 2:684.
26. Truswell AS, Mann JI (1971): Epidemiology of serum lipids in Southern Africa. Athero 16: 15–29.
27. Tulloch JA, Patel KM (1969): Studies of normal carbohydrate tolerance in the Ugandan African. Trans R Soc Trop Med Hyg 63:644–649.
28. Walker ARP (1974): Studies on sugar intake and overweight in South African Black and White school children. S Afr Med J 48:1650.
29. Wapnick S, Kanengoni E, Wicks ACB, Jones JJ (1972): Can diet be responsible for the initial lesion in diabetes? Lancet 2:300–301.
30. Wilmsen EN (1978): Seasonal effects of dietary intake on Kalahari San. Fed Proc 37:65–72.

Malnutrition: Determinants and Consequences, pages 447–455
© 1984 Alan R. Liss, Inc., 150 Fifth Avenue, New York, NY 10011

Regional Strategies for the Improvement of Nutrition in the Western Hemisphere

Carlyle Guerra de Macedo, MD, MPH, and
Carlos Hernán Daza, MD, MPH
Pan American Sanitary Bureau, Pan American Health Organization, WHO,
Washington, DC 20037

INTRODUCTION

At its XXVIII Meeting in October 1981 the Directing Council of the Pan American Health Organization (PAHO) adopted a Plan of Action to implement the Regional Strategies of Health for All by the Year 2000 [PAHO, 1980]. This is a momentous political decision and, indeed, a prime social target that commits the member governments and PAHO to implement all measures needed for the attainment of levels of health that will permit every individual in the Americas to lead a socially and economically productive life [PAHO, 1982].

The challenge now is how and by what means to make this apparently idealistic but imperative goal a practical reality, particularly for the segments of the population that have been traditionally kept outside the mainstream of social and economic progress in the region.

Health and good nutrition are essential to the quality of life, and any government action for their sustained improvement will necessarily require the effective participation of all development sectors — both public and private — including the scientific and academic communities, which were so well represented at the Western Hemisphere Nutrition Congress.

Progress toward this high social goal will obviously require a fundamental change in the conception and operation of health services and systems and, at the same time, the advancement of other sectors directly related to the social sphere. In other words, a more coherent, comprehensive, and balanced development is needed to assure the economic and social advancement of the countries in the Americas [PAHO, 1980].

The Regional Plan of Action sets three main operational objectives to ensure that the health sector will make its specific contribution to the reduction of social inequalities and hence to the improvement of the quality of life. These objectives are:

1. Reorganization and expansion of health service systems so as to improve their equity, efficiency, and effectiveness.
2. Promotion and improvement of intersectoral linkages and cooperation.
3. Promotion and improvement of regional and interregional cooperation.

These objectives are consistent with the overall strategy and are intimately bound up with the improvement of nutrition in the Western Hemisphere. As progress is made toward their fulfillment, the quality of life will improve, and with it the health and nutritional well-being of the population.

On the other hand, the governments of the Americas have adopted primary health care as the principal strategy for the attainment of Health for All by the Year 2000, which in the definition adopted by the World Health Organization [PAHO, 1982; WHO, 1978] is "essential health care based on practical, scientifically sound and socially acceptable methods and technology, made universally accessible to individuals and families in the community through their full participation and at a cost that the community and country can afford to maintain at every stage of their development in the spirit of self-reliance and self-determination. It forms an integral part both of the country's health system, of which it is a central function and main focus, and of the overall social and economic development of the community. It is the first level of contact of individuals, the family and community with the national health system, brings health care as close as possible to where people live and work, and constitutes the first element of the continuing health care process."

Since nutrition is a basic component of primary health care, which in turn is closely linked to social development, any strategy for improving the availability and consumption of foods and the nutritional status of the population should be framed in a context of broadly intersectoral social and economic plans in which the health sector has a well-defined role and responsibility [WHO, 1981a].

Therefore, there being no single sectoral solution for solving the problems of hunger and malnutrition, the strategies adopted by the governments of the Americas clearly emphasize the role that the health sector must play in nutrition by providing services through its care delivery facilities in the community by the primary care approach and exercising vigorous leadership in promoting the involvement of other sectors in the formulation, implementation, and evaluation of food and nutrition policies and programs.

TRENDS IN FOOD AND NUTRITION

Despite the scientific progress and technological advances made in the field of food and nutrition during the last decades, malnutrition is still a major health problem in the Western Hemisphere, not only in terms of high morbidity and mortality but also as an inhibitor of the social and economic progress that improves the quality of life.

Hidden hunger, undernutrition, and specific deficiencies are widespread in Latin America and the Caribbean. On the other hand, malnutrition related to excessive food intake is becoming a health problem for some population groups, even in countries where nutritional deficiencies are still prevalent. The connection between dietary practices and obesity, late-onset diabetes, cardiovascular diseases, and some forms of cancer is a matter of public health concern.

Although the food situation and the nutritional status of the population have indeed improved in some countries, in others no measurable progress has been made during the last decade. This is also true in geographical areas within a single country. The paradox of the food and nutrition problem lies in the existing gap between available knowledge, technology, and resources and the actual commitment to and implementation of effective programs at the national level.

In general, the food and nutrition situation in Latin America and the Caribbean is characterized by a manifestly unbalanced distribution and consumption of basic foods, especially among the lowest-income groups. In addition, there are persistent environmental and sociocultural factors, especially the diarrheal and acute respiratory infections, which impede the proper utilization of foods and their nutrients at the cellular level; these factors can be greatly reduced by preventive measures and improvement of the environment [PAHO, 1980].

Of greatest significance and consequence are five nutritional deficiencies: energy, protein, iron, iodine, and vitamin A. Deficient intake of energy and protein coupled with a high incidence of infectious diseases leads to stunted growth in children and to high mortality. Moderate and severe malnutrition resulting in clinical marasmus and kwashiorkor, accompanied in some cases by psychomotor impairment, afflicts every year about half a million children under 5 years of age.

Iron-deficiency anemia is found in about half of pregnant and lactating women and at least one-fourth of children of all ages. Endemic goiter remains highly prevalent in some countries and is often associated with cretinism. Vitamin A deficiency is also prevalent in some countries.

The above figures are gross estimates and do not reflect the significant variations that occur not only between countries but between regions or areas within a country, particularly among the lower-income groups, in which the energy and protein intake is estimated at 20% below the recommended level.

In countries with well-established health services, the incidence of severe malnutrition in children has significantly decreased, but the prevalence of mild to moderate cases has shown less significant improvement. In rapidly urbanizing areas, infant malnutrition has extended into the first months of life, probably because of early interruption of breast feeding and improper weaning practices.

This situation contrasts with the countries' potential for feeding themselves in the form of land and untapped natural resources, which they have in sufficient measure, plus an abundance of labor for converting them into goods and services.

In general terms, while there has been no significant change in the food and nutrition situation during the last decade owing to the persistence of these deficiencies, it is clear that the severity of energy-protein malnutrition has diminished in some countries. Moreover, in some countries there has been progress in food production, though not at the pace needed to meet the demands of a steadily growing population.

The existence of malnutrition in the region despite an apparently adequate general availability of food indicates that it will not be enough merely to increase agricultural production, and that the countries need to direct their efforts towards intersectoral responses to the problem, including increasing the real income of the poor, developing efficient systems for distributing food to them, providing improved comprehensive health protection for them, and raising their social and educational levels.

In spite of the fact that the health sector receives the direct brunt of malnutrition and undertakes specific measures to overcome it, the characteristics of the problem necessitate the adoption of intersectoral approaches to its solution, which should be the basis for a national food and nutrition policy. These policies should be oriented to the solution of problems of food availability and consumption in the light of the factors that determine the biological benefits of foods and the habits that determine whether a recommended diet is consumed.

FOOD AND NUTRITION STRATEGIES

An effective articulation of all relevant sectors has long been recognized as a need in the countries of the region, as a fundamental strategy for achieving a satisfactory nutritional status for the whole population, and for controlling the nutritional deficiencies of large numbers of people in rural areas and the fringes of large cities [Daza and Rodríguez, 1981].

Many attempts have been made to develop effective intersectoral articulation in solving food and nutrition problems. Some have sought it through coordination at the highest level of the national planning process, and others have been confined to small geographic areas and populations. Both approaches have been useful for the acquisition of methodological experience and empirical knowledge of how to deal with food and nutrition problems.

In the early sixties several countries, with the stimulus and support of PAHO/WHO, FAO, and UNICEF, initiated a multisectoral approach to food and nutrition problems through the so-called "Integrated Aplied Nutrition Programs," whose basic purpose was to solve the health and nutrition problems most prevalent in rural areas on the basis of the promotion of community involvement and the coordination of the sectors closely concerned with food and nutrition: health, agriculture, and education. These experiences laid a sound foundation for an approach to the problem through its different causes, and contributed to the design of community strategies for its solution.

Beginning in 1970, an important movement emerged in the region to promote the formulation and implementation of national food and nutrition policies, which have been defined as a set of coherent principles, objectives, priorities and decisions adopted by a government to give the population access to and the capacity to consume basic foods, and other services essential to the attainment of nutritional well-being.

Concurrently with the promotion of food and nutrition policies, several countries have established national coordinating commissions, councils, or committees of high officials representing the sectors most directly involved. However, with very few exceptions these coordinating bodies have not succeeded in the adoption and implementation of food and nutrition policies, and formal declarations have not necessarily eventuated in specific actions.

There have been attempts to institutionalize the intersectoral planning process by setting up multidisciplinary groups responsible for analyzing the food and nutrition problems in the national planning agencies. Experience so far indicates that the introduction of this additional technical capability into the national planning process has not been accompanied by any significant improvement in sectoral relations, which are basic for the incorporation of nutritional considerations into social and economic policies and plans. This is an area in which detailed analysis is needed if coordinating mechanisms are to be effective in combating hunger and malnutrition.

It is also known that a sound social and economic development process requires the definition of consistent levels of well-being in terms of health, food, housing, education, production, employment, income, consumption, social involvement, etc, for the society as a whole and for the most neglected population groups in particular.

From this point of view, the analysis of intersectoral relations goes beyond simple coordination between sectors and institutions for the achievement of partial objectives, and reaches into the very core of more comprehensive social programming.

In this perspective it is clear that successful implementation of the strategies for the improvement of nutrition will greatly depend on a political decision to close the gap between the basic needs of the population and the available resources. Since the national resources allocated to the social sectors — including health and nutrition — are traditionally insufficient, it is imperative that the strategies contribute to self-reliance through the optimization of resource productivity, the use of low-cost technologies appropriate to the sociocultural context, and the effective articulation of the sectors concerned [Daza and Rodríguez, 1981].

The Pan American Health Organization is assisting its member governments in the development, adaptation, and use of appropriate methods for the promotion of proper nutrition and the reduction and prevention of nutritional deficiencies [PAHO, 1982].

The regional strategies call for measures to increase the availability and consumption of basic foods, combined with specific activities for the prevention and remedying of malnutrition, with special emphasis on the most vulnerable population groups, and for the reduction of malnutrition and promotion of an optimum nutritional status for the population through integrated intersectoral approaches. Particular attention is given to the following policies:

1. Establishing food and nutrition surveillance systems, the identification of useful indicators, techniques, and operational schemes for the ongoing evaluation of nutritional status, and screening of populations at risk.

2. Monitoring the effectiveness of food and nutrition policies and programs and, when necessary, developing new policy aims, clearly defining the role of the health sector in assessing the nutritional implications of sectoral strategies related to income, employment, the production and distribution of basic foods, prices and subsidies, etc, particularly those affecting low-income populations in urban and rural communities.

3. Strengthening the nutrition component of primary health care, including the early detection and treatment of malnutrition, the promotion of maternal and child nutrition, and promotion of breast feeding and better weaning practices.

4. Implementing food fortification programs for the prevention and control of iron deficiency anemia, endemic goiter, and vitamin A deficiency in countries where those specific deficiencies are prevalent.

5. Designing and conducting effective food and nutrition education activities at the community and national level.

6. Strengthening the nutrition training of specialized and general health personnel, including the development of expertise and capabilities in nutrition at the planning, monitoring, and implementation levels.

7. Promoting and supporting action-oriented research in food and nutrition for the development, field testing, and extended use of appropriate technologies for the application of measures to control malnutrition that are effective within local constraints and make use of available resources.

8. Contributing to the development and dissemination of new knowledge in nutrition and the adoption of appropriate technologies in food and nutrition.

9. Promoting collaboration with other international organizations, bilateral agencies, and nongovernmental groups concerned with the production, distribution, and safeguarding the quality of food; dietary practices; and improvement of the nutritional status of the most vulnerable population groups.

TRAINING AND RESEARCH PRIORITIES

There is no doubt that the strategies for the improvement of food and nutrition in the region should include not only economic measures to combat poverty but also measures to deal with nutrition and health problems specifically. This implies that an understanding of the problems and their possible solutions must be effectively impressed on high-ranking decision-makers in government and on needy populations alike [WHO, 1976].

Hence, training and education are basic elements of any program for nutritional improvement, and the effectiveness of existing training programs should be reviewed. There is often no adequate structure to absorb trained professionals and make use of their expertise, and when food and nutrition programs are being formulated, careful consideration should be given to the functions required and to the numbers of personnel needed to perform them, and training schemes should be developed. There is a great need for personnel at the operational level, ie, of those concerned with the delivery of food and nutrition services to the community, and major emphasis should be placed on the training of multipurpose workers, particularly for employment in primary health care services [WHO, 1981b].

In regard to research, the root causes of malnutrition are recognized to be social and economic, and research on them should have high priority.

Reliable information is needed on who is malnourished and how severely, what outcome may be expected from a given degree of deprivation, and whether or not the situation is changing. To obtain this information, better functional indicators for diagnosing nutritional status of populations must be devised, along with methods for identifying the primary determinants of malnutrition in particular groups. The usefulness and significance of various indexes of nutrition and health status need to be determined, and research should be directed towards the development of simple and efficient "early warning" indicators for identifying the populations at risk.

More information is needed on nutrient requirements, the range of individual variability, and body storage capacities for energy and nutrients, particularly those known to be commonly implicated in deficiency diseases. The objective here in regard to planning is to establish scales of risk of dysfunction in relation to different levels of intake, which, coupled with other indicators, would provide scales of intensity of need for nutritional measures.

More and better data on food intake are required as well as improved information on the nutrient composition of foods, including estimates of ranges of content and effects of alternative production, processing, and preservation methods. The constraints imposed upon food consumption by such factors as bulk, palatability, and social and cultural influences should be determined. An analysis needs to be made of the errors incurred by different techniques for assessing the food intake of individuals, and of young children in particular, with a view to more accurate quantification of the pattern of distribution of available food within the household.

Systematic research is needed on the nutritional and income distribution implications of policies for food production and supply, food distribution, and public health. The effects of such policies must be examined in detail to ensure that the desired results are achieved for the target deprived population [WHO, 1976].

Studies of the organizational aspects, impact and cost of action programs are also needed. Examples include child nutrition rehabilitation at home and in centers, supplementary feeding of mothers and children, and periodic administration of nutrients for the prevention of anemia and vitamin A deficiency. The mechanisms for and effectiveness of providing nutrition, health, agriculture, and education inputs as integrated packages in contrast to vertical and independent programs should be studied at the community level.

Finally, important areas of research are the policy-making process and the organizational aspects of food and nutrition programs, which might be of interest to political and social scientists. An example is the operation of planning and administrative structures and the extent to which political constraints upon effective planning and decision making modify and are modified by the organizational structure. The dynamics of the planning, policy-generating process need to be analyzed, and the degree to which lack of adequate communication between planners and nutritionists constitutes a barrier to the adoption and implementation of nutrition-oriented programs should be evaluated.

The contribution of the health sector to the search for feasible solutions and their application to reduce hunger and control malnutrition in the Western Hemisphere depends in great measure on the creativity and dedication of the health profession, working in conjunction with related disciplines, particularly food and nutrition scientists, educators, and social and economic planners.

In this endeavor, the Pan American Health Organization will continue its cooperation with member governments, the academic and research community, and other interested groups. Moreover, the active contribution and participation of the nutrition science community as represented in the Seventh Western Hemisphere Nutrition Congress are essential to strengthen PAHO's role and leadership at the international level for the promotion and support of optimum nutrition in the population of this Hemisphere.

REFERENCES

Daza CH, Rodríguez N (1981): Intersectoral approach to health and its relation with food and nutrition planning. In Aranda-Pastor J, Saenz L (eds): "Proceedings of an International Conference on the Process of Food and Nutrition Planning" held in Antigua, Guatemala. Guatemala City: INCAP.

PAHO (1980): "Health for All by the Year 2000: Strategies." PAHO Official Document No. 173.

PAHO (1982): "Health for All by the Year 2000: Plan of Action for the Implementation of Regional Strategies." PAHO Official Document No. 179.

WHO (1976): "Food and Nutrition Strategies in National Development." Ninth report of the Joint FAO/WHO Expert Committee on Nutrition. Technical Report Series No. 584.

WHO (1978): "Alma-Ata 1978. Primary Health Care: Report of the International Conference on Primary Health Care, Alma-Ata, USSR, September 6–12, 1978." "Health for All" Series No. 1.

WHO (1981a): "The Role of the Health Sector in Food and Nutrition." Report of a WHO Expert Committee. WHO Technical Report Series No. 667.

WHO (1981b): "Guidelines for Training Community Health Workers in Nutrition." WHO Offset Publication No. 59.

Malnutrition: Determinants and Consequences, pages 457–469
© 1984 Alan R. Liss, Inc., 150 Fifth Avenue, New York, NY 10011

Food and Agricultural Technology in Combating Malnutrition

Joseph H. Hulse

International Development Research Centre, Ottawa, Canada K1G 3H9

This chapter will address: a) progress in agricultural development and food supply in the developing regions; b) some important obstacles to agricultural and nutritional improvement; and c) some recommended opportunities for future food and agricultural technological improvement.

To present the subject proposed solely in terms of food and agricultural technology would risk an overly simplistic, even distorted, picture of the difficulties that face the developing countries and the means by which to improve their welfare. First, therefore, it is necessary to set the subject in a broader international economic context.

FOOD, PEOPLE, AND RESOURCES

Though the early English poet John Donne wrote that "No man is an island" and his contemporary George Herbert told us that "Man is one world", to all intents and purposes, the present inhabitants of North America and northern Europe live in a world and on social and economic islands vastly different in human health, welfare, opportunities, and resources from those of their contemporaries in Africa, Asia, and Latin America. The data presented in Table I amply illustrate how the privileged minority own most of the world's important resources and control most of its wealth. In addition to the statistics quoted, the developed countries undertake more than 90% of the world's research and publish 89% of all its books. Furthermore, the developed countries enjoy an annual positive balance of more than US $300 billion in their trading transactions with the developing countries.

Table II shows how, towards the end of the decade, the population in the developing countries will increase from roughly three-quarters to four-fifths

TABLE I. Distribution of Selected World Resources, 1980, by Developed and Developing Nations

	Developed	Developing
World population (%)	27	73
World agricultural production (%)	62	38
World cereal production (%)	88	12
World commercial energy (%)	62	38
Energy in agricultural systems (% national consumption)	17–30	60–90
Average daily calories per capita	3,300	2,200
Arable land 2000 AD (hectares per capita)	0.46	0.19

TABLE II. Distribution of World Population, 1980 and 2000, by Developed and Developing Nations

	1980		2000	
	$\times 10^9$	%	$\times 10^9$	%
World	4.4	100	6.2	100
Developed	1.2	27	1.3	21
Developing	3.2	73	4.9	79

of the world's total. Of particular demographic interest is the increasing proportion of elderly people in the developed countries and of younger people in the developing countries. For example, over the past 5 years the number of Canadians under the age of 15 has decreased by 7% and the number of those over 65 years of age has increased by 18%. The present median age in Canada is 29 years; it is forecast that it will reach 36 by the end of the century. In 1950 in the United States there were 16 workers for each pensioner. By 1982 the ratio had fallen to 3 workers for 1 pensioner and by the end of the century there will be only 2 workers for each retired person if the present age of retirement is retained.

Since older people eat less than active young people, major food producers such as Canada, the United States, and Australia will consume relatively less whereas the poorer nations with large proportions of young people will demand more. In addition, it is anticipated that the proportion of urban to rural populations in developing countries will significantly increase. The urban population of Latin American countries is expected to exceed 60% by the end of the century.

It requires little diagnostic skill or intuitive imagination to propose that the royal road to nutritional sufficiency lies in, first, higher food crop production;

TABLE III. Arable Area Per Capita, Actual and Projected (trend)

Countries	1951–1955	1961–1965	1971–1975	Projected 1985	Projected 2000
Industrialized	0.61	0.56	0.55	0.50	0.46
Centrally planned	0.45	0.39	0.35	0.30	0.26
Less developed	0.45	0.40	0.35	0.27	0.19
World	0.48	0.44	0.39	0.32	0.25

Note: Arable area includes land under temporary crops (double-cropped areas are counted only once), temporary meadows for mowing or pasture, land under market and kitchen gardens (including cultivation under glass), and land temporarily fallow or lying idle.
Source: "The Global 2000 Report to the President," Vol 2; "The Technical Report." Prepared by the Council of Environmental Quality and the Department of State (1981).

second, putting more land under cultivation; and third, and perhaps most important, devising and gaining acceptance of more efficient systems of food conservation and distribution. The most primitive of known terrestrial and aquatic species, when left undisturbed, appear to maintain and protect their essential life-support systems. Human animals seem almost unique in the willful degradation of their most essential and unrenewable resources: arable fertile land and uncontaminated water.

LAND RESOURCES

Table III shows the serious loss in arable land per capita the world over during the past 25 years. Table IV presents the population pressures on arable land and illustrates the very serious situation that some countries will be faced with by the end of the century. Arable land formerly irrigated from the Nile in Egypt has been so overrun by urban spread that the American University and several other Egyptian institutions are investing extensively in research to rehabilitate the surrounding desert for crop, animal, and forest production.

Table V illustrates the irresponsible depredation of arable land throughout the world, particularly in the developed countries. Only 3% of the total earth's surface is considered arable. Of the 15 million hectares lost annually, nearly half (7 million hectares) is attributable to urban spread, 3 million hectares of which occurs in the developed countries.

The total loss to urban spread could on a conservative estimate produce sufficient cereal calories for about 68 million adults per annum. The average annual increase in world population amounts to about 70 million persons per year. It would seem, therefore, that our most urgent priority ought to be to protect and conserve the land already available from further destruction. Reclamation of once fertile land that has been destroyed or debased, even where

TABLE IV. Population Per Arable Hectare in Selected Countries, 1975, 1985, and 2000 AD, Assuming No Change in Population Growth Rate

	Arable hectares (millions)	Population, 1975 (millions)	Population per arable hectare, 1975 (persons)	Annual rate of natural increase 1965–1975 (%)	Population, 1985 (millions)	Population per arable hectare, 1985 (persons)	Population, 2000 AD (millions)	Population per arable hectare, 200 AD (persons)
Mexico	28	60	2	3.5	85	3	136	5
Korea	2.4	34	14	2.0	41	17	54	22
India	167	608	4	2.0	741	5	983	6
China	129	823	6	1.7	974	5	1,241	10
Kenya	1.8	13	7	3.3	18	7.5	28	15
Tanzania	6.1	15	2.5	2.8	20	3.5	30	5
Egypt	2.9	37	13	2.3	46	16	63	22
All LDCs[a]	670	1,900	3	2.5	2,400	3.5	3,343	5

[a]Less developed countries.

Sources: Data on arable hectares are from FAO Production Yearbook (1980). Arable hectares includes land used for both annual and permanent crops. Population levels and rates of natural increase are from "World Population Growth and Response" (1976), Population Reference Bureau, Washington, DC.

Ratio of man to land extrapolated.

TABLE V. Annual World Loss of Arable Land

	Hectares ($\times 10^6$)
Urban and industrial spread	7.0 (DC^a = 3.0)
Mineral exploitation	1.0
Erosion	3.0
Desert spread	2.0
Chemical damage (salinity, etc)	2.0
Total	15.0

Potential cereal production from 15.0 million hectares is equivalent to the energy needs of 68 million adults. Annual average population increase to 2000 AD = 70 million.
[a]DC = Developed Countries.

this is possible, costs considerably more than conservation of what is already under the plough. The cost of bringing despoiled, marginal, or uncultivated land under the plough varies greatly according to circumstances. Cultivation of savanna pasture costs about $50/hectare, whereas cultivation of the tropical rain forest may approach $1,000/hectare.

FOOD PRODUCTION AND DEMAND

Table VI indicates the increases in agricultural production necessary to meet forecast demands by the end of the century. Whether achieved by expanding the land under cultivation or by higher yields per unit of land area, FAO estimates that close to a doubling of output will be necessary to meet minimum human demands by 2000 AD.

One's hope must inevitably be conditioned by what is evident in Table VII, where the food production indices in 1979 are compared with a baseline averaged over the period 1961–1965. The most encouraging production increases are to be found among the nations of Southeast Asia where, for example, Burma, the Philippines, and Indonesia increased their cereal production by more than 60%. Improved cropping systems practiced by these nations, added to those of South Korea and northern India, contributed notably to the 37% increase in overall cereal production in the decade of the 1970s. The prospect for many African nations is considerably more bleak.

Table VIII demonstrates the growing dependence of the developing countries upon cereal exports from North America. Table VIII does not reveal the grossly disproportionate balance of trade between the developed countries, particularly those of North America, and the less-privileged regions. Close to 40% of all exports and about one-third of all farm products exported from the United States go to the developing countries. The United States exports to developing countries at least double what it exports to the European Economic

TABLE VI. Production Increases Required to Meet Minimal LDC Needs in 2000 AD

		% Increase 1971–1980
Total cereals	× 2	37
Coarse grains	× 2	31
Root crops	× 2	
Vegetables	× 2.5	
Vegetable oils	× 2.5	
Fruit	× 2.5	
Milk	× 2.25	
Meat	× 2.5	

TABLE VII. Food Production Indices in Various Regions of the World (1961/65 = 100)

	Total production			Per capita production		
	1970	1975	1979	1970	1975	1979
World total	123	135	147	107	108	110
Developing countries						
Latin America and the Caribbean	129	152	173	107	110	113
Africa[a]	117	120	134	98	96	88
West Asia	122	154	168	102	110	108
South Asia	128	140	146	110	107	103
East Asia[b]	129	155	175	108	116	120

[a]Except South Africa.
[b]Except Japan.
Source: Second Review, CGIAR (1981).

Community (EEC). Exports from the EEC to developing countries are roughly three times what the EEC exports to other developed countries.

Most of us in North America can justifiably complain of the erosion in the purchasing power of our disposable income over the past several years. Table IX illustrates the enormous burden borne by the developing nations from the increase in world oil prices, the excessive investment in armaments, and the general destabilization of their former patterns of economic growth and development. Table IX clearly indicates that the developing countries, especially those without petroleum resources, have borne a disproportionate cost of the destabilization of the world's economy. The crippling increased cost of food imports illustrated in Table IX if continued will inevitably seriously reduce the capacity of the developing countries to import fertilizers, machinery, and other imports essential to increased food production and improved agricultural technologies.

TABLE VIII. Net Trade in Cereals (metric tons) by Selected Geographic Regions

	1968	1978
North America	49	113
Africa	(2.6)	(10.8)
Latin America	1.4	(4.3)
Northeast and West Asia	(4.4)	(14.0)
South and Southeast Asia	(11.8)	(11.1)
All LDCs Developing Countries	(17.6)	(40.4)
USSR group	(0.4)	(28.7)

Data in parentheses are negative values.

TABLE IX. Cost of Living Increases by Developed and Developing Nations

	1971	1980
Average inflation rate (%)		
Developed	5.3	12.7
Developing	4.5	19.2
Average increase of consumer food prices (%)		
Developed	4.6	9.4
Developing	4.0	22.3

Though recent estimates forecast sizeable grain crop surpluses in North America and growing butter mountains and milk lakes in Europe, because of their unfavorable balance of trade, most of the food-deficient developing countries do not possess the disposable foreign currency with which to buy the food they need. Thus, in spite of its concomitant and unsatisfactory consequences, food aid on concessional terms will be necessary for many years to come.

The developing countries that are not oil producers rely on the export of primary products for 60% of their income. In consequence of the depressed industrial growth in North America, Europe, and Japan both the prices for and the total volume of raw material exports have fallen, resulting in loss of income and a disturbing rise in the foreign debt load of many Third World nations. Developing countries thus have been forced to impose austerity measures and to reduce their imports from the industrialized countries. It was recently stated (Globe and Mail, Toronto, Canada, 6 August 1983) that Mexico's cessation of imports from its northern neighbor added more US workers to the ranks of the unemployed than the recession in the automobile industry.

TABLE X. Armaments Versus Agricultural Investment ($US billion)

	1980	1982	% Increase	$US/capita, LDCs 1982
Investment in armaments (worldwide)	450	650	44	200
Aid for food and agriculture (bilateral and multilateral)	11	11	0	3

TABLE XI. Official Development Assistance (ODA) As Percentage of GNP

Nation or region	%
OPEC countries	1.46
UK	0.44
Canada	0.43
Australia	0.41
Japan	0.26
USA	0.20
OECD countries (average)	
1965	0.5
1981	0.32
Accepted target	0.7

Data are for 1981, except as noted.

INVESTMENT IN DEVELOPMENT

It would appear self-evident that the greatest need now and for the foreseeable future is to protect the world's limited and fragile productive resources and to invest significantly more in research and development destined to increase food production by conventional and traditional agricultural technologies. What significant improvement in food resources, if any, may be derived from the as yet unfamiliar derivatives of biotechnology and genetic engineering is probably many decades into the future. Notwithstanding what appears to be self-evident, the politicians who guide the destinies of developed, developing, and least-developed countries seem singularly undisposed to give priority of investment to food and agricultural research and development.

Table X shows that in the first two years of the 1980s, worldwide investment in armaments increased by 44% and is now equivalent to $200 per annum for every man, woman, and child in the developing countries. Over the same period multilateral and bilateral investment in food and agricultural development remained static in actual expenditures and therefore significantly declined in constant dollars, the present investment being roughly equivalent to $3 per year per person living in the developing countries.

In dismal contrast to the investment in the proliferation of armaments, Table XI gives the Organization for Economic Cooperation and Development (OECD) assessments of overseas development assistance to developing countries as a percentage of the gross national product of the wealthier nations. Shown in Table XI is the relatively high contribution of the OPEC countries (roughly 1.46% of their GNP) and the virtually nonexistent contribution to economic development, as distinct from the delivery of armaments, by the Soviet bloc.

Are there any contemporary developments that encourage us to believe that those who survive beyond our lifetime can be adequately fed? If all known existing agricultural technology were supported by a half of what is invested in armaments, we would need have little concern for the welfare of generations of humankind beyond us.

INTERNATIONAL AGRICULTURAL RESEARCH

One of the most imaginative collaborative research ventures has resulted in the family of International Agricultural Research Centres (IARCs) supported by the Consultative Group on International Agricultural Research (CGIAR). The IARCs maintain an immense germplasm base from which new and more productive genotypes, adaptable to a wide range of agroclimatic conditions and possessed of desirable functional and nutritional characteristics, can be derived.

Many advances in plant breeding have evolved over the life of the International Rice Research institute (IRRI). One of the earliest high-yielding rice types, IR8, was the progeny of two parents. The more recent IR36, derived from a more diverse ancestry through genetic selection and gene pyramiding combines a high-yield potential with a broad spectrum of disease resistance.

It would appear less difficult to derive food plants possessing superior characteristics than to persuade farmers, particularly those operating close to a subsistence level, to grow them. Over the last decade, agricultural scientists have gradually come to understand that productive research begins not on the experimental station but in the farmer's field. Before seeking to bring about technical, economic, or social improvement, the research scientists must first understand what already exists: what are the technical, social, and economic opportunities and constraints by which the rural communities and individual farmers are controlled and conditioned. It is this realization that has given rise to a new methodology in farming systems research.

Current concepts of farming systems research recognize the necessity first to understand the nature of the farming systems that exist; to comprehend the farmer's resources, opportunities, and constraints before embarking upon research to bring about improvement. In effect this calls for a close working relation between research workers and farmers, since much of the research is carried out in farmers' fields under the farmer's management.

THE VALUE OF THE FOREST

It has been estimated that the area of tropical forest destroyed every year is equal to half the size of the United Kingdom. Furthermore, a high proportion of the trees cut down are not used for human benefit. Trees are immensely useful plants providing, according to species, fuel, food, feed, fodder, and fertilizer. Tree plantations stabilize soil conditions and prevent erosion; they can provide shelter for animals and, as windbreaks, protect cultivated crops from desiccating winds and blowing sand.

In 1982 the International Development Research Centre (IDRC) began a network of social forestry projects in semiarid Africa that now includes 15 countries where trees grown by small-holder farmers and rural village communities provide various combinations of the uses and benefits listed above. In several remote areas of the People's Republic of China, IDRC is supporting the production of the indigenous Paulownia, which produces a favorable microclimate when grown in association with various other crops, provides fuel for rural and urban communities, and is an important construction material for buildings, furniture, and, because of its unique physical stability, for musical instruments.

Elsewhere in China, research on bamboo has identified species capable of producing culms 25 m in height and 18 cm in diameter in 1 year. The program is also selecting bamboo types capable of withstanding frost, thus permitting expansion of bamboo into more northerly regions.

IDRC was largely instrumental in bringing into being the International Council for Research on Agroforestry, with its headquarters in Nairobi.

POSTPRODUCTION PROBLEMS

Though agricultural scientists have made notable progress in recent years in seeking to comprehend the nature, opportunities, and constraints of existing farming systems before embarking upon research to improve them, a comparable approach is less evident among scientists and technologists who seek to improve existing, or to testablish new, agroindustrial enterprises. Disproportionate effort seems to be invested in laboratory and pilot plant research, the invention and elaboration of novel products and processes. Often, however, the most urgent need is to begin with a comprehensive quantitative determination and analysis of actual and potential markets in relation to the financial, material, technical, and human resources available to the industries that exist.

The linear concept of developmental research, ie, starting in a laboratory and continuing through a pilot plant before considering the market demand, seems often accompanied by an equally unproductive expectation from the transfer of technology. Food and agricultural technologies are conditioned by the physical, social, and economic environments in which they are to be applied and by the markets they must serve, all of which need to be thoroughly evaluated before technological research and development are started.

The introduction of new foods derived from familiar plant and animal material resources generally calls for sizeable investments in market research and development. Future derivatives of such embryonic biotechnologies as the genetically manipulated microbial transformation of agricultural wastes and by-products will present a whole new generation of difficulties and hazards. Though some accepted techniques exist by which to determine the chronic or acute toxicities of known chemical additives or contaminants, it is doubtful if any reliable biological methodology is available by which to establish the safety and wholesomeness of "novel" foods derived from unconventional raw materials or by processes of transformation for which no prior long-term human experience is recorded.

It would therefore seem sensible to give greatest immediate priority and investment to the conventionally accepted systems of food and agricultural development. Research to produce foods from novel and unfamiliar biotechnologies must be preceded by the elaboration of reliable biological methods by which to evaluate their safety and wholesomeness when consumed regularly and over long periods by human beings.

Under no circumstances should the least privileged people in the developing countries be presented with the products of inadequately evaluated biotechnologies that would not be acceptable to food and drug administrations in the more privileged and economically developed countries.

POVERTY AND MALNUTRITION

Though science and technology have made, and will continue to make, outstanding contributions to social and economic progress, they are not the sole determinants of nutritional adequacy. Nutritional deficiencies are the historical and contemporary companions of poverty. Studies in India demonstrate that the poorest people spend close to 80% of the first increments to their depressingly low incomes on essential foods.

The eradication of chronic poverty requires a greater equity in trading relations between the rich and the poor nations, a drastic reduction in the peddling of armaments, and a much greater investment in agricultural development.

AGRICULTURE: THE LEADING EDGE OF DEVELOPMENT

Historically, from the time of city states of the Tigris and Euphrates, agricultural development has provided the leading edge of national economic growth. Bearing in mind the dominance of the agricultural sector in the economies of most developing countries, it seems axiomatic that future economic progress will be heavily dependent upon agricultural development. It would therefore appear logical that the highest priority be given to strengthening the national agricultural systems of the developing countries. Agriculture and agroindustries provide both food and employment; employment and food in excess of subsistence needs generate the disposable income that is a first essential of economic growth.

The need for opportunities for imaginative scientific cooperation between food and agricultural scientists in developed and developing countries has encouraged several governments and international agencies to provide the means to support such cooperation. The International Council of Scientific Unions (ICSU) has created an International Commission to identify the opportunities and the means of realizing more productive cooperation in basic research related to agriculture, forestry, and aquaculture in the Third World.

Such programs need to be truly cooperative and not a domination of the developing country scientists and technologists by the expatriate agents of bilateral or multilateral assistance. The IDRC was created to encourage and support the scientific efforts of people and institutions in developing countries. It is the IDRC philosophy that, given adequate resources and encouragement, scientists, technologists, and farming and agroindustrial communities of the developing countries will be better able to provide for their own people's long-term nutritional needs than will large numbers of imported expatriate experts. More productive agricultural technologies and more efficient postproduction systems of preservation and distribution must be developed and put into effect in full cooperation with the communities who are to use and benefit from them. Such cooperation is generally more effectively realized by those who are familiar with these communities, people who speak the same language and inherit similar traditions.

Most urgent and essential, however, is the need for a dramatic shift in political priorities and political will in all countries: an understanding and acceptance that ploughshares must be given precedence over swords; that bread is more important to human survival than bombs; that "one man's hunger is every man's hunger."

BIBLIOGRAPHY
Author's Note

The tables and data presented are derived from several sources. The following references include the principal sources together with more detailed discussions of the subjects addressed.

Bunting AH (1981): Changing perspectives in agriculture in developing countries. J Agric Econ, September 1981, p 287.

Second Review of the Consultative Group on International Agricultural Research (November 1981). Washington: World Bank.

Food and Agricultural Organization (1980): "FAO Production Yearbook."

Food and Agricultural Organization (1981): "Agriculture: Towards 2000."

Hulse JH (1977): Research management. In "Agricultural Research Management," Vol 2. Los Baños, Philippines: Southeast Asian Regional Research Centre for Graduate Study and Research in Agriculture.

Hulse JH (1981): "World Food Resources — An Overview." Parkville, Victoria: Australian Academy of Technological Sciences, pp 15–41.

Hulse JH (1982): Research and post-production systems. In Manassah JT, Briskey EJ (eds): "Advances in Food Producing Systems for Arid and Semi-Arid Lands." New York: Academic, pp 1127–1178.

Hulse JH (1982): Food science and nutrition: The gulf between rich and poor. Science 216 (4552):1291–1294.

Hulse JH (1982): Food science for richer or for poorer, for sickness or for health. Proc Br Inst Food Sci Technol, Vol 16, Nos. 1, 2.

Independent Commission on International Development Issues (Brandt Commission) (1980): "North-South: A Programme for Survival." Cambridge, Mass: MIT Press.

Independent Commission on International Development Issues (Brandt Commission) (1983): "North-South: Common Crisis Cooperation for World Recovery." Cambridge, Mass: MIT Press.

International Development Research Centre (1981): "A Decade of Learning." IDRC 170e. Ottawa, Canada.

International Bank for Reconstruction and Development (1982): "World Development Report." Cambridge: Oxford University Press.

Kennedy ET, Pinstrup-Anderson P (1983): "Nutrition Related Policies and Programs." Washington, DC: International Food Policy Research Institute.

Swaminathan MS (1983): "Agricultural Progress — Key to Third World Prosperity." Third World Foundation Lecture. Beijing, China.

"World Population Growth and Response" (1976): Washington, DC: Population Reference Bureau.

Malnutrition: Determinants and Consequences, pages 471–475
© *1984 Alan R. Liss, Inc., 150 Fifth Avenue, New York, NY 10011*

Socioeconomic Development and Nutrition in Latin America

Mauricio Herman, PhD
Social Development Division, Inter-American Development Bank,
Washington, DC 20577

It is extremely difficult to present, in the space permitted, a comprehensive review of the interrelationships between socioeconomic development and human nutrition problems. Others have addressed the effects of adequate nutrition on socioeconomic development, such as improvement of health indicators and reduction in the incidence of some diseases. Other effects include increase of economic activity and productivity levels, and as a result, of individual and family income; and also prevention of the negative effects of malnutrition on the mental development of children and the consequent impact on long-term human potential.

I have chosen to focus on the reverse side of the coin, that is, a discussion of the effects of the stages of socioeconomic development on the levels of nutrition. In this context, it would seem appropriate to start with a couple of basic propositions derived from statistical and econometric studies carried out in recent years. The first one is that, at the microeconomic level, family income is a major determinant of the quantity and quality of foods consumed. The second is that, at the macroeconomnic level, there is no clear relationship between per capita income levels and the degree of income concentration in the various countries of the world.

If we accept these two basic propositions, we must with logical rigor conclude that hunger and malnutrition basically originate in family poverty, and that the latter is due to poor distribution of wealth and income.

Actually, food production in Latin America is sufficient to satisfy the nutritional needs of its population. Poverty, not lack of food, is the root of hunger in the region, and this is the basic reason why I am postulating that, in the Latin American subcontinent, hunger and, more significantly, malnutrition have unequal distribution of wealth and income as their primary cause. What is terrifying in its implications, moreover, is the fact that accelerated economic growth does not necessarily result in changes in the patterns of income distribution. Therefore, even if the economic growth rates of Latin America return to the high levels registered in the last two decades, the existing distribution of wealth and income in the subcontinent will continue to generate human nutrition problems that cannot be solved by any one sector in particular. The ultimate answer does not lie in partial actions to be undertaken separately by the health authorities or in technological "break-throughs" to be achieved in nutrition research, or even in greater production or better yields of food crops, but in attaining a higher stage of socioeconomic development in the countries of the region.

The Inter-American Development Bank, from its very inception, recognized that the economic and *social* development of its member countries was to be its basic mandate, and in its 23 years of existence has channeled almost US$23 billion in loans and technical assistance operations to Latin America and the Caribbean.

Particularly significant, however, is not the absolute amount of lending but the Bank's emphasis on the social sectors and its increasing concern with the needs of low-income groups.

For many years now, at least half of the Bank's operations have had to be directed towards low-income beneficiaries. Social infrastructure projects (environmental and public health; education, science, and technology; urban development) represented over one-fourth of the Bank's lending for 1982 — which reached a record of US$2.7 billion — and have averaged around 18% since 1961.

Special mention should be made also that, as of December 31, 1982, the Bank had lent about US$5.1 billion for agriculture and fisheries development. The Bank has been the region's principal international source of financing for the food sector. The loans provided for fishing projects, for example (US$361.5 million as of the end of 1982), should generate over 2.5 million tons of catches annually, contributing substantially to a greater availability of valuable animal proteins for Latin American diets.

Regarding nutrition in particular, the Bank has established the following operational policy.

The primary objective is to reduce the incidence of malnutrition, especially within low-income groups. For this purpose it is considered important to assist countries in developing their capacity to determine the types, causes, and incidence of malnutrition, and formulate programs to remedy these deficiencies, as well as to monitor and evaluate the impact and the more lasting effects of such measures.

The Bank believes that the nutritional status of the population should be taken into account in defining food policies and in agricultural and rural development programs. It is recommended that countries establish nutrition policies based on quantitative evaluation of needs in terms of food production types and levels; define specific goals with regard to the desired levels of national food production and food imports; adopt measures to stimulate food production and distribution at reasonable cost and generally acceptable standards of quality and safety; and give particular attention to those segments of the population most adversely affected by malnutrition (expectant and recent mothers and children under 5 years of age). Such policy may need to include action programs for groups within the society that lack the means of acquiring the essential components of a minimal diet, even at reasonable prices.

Within the framework of these general concepts, the specific objectives are the following:

1. To assist countries, where pertinent in projects, in identifying nutrition problems and the causes thereof and in taking the proper actions needed to solve them, including the mobilization of resources to identify, prepare, and implement projects and programs to reduce malnutrition.

2. To encourage the introduction of nutritional considerations in those types of projects where it would be particularly appropriate as a complementary or associated element of the project or program—ie, agriculture, health care, education, integrated development, fishery, and food-related industry, etc.

3. To foster the development and adaptation, transfer, and use of suitable technology to improve food problems and relieve malnutrition.

4. To strengthen and support national and international institutions operating in the nutrition sector and promote regional cooperation, particularly in aspects of manufacture and marketing of low-priced food supplements.

5. To support projects designed to determine the socioeconomic feasibility of production and marketing techniques for nontraditional processed foodstuffs that make sufficient use of locally produced raw materials.

FIELDS OF ACTIVITY

The Bank favors the financing of projects for direct improvement of the nutritional status of disadvantaged population groups. Within this central orientation, the following examples are eligible for Bank financing.

1. Projects featuring technological or socioeconomic research and training in new methods for production, preservation, and distribution of food products, particularly low-priced, mass-produced items.

2. Projects for production, preservation, and distribution of basic and processed low-cost food items consisting, insofar as possible, of local raw materials that can be used in public programs or marketed commercially. This in-

cludes fortification of generally consumed basic foods, development of new food products with high nutritional content, and reduction of losses that affect food products at all stages of the marketing and distribution channel.

3. Projects that support development and implementation of public programs designed to: a) distribute food to disadvantaged population groups (school breakfasts, special prenatal and postpartum diets for mothers, food for the elderly, etc); b) change dietary habits and introduce new foods into the family diet through utilization of the mass media; c) supply nutrition education through rural extension services, schools, adult education, and mass communication systems; d) train technical and other types of personnel to carry out nutrition programs; and e) establish facilities for proper storage and preservation of essential foods and disseminate knowledge of food preservation technology.

4. Projects to strengthen institutions concerned with nutritional research, the definition of policies, and implementation of programs in nutrition and those for the development and adaptation of food technology. As a means of determining the positive or negative effects on human nutrition of agriculture, fishery, marketing, education, health care, and industry projects, it is important to help establish and improve information systems and develop the capacity to conduct basic studies for nutrition policy formation and applied research.

In considering operations to be carried out in various activity sectors, wherever particularly appropriate, the Bank may cooperate with countries to introduce nutrition components, especially in integrated urban and rural development, agriculture, agroindustry, fishery, public health, and education projects. Where there is apparent reason for concern, the Bank may recommend that countries give special consideration to possible adverse nutritional consequences that may result from projects and programs in various sectors and seek measures to correct them.

To support national efforts to define nutrition policies, investment programs, plans and projects, the Bank may, at the request of the countries, authorize adequate technical cooperation resources. In using such resources, preference will be given to activities that contribute to publicizing an awareness and understanding of nutritional problems, institutionalization of action programs, formulation of preinvestment and investment projects, staff training, and conducting of research, the results of which are vital for programming in the field of nutrition and food.

There is no panacea that will solve the widespread malnutrition problems in Latin America and the Caribbean. Traditionally the health sector has carried most of the responsibility for amelioration of malnutrition. It is clear, however, that in this regard, preventive medicine implies carrying out supplementary feeding of such vulnerable groups as mothers and children. At the same time, agricultural and fishery production, and food marketing programs, need to be implemented in order to obtain a supply sufficient in quality and quantity to meet nutritional requirements of the population. Furthermore, an all-out attack on the causes of poverty must be at the center of any socioeconomic development strategy. For development is a much broader term than growth; it signifies not only a quantitative increase but also qualitative modifications, with the satisfaction of basic human needs — both physiological and spiritual — as the ultimate societal goal. All of us, no matter what our nationalities or fields of professional specialization, must bear a share of this responsibility towards present and future generations.

Malnutrition: Determinants and Consequences, pages 477–478
© *1984 Alan R. Liss, Inc., 150 Fifth Avenue, New York, NY 10011*

Summation

José María Bengoa, MD
Nutrition Unit, World Health Organization, Geneva, Switzerland

I should like to stress several points that emerged in the Seventh Western Hemisphere Nutrition Congress, and to give a personal impression about where we are at present as far as the social problem of malnutrition in the American Hemisphere is concerned.

The *first* point is that in the decades of the sixties and seventies, important advances were made in reducing both mortality in young children and incidence of the most severe forms of protein-energy malnutrition in all countries of the hemisphere.

Second, it is too early to know the impact that the present international crisis is going to produce. For this reason, we have to watch carefully, through an appropriate surveillance system, the main economic, agricultural, and health indicators related to nutrition.

Third, it is clear that the main concerns at present are the chronic forms of malnutrition and the functional development of human beings, particularly as related to performance and physical activity, rather than acute forms of malnutrition. In addition, scientific information has been presented to emphasize the role of micronutrients in human nutrition. In this respect, I wish to call your attention to the importance that the INFOODS (International Network of Food Data Systems) project will have in the near future in facilitating the interpretation of nutritional data.

Fourth, in the Seventh Congress, the concept of *poverty* was used frequently to explain the nutritional situation in the hemisphere. In previous meetings we were afraid to use this term so openly. I think this is an important advance, and in the future, we will have to be much more involved in the poverty problem than in the past.

Fifth, we have to welcome the efforts of the health sector, particularly in the area of primary health care, in taking full responsibility in the field of nutrition, which was neglected for many years.

Sixth, in spite of the few papers presented on agricultural issues, planning for adequate food production and food distribution still remains an indispensable component of basic strategy in the fight against malnutrition. Perhaps the priorities should be to concentrate on the eight or ten basic foods that provide 90% of the caloric intake in Latin America.

Seventh, one must stress once again the need for more research and training facilities, not only in the medical field, which is relatively well covered, but also in the economic, agricultural, and social sciences.

Eighth, some mechanisms must be developed to facilitate the transfer of scientific information in nutrition to the policy-makers in each country. It is obvious that at the present time, policy-makers are often still basing their decisions on concepts developed 20–30 years ago and it is absolutely essential to bring them up to date. This is even more important in view of the fact that the field of nutrition has been invaded by an increasing amount of misinformation directed at the public through the mass media with very large financial support. This issue must be faced by improving the quality of the dissemination of scientific information in nutrition.

Finally, and above all, we have to stimulate more innovative ideas in order to overcome one of the more dramatic problems that faces mankind: *hunger*. For this, two major objectives are required: peace, peace everywhere; and justice, justice for everyone.

Index